SURGERY AND PATHOLOGY OF THE MIDDLE EAR

The Antwerp Conference was organized by the Belgian Society of ORL-HNS and the Politzer Society, in association with the International Society of Audiology, under the auspices of the Council for International Organizations of Medical Sciences (CIOMS) and the International Federation of Otorhinolaryngological Societies (IFOS)

SURGERY AND PATHOLOGY OF THE MIDDLE EAR

Proceedings of the International Conference on 'The Postoperative Evaluation in Middle Ear Surgery' held in Antwerp on June 14-16, 1984

●

Edited by Jean F.E. Marquet

●

1985 **MARTINUS NIJHOFF PUBLISHERS**
a member of the KLUWER ACADEMIC PUBLISHERS GROUP
BOSTON / DORDRECHT / LANCASTER

Distributors

for the United States and Canada: Kluwer Academic Publishers, 190 Old Derby Street, Hingham, MA 02043, USA
for the UK and Ireland: Kluwer Academic Publishers, MTP Press Limited, Falcon House, Queen Square, Lancaster LA1 1RN, UK
for Belgium: Medical Media International, Av. van Becelaere 28 b, b.8, B-1170 Brussels, Belgium
for all other countries: Kluwer Academic Publishers Group, Distribution Center, P.O. Box 322, 3300 AH Dordrecht, The Netherlands

Library of Congress Cataloguing in publication data

International conference on the postoperative evaluation in middle ear surgery (1984: Antwerp, Belgium)
Surgery and pathology of the middle ear.

1. Middle ear – surgery – congresses. 2. Middle ear – surgery – complications and sequelae – congresses. 3. Middle ear – diseases – congresses. 4. Middle ear – surgery – data processing – congresses. 5. Middle ear – surgery – complications and sequelae – data processing – congresses. I. Marquet, Jean F.E. II. Title. [DNLM: 1. Diagnosis, surgical – congresses. 2. Ear, middle – pathology – congresses. 3. Ear, middle – surgery – congresses. 4. Postoperative complications – diagnosis – congresses. WV 230 I592s 1984] RF126.I55 1984
617.8′4 85-346

ISBN-13: 978-94-010-8715-5 e-ISBN-13: 978-94-009-5002-3
DOI: 10.1007/978-94-009-5002-3

Book Information

Joint edition published by: Martinus Nijhoff Publishers, Dordrecht and Medical Media International, Brussels

CONTENTS

SYMPOSIUM II - RECONSTRUCTIVE SURGERY

Chairman: E.H. Huizing

SYMPOSIUM III - SURGICAL PROCEDURES

Chairman: G. Lacher

PLENARY SESSION

PANEL II - MIDDLE EAR PATHOLOGY

Moderator: G. D. L. Smyth

SYMPOSIUM IV - POSTOPERATIVE COMPLICATIONS

Chairman: U. Fisch

SYMPOSIUM V - PATHO-ANATOMY

Chairman: L. Manolidis

SYMPOSIUM VI - PATHOPHYSIOLOGY

Chairman: M. Sakai

PLENARY SESSION

PANEL III - FUNCTIONAL EVALUATION

Moderator: H. Diamant

SYMPOSIUM VII - COMPUTER PROCESSING OF DATA

Chairman: G. Gates

SCIENTIFIC EXHIBITION

Abstracts are published for contributions
not received on time.

FOREWORD

Dear colleagues,
Promotion of the development of ENT is one of the most important tasks of IFOS (International Federation of Otorhinolaryngology). Apart from organizing the World Congresses it supports different international and regional meetings, organizes symposiums on well-determined subjects, etc.

Since the last World Congress in 1981, in addition to the Danube Symposium in 1982 and the Congress of ENT Societies in Asia-Oceania in 1983, an international symposium was organized in Antwerp by the Belgian ENT Society on evaluation problems of middle ear surgery. This is a very controversial question on which there is no concensus. During a four-day meeting many anatomical and pathological aspects, operative methods, possibilities of the evaluation of the results with computers, were widely discussed.

You will find all the lectures presented in this book. I am convinced that these papers will prove to be a good basis for further discussion and hope that finally we shall achieve an international agreement on the evaluation of our results in middle ear surgery.

My thanks go to Professor Marquet for organizing the meeting and for publishing the papers.

Professor Dr. L. Surján
President of IFOS

WELCOME

Dear colleagues and especially dear Professor Marquet,
In my function as pro-rector of the University of Antwerp I am very proud of welcoming you to the opening of the International Conference on "The Postoperative Evaluation in Middle Ear Surgery".
It gives me the opportunity to stress the importance of this congress and to honour Prof. Marquet.

As a pediatrician I can only confirm the words of Dr. Charles Bluestone as he writes that "otitis media is the most frequent diagnosis made by physicians who care for children". Many children have recurrent and chronic middle ear disease that requires repeated antimicrobial therapy and surgical intervention.
Although there is a considerable body of evidence to guide our therapeutic approach, there are still many gaps in our knowledge of the disease. Therefore, it is of the utmost importance to have objective randomized clinical trials of medical and surgical therapy.

Good postoperative evaluation of middle ear surgery could prevent situations such as those described by Nick Black in the Lancet of 14 April 1984 under the title "Surgery for glue ear - a modern epidemic: Analysis of routine hospital statistics confirms anecdotal reports of an epidemic surgery for glue ear. The surgical rate rose by 74 % in the Oxford region between 1975 and 1981. The peak ages for surgery are 5-7 years and the rates are high in social class I and low in class V. Although the prevalence of glue ear is hard to ascertain, the current surgical epidemic probably reflects an increase in *apparent* prevalence rather than a real increase in morbidity". I am quite sure that good evaluation of the results of middle ear surgery for chronic ear disease, based upon a definite schedule, will establish the most objective guidelines for all physicians to treat their patients in the most adequate way.

I would like to take the opportunity of this welcoming speech, to honour Prof. Marquet as a doctor, a researcher and a teacher. Homer wrote in the 17th book of the Odyssey: "Who pray of himself ever seeks out and bids a stranger from abroad unless it be those who are masters of some public craft, a prophet or healer of ills, or a builder, or a divine musician, for these men are bidden over the boundless earth". These masters of the public craft or healing are even more mobile today than they were a few millenia ago. Little has changed except the boundless earth, now shrunken and bounded. Prof. Marquet belongs to these great masters of healing, bidden over the boundless earth.

H. Osmond defines the medical authority as consisting of three types: sapiential, moral, and charismatic, combined in a particular manner. He called this "Aesculapian authority". By sapiential authority, Osmond means the right to be heard that is derived from knowledge or expertness. Such authority resides in the person and not in any position that he may occupy. A person with this kind of authority may advise, inform, instruct, and direct, but not order. Doctors possess sapiential authority because of their knowledge of medicine.

The view that is most common, and perhaps most widely held by non-physicians is that there is something inherently contradictory between science and humanity, between technology and compassion. If this were indeed the case, it would be almost inevitable for humanity to regress as science marches ahead. I believe this view to be a dangerous one with far-reaching consequences of anti-intellectualism and anti-science. Technology and science are here to serve us. The much maligned and expensive CT scan, the example of medical technology par excellence, has not dehumanized medicine. On the contrary, it has been a tool of unparalleled compassion. Its use has spared patients many more difficult, painful, and dangerous procedures. Technology is just a means to an end. In a perverse manner of speaking, compassion too is just a means to an end. In the field of medicine, both technology and compassion have healing the patient as a goal; we can ignore either only at the peril of producing poor medicine. We need physicians who are both compassionate and competent. Everybody who knows Prof. Marquet, has been under the impression of his scientific competence and compassionate attitude.

The second ingredient of Aesculapian authority is moral authority, the right to control and direct that is derived from the rightness and goodness according to the ethos of the enterprise. The moral authority of doctors, which is expressed in the Hippocratic oath, stems from their doing what is expected of them as doctors and their concern with the good of the patient. To seek the welfare of his patients has always been considered by Prof. Marquet as his primordial task. Practising scientific medicine to help people, who are suffering and are in pain, has given meaning to his life.

The third ingredient in Aesculapian authority is charismatic authority. There are too many unknown and unknowable factors in illness for medicine to rest entirely on sapiential authority. For this reason, the doctor still retains some of his original priestly rôle.

F. Ingelfinger, ex-editorialist of the New England Journal of Medicine, in his last George W. Gay lecture, puts the following question about the personal encounter between physician and patient: is it marked by authoritarianism, paternalism, and domination? My answer is not only "yes" but also that a certain measure of these characteristics is essential to good medical care. In fact, if you agree that the physician's primary function is to make the patient feel better, a certain amount of authoritarianism, paternalism, and domination are the essence of the physician's effectiveness. Everybody who comes in contact with Prof. Marquet, either as a patient or as a colleague, comes under the impression of his charismatic authority, by what Ingelfinger calls his beneficial arrogance. Knowledge, moral authority and a certain measure of paternalism are the ingredients which make Prof. Marquet a "good doctor". I personally believe that this is the greatest honour that we can pay him.

Besides being an excellent clinician, Prof. Marquet is also a great teacher. To be a good teacher one must practice what one teaches. This requires, working with students and house staff, caring for one's own patients and maintaining a continual presence on the firing line, in the trenches of the clinic, emergency room, and wards. Patient care, so necessary for effective student and resident teaching, always takes precedence for Prof. Marquet. I believe that this is the most important factor in his being a great teacher of clinical medicine.

Dear Professor Marquet,
We are glad that you are a member of our faculty; we are happy that you have gathered so many brilliant scientists and famous clinicians at an international meeting in our very young University. I hope and I am sure that under your chairmanship this Conference will be very successful.

Dear colleagues,
I also hope that the accommodation of our University will fulfil your needs and that the attractiveness of the town of Antwerp, with its rich cultural patrimony will make your journey to the Low Countries a very pleasant trip.

Pro-Rector R. Clara
University of Antwerp, Belgium

PLENARY SESSION

International Nomenclature of Diseases (IND)

Z. Bankowski

The title of the conference is "Postoperative Evaluation in Middle Ear Surgery" and I would like to emphasize the word "evaluation". In the process of evaluation we always compare. In order to be able to compare and thereafter to evaluate, it is obvious that the terminology used by all those who participate in the process of evaluation should be standardized. One of the main purposes of your conference is "to produce a truly international standard for reporting and computer processing of the results of middle ear surgery". Therefore, the main aim of the conference is not only to exchange views and opinions of the scientific and technical aspects of middle ear surgery, but to make a step forward in the standardization of terminology and to try to improve communication in otology and medicine at large.

Improperly used terms have always constituted an obstacle to communication in medicine, but the absence of standardized terminology has become a major problem in recent times. Up until about fifty years ago, any specialist could be expected to master the terminology in his own field of interest and keep up with the relevant literature. Today, however, new developments in medical science have completely changed the situation, giving a new dimension and immediate urgency to the problem of communication, storage, and retrieval of biomedical information.

The first development is the dramatic increase in the number of biomedical research workers, resulting in an almost geometrical rate of increase in the number of publications and a "terminological explosion".

The second, perhaps no less important, is the multidisciplinary approach to research. In the past, specialists tended to carry out research in isolation, using their own methods of observation and experimentation and their own terminology; the present approach to research, however, brings the specialist in touch with fields other than his own and with a terminology that he does not fully master.

The third development, which also has far-reaching consequences, is the enormous growth in the international exchange of information in all fields of medicine.

The disorder in terminology also raises great obstacles to the efficient communication of information because: a reader (or listener) is often unfamiliar with a term used by a writer (or speaker) and may himself use a different term for the same concept; a reader (or listener) may understand a term used by a writer (or speaker) in a different sense from that intended.

Editors, abstractors, translators, and interpreters may be considered as special kinds of writers and speakers — and the absence of standardized terminology renders their work much more difficult and costly. In this context, it is important to emphasize that nowadays most scientists act, at one time or another, as translators, writers, editors, or interpreters, by writing accounts of meetings they have attended, by abstracting papers written by colleagues in languages other than their own, by using literature in various languages in their own writings, or in a variety of other ways. Because there is no standardized terminology, they select the terms arbitrarily and such improvised neologisms find their way into publications and are used in turn by other writers. By this process the number of synonyms keeps growing, constantly increasing the existing confusion.[1]

The preparation of internationally agreed names of diseases is one step forward to improve the communication in medicine.

Before presenting the joint CIOMS/WHO project for the preparation of the International Nomenclature of Diseases, I would like to clarify certain points which have been the cause of confusion and have stood in the path of similar attempts in the past.[2] To begin with, one should clearly differentiate three concepts, namely medical terminology, classification of diseases and disease nomenclature.

Medical terminology is a collection of terms that apply to specific concepts in medicine arranged systematically, and usually without definitions. These terms may apply to diseases, to symptoms, to parts of the body, to therapeutic procedures, to surgical appliances, to laboratory tests and reagents.

Classification of diseases is a list of diseases, arranged systematically in accordance with their characteristics and interrelationships. Most existing classifications are forced to use a combination of criteria such as pathology, aetiology, topography, symptomatology, etc. and none of them are satisfactory.

Nomenclature of diseases is a systematically arranged list of names of all diseases, usually (but not necessarily) without definitions. Thus, the nomenclature of diseases refers to the names under which the various diseases are recognized.

It has been long recognized that the increasing confusion in disease nomenclature constitutes a barrier to communication and to the storage and retrieval of information. Few diseases have a single recognized name: most have several different - sometimes widely different - names, and some have thirty or more. Many of these names are strict synonyms; others, however, are not, but may represent only a single clinical manifestation of a given disease rather than the disease itself. The confusion is aggravated by the fact that the same name, or very similar names, may be applied to two or more different conditions, or be used in different ways by different authors. Moreover, very similar names may be used in different senses in different languages.

The main purpose of the International Nomenclature of Diseases[3] is to develop, through consensus of a large international group of experts, a single recommended name for every disease of man. The main criteria for selection of this name are that it should be specific, unambiguous, as self-descriptive and as simple as possible. Each recommended name will be accompanied by:

- ☐ a brief but fully adequate definition, in order to identify the disease unambiguously;
- ☐ a complete list of other names (synonyms) that have been applied to the disease and that are used in the medical literature (these lists are invaluable for information retrieval);
- ☐ when appropriate, linguistic notes that will clearly explain why a particular name is recommended in preference to others and any other factors that will be helpful to the reader.

A second objective of the IND is to facilitate the efficient storage and retrieval of medical information. Bibliographic information storage and retrieval systems are another area where an internationally agreed disease nomenclature would make a lasting impact. There are already a number of systems operational in the medical and health sciences and the field is still in rapid expansion. A major problem in using them is the lack of standardization of their respective indexing and retrieval vocabularies. By the standardization of terminology and the inclusion of complete lists of synonyms, the IND will provide a remedy for this situation.

A third objective of the IND is to serve as a complement to the WHO International Classification of Diseases (ICD). This calls for a brief explanation of the difference, and the relationship, between the two. The ICD is designed for the statistical classification of diseases for purposes of health statistics, and it is not a nomenclature: that is, the terms used in the ICD are not recommended names. The IND, on the other hand, is a nomenclature, and not a classification: it is a list of recommended names for diseases, without any attempt to specify the manner in which those diseases should be classified for the purposes of statistical reporting. The names recommended in the IND will be used, as appropriate, instead of the present ICD names when the Tenth Revision of the ICD is prepared for implementation.

The technical preparation of each volume of the IND is undertaken by a consultant, or group of consultants, engaged by CIOMS especially for that volume. The phases in which the preparation is carried out are as follows:

Phase I: *Preparation of first draft.* The consultant(s) prepares a first draft of the volume on a specific group of diseases (e.g. all bacterial diseases, diseases of the respiratory system, or diseases of the gastro-intestinal system). In preparing this draft, all existing international terminologies are considered; standard authoritative textbooks and journals are studied; reference is also made to standard dictionaries, classifications, and other reference works.

Phase 2: *Review of first draft.* A printout of the first draft is distributed for review to an extensive panel of approximately 50-60 experts throughout the world. These experts are invited to comment on all aspects of the first draft, especially the recommended names.

Phase 3: *Preparation of second draft.* When all the comments on the first draft have been received from the reviewers, the consultant(s) prepare a second draft, taking these comments into account.

Phase 4: *Review of second draft.* A printout of the revised draft is distributed to the same reviewers for their final comments.

Phase 5: *Preparation of final text.* On the basis of the comments received from experts after review of the second draft, a final text is prepared. An alphabetical index of all recommended names and synonyms is prepared and added to the text, which is then set up in final form for printing.

Phase 6: *Printing and publication.* The final text is published and distributed through WHO Distribution and Sales Service.

It should be emphasized that the International Nomenclature of Diseases is proposed and agreed upon by a large internationally recognized panel of experts and specialists in different disciplines of medicine and they themselves recommend the terms which should be used. The main rôle of CIOMS and WHO is essentially to coordinate and facilitate this important but extremely difficult task.

This conference - its debates and conclusions - will certainly be a most important step toward the improvement of terminology in your discipline. It is particularly important that this conference is organized under the auspices of two international societies of highest professional reputation, namely the International Federation of Otorhinolaryngological Societies and the International Society of Audiology.

I would like to take this opportunity to invite all of you, individually and as CIOMS members of your respective society, to collaborate in the preparation of the international nomenclature of otorhinolaryngological diseases. It is the hope of both CIOMS and WHO that the International Nomenclature of Diseases will facilitate communication between health workers throughout the world by providing a truly international language of dis eases and thus eliminating the barriers to communication which at present hamper efforts to improve the health of mankind.

References:

1. MANUILA A., BANKOWSKI Z., KUPKA K., LOWE D.A. Introducing the International Nomenclature of Diseases (IND), *Progress in Medical Terminology*, ed. A. Manuila, published by S. Karger, 1981
2. Medical Terminology and Lexicography. Proceedings of an International Group of Experts, Paris 1965, published by S. Karger, Basel, New York 1966.
3. Project Proposal for the Preparation of an International Nomenclature of Diseases, CIOMS document CIOMS/IND/82/1, 1982, unpublished.

Postoperative evaluation of middle ear surgery

J.F.E. Marquet

Introduction

The evaluation of the results of middle ear surgery for chronic ear diseases is essential and necessary in order to make progress. This task is difficult because there are so many data to be considered. Therefore, a definitive standard of assessment that can be accepted worldwide is urgently needed.

Correct evaluation and analysis of the results in chronic ear surgery provide the most accurate information for improvement of surgical procedures. The "postoperative state" (POS) of the surgically treated ear is the only term to be used in such an evaluation.

Who is concerned with the evaluation of the POS?
— The surgeon, in order to assess his work and the work of his team, including the other disciplines involved, but also in order to compare his study with others,
— the patient, of course, has the right to be informed about the proposed or available surgical techniques, and
— national or international professional organizations requiring standard reporting of results.

The main qualities of the POS evaluation are honesty, efficiency and uniformity.

Definition of "number"

When collecting a number of cases to be evaluated, analysed and reported, it is essential to define the term "number" versus the term "case". Therefore, we have adopted the symbol (N) when only the number of patients is considered, each patient having his particular number, and the symbol (n) for the number of surgical cases, this being a composite number indicating the year and month, together with a final number indicating the numerical position of that case during that month. Knowing the previous "surgical case" numbers and the subsequent case numbers, the entire history of the patient can be reconstructed.

Timing of POS (POS evaluation) (t)

Time intervals between successive POS evaluations should be universally similar. In our department, evaluation is done: preoperatively, immediately after surgery, within 8 days after removal of the packing, after 2 months, after 6 months and then yearly and every 5 years. These 5-years reports are not the simple mathematical addition of the cases seen during the last 5 years, but a series of cases all followed up during 5 years.

Statistical evaluation

Only well-defined terms and correct statistical methods should be used when recording statistical reports.

One has to remember that both the number of patients (N) and the number of cases (n) decrease after each period of time elapsed, as a certain number of patients disappear from follow-up because of death, personal factors, neglect of the follow-up etc. Only those cases checked after the specified period must be considered. The number (Nt) or (nt) will always be less than the initial number (Nto) and (nto).

The follow-up

A normal follow-up is represented by the number of patients (Nt) or the number of surgical cases (nt) checked at the end of each year. The quality of a follow-up may be estimated by a ratio or a percentage, e.g. Nt/Nto.

The data

Because there is a large amount of data to be recorded for surgical evaluation, a choice has to be made:

☐ *Preoperative data:*

Personal identification and preoperative diagnosis.

☐ *Peroperative data:*

General information concerning surgery: duration, technique of anaesthesia, names of surgeon and assistant. Diagnosis as result of the surgical and histopathological findings; immediately after surgery, the surgeon's opinion about the possibilities of recurrence and progress should be recorded.

Surgical procedure (here only standard data should be recorded):

— the incision should be well described,

— the approaches to the middle ear cleft must be well defined,

— eradication of pathology: as it is important to know which tissues have been removed, replaced or substituted, the surgical attitude towards drum remnants, fibrous annulus, bony walls and ossicular chains must be correctly described,

— restoration of the sound transmission system: considering the variety of possible combinations at this stage of surgery, we strongly advocate the use of the ossicular formula, based on an ossicular code, which we introduced and have routinely used for more than 15 years. The use of such a formula makes discussion of the subject easier and more comprehensive and allows a brief and thorough description of all the possible combinations especially for computer use as only 14 squares are necessary in order to tabulate every aspect of the formula. This tympano-ossicular formula is clearly illustrated on the poster "Classification of allografts in middle ear surgery" by D. Keusters, C. Van Laer and J. Marquet (cfr. p. 371).

☐ *Postoperative data:*

POS should be recorded and evaluated with respect to the anatomical status, the healing of the ear and the functional result. By definition a POS attaining the expected goal with respect to a defined technique concerning the anatomical (A) restoration, healing (H) and function (F) of the ear, is to be considered as a normal result.

— The anatomical POS states the result obtained with respect to the anatomical goal of the used technique which should be described according to the preservation, destruction or replacement of essential anatomy.

— The healed POS are the data recorded in respect of the healing after giving due consideration to the preoperative pathology.

— The functional POS represents the audiometric results but vestibular functions should also be considered. The commonly used methods are the measurement of the hearing level, the air-bone gap, the speech discrimination test and tympanometry and each method has its advantages but all of them are necessary to obtain a complete and correct functional POS. Unfortunately, many different recording techniques and reporting methods are used and consequently, this is the field in which standardization is urgently needed.

Complications

Complications should not only be described but their causes should also be analysed. The evaluation of complications is perhaps the most difficult task for it requires standardization of definition and causes, as well as an accurate statistical record.

☐ The definition of "complications" requires a correct and standard description of the POS which is not in agreement with the expected goal concerning anatomy, healing and function.

☐ The study of their causes or aetiology should be stated; the main aetiological factors to be described are surgical faults, residual pathology, recurrent pathology and postoperative problems.

☐ Their statistical study also requires further definition which must be reported correctly.

Timing

The time interval between surgery and the development of complications should be observed and reported; immediate complications according to an agreed formula within the first postoperative days; primary complication (appearing within the first postoperative year); late complications appearing at a minimum of one year after surgery; secondary complications appearing after a primary healed POS.

Numbers reported

A choice has to be made and specified in each report.

☐ First (see above) the difference between the number of patients (Nt) and the number of surgical cases (nt).

☐ To avoid confusion, it is essential to report accurately, e.g. does the population number concern the total number of patients (Nt) or the total number of cases (nt) or only the total number of patients or of cases having complications (Ct) or (ct). Both methods have their advantages and value. If the total number (Nt) or (nt) is considered, it generally concerns a study of the evaluation of similar techniques. If the total number of complications is considered, it generally concerns an evaluation of the complications themselves with respect to the pathology.

Other relevant data

— Auditory tubal function,
— Packing technique,
— The general health of the patient,
— Anaesthetisation technique,
— Radiological evaluation.

Conclusions

The suggested framework regarding postoperative evaluation of middle ear surgery has been limited to our personal view of the problem and our personal experience.[1] By bringing together the varied views here at this conference in Antwerp, we hope to be able to set up a framework that can be accepted as a basis for standardization.

Reference:

1. MARQUET J., GRAFF A. Postoperative evaluation in middle ear surgery, Audiology 21, 20-32, 1982.

Surgical anatomy of the middle ear

ABSTRACT

Y. Guerrier

TYMPANIC CAVITY

- Descriptive study

— Walls osseous, 11, labyrinthine wall - 12, jugular wall - 13, tegmental wall - 14, lateral wall - 15, carotid wall - 16, mastoid wall.

— Walls membraneous, 17, tympanic membrane.

— Contents, 18, auditory ossicles - 19, ossicular articulations - 110, ossicular ligaments - 111, ossicular muscles - 112, mucous membrane and mucosal folds.

- Topographical study

— 131, Atrium - 132, epitympanum - 133, protympanum - 134, hypotympanum - 135, retrotympanum.

MASTOID ANNEX

- 21, Mastoid process

— 221, Tympanic antrum - 222, aditus ad antrum - 223, mastoid cells.

AUDITORY TUBE

- 31, Osseous portion

— 311, Walls - 312, ostium - 314, isthmus.

- 32, Cartilaginous portion

— 321, Tubal cartilage - 322, membranous lamina

- 33, Mucous membrane
- 34, Tympanic ostium.

FACIAL NERVE AND FACIAL CANAL

TYMPANIC NERVE

VASCULAR SUPPLY OF THE MIDDLE EAR

PANEL I

Middle ear surgery

Moderator: M.M. Paparella

Moderator's comments

I am fortunate to have had the privilege of moderating this panel on middle ear surgery with such pioneering experts representing various countries of the world. Middle ear surgery in this regard refers to surgery of the middle ear cleft. The middle ear cleft is defined as the Eustachian tube, the middle ear proper, and the attached mastoid air-cell system. Topics selected in this program are timely and of interest, but certainly do not represent the many other hundreds of diseases and procedures of the middle ear cleft that might also be discussed, perhaps at other symposia.

Dr. van den Broek discusses the classic incisions for approaches to the mastoid, particularly for chronic mastoiditis. These classically described incisions, with very little modification, are currently used today according to personal preference. He further correctly stresses the importance of adequate exposure with secondary attention to cosmetic closure. Throughout the years, I have noted in teaching residents and fellows that a common mistake is made when incisions are too limited and inadequate exposure results. Since this is so, whether we are using an endaural or a postauricular approach, we always stress a wide exposure to the middle ear and mastoid. An exaggerated canalplasty, whereby first the posterior bony canal wall and then the anterior and inferior canal walls are drilled down, helps initiate exposure to the middle ear when doing chronic mastoid surgery, and it also provides a gateway for either a closed or open-cavity technique.

We are all grateful to Dr. Shea for having introduced us to stapedectomy 28 years ago. As he states, this procedure has now become adopted throughout the world and, although techniques and results vary somewhat, there is no question that this has become the desired operation for otosclerosis when applicable. The modifications of Dr. Shea's former technique are nicely itemized in his presentation in this symposium. He, with others, finds that the small fenestra is better than the large fenestra, not only for optimal hearing results, but also to avoid labyrinthine complications. He touches upon a very important point, namely whether all otolaryngologists should be performing stapedectomies. There have been several papers delivered at recent meetings in the United States which indicate that because of limited patients and training opportunities for residents, only certain individuals with adequate experience should continue to do this operation.

I think his advice is wise, because the surgeon doing an occasional stapedectomy will have a complication rate for dead cochleas much higher than would be acceptable. Surgeons who perform stapedectomies tend to have their own personal preferences. I essentially do three stapedectomy procedures, depending upon pathological and anatomical considerations. One needs not only to be concerned about otospongiotic pathology but anatomical characteristics of the oval window, the promontory, the facial nerve, the incus, etc. that will all play an important rôle in making the decision on which procedure to employ. I still, for certain patients, will perform a complete stapedectomy with a custom-made wire/connective tissue graft. We have done this for many years, and the results continue to be good to date, with a very small incidence of high-tone sensorineural loss. If the otosclerotic fixation of the footplate is limited, either anteriorly or posteriorly, I will still employ a partial stapedectomy, typically an anterior crurotomy, in which case the incudostapedial articulation as well as the stapedial ligament are preserved. If the oval window is small or if there is obliteration, or depending upon other pathological or anatomical characteristics, we more frequently will use a piston-type prosthesis through a small fenestra as described by Dr. Shea and others.

Dr. Rivas refers to the classically described types of mastoidectomy and updates them in terms of some of the procedures done currently. His term "mastoidoplasty" is an interesting one, although somewhat confusing; in my clinic, I essentially never do a radical mastoidectomy as classically described, since I use grafting techniques and Silastic in the middle ear cleft, and never obstruct the Eustachian tube with tissue. Dr. Rivas stresses the important principles of first removal of pathology and second the consideration of preservation or restoration of cochlear function.

Dr. Jansen has been one of the first pioneers for the recently described closed-cavity technique of intact-wall tympanomastoidectomy. On several occasions and again in this symposium, he has described the indications as well as the careful technique required to eradicate disease while preserving the posterior bony wall for patients with chronic otitis media and mastoiditis. This technique is a sophisticated and contemporary modification of the classically described simple mastoidectomy. In this instance, the suprapyramidal recess is opened for exposure to the middle ear and the posterior canal wall is thinned down. We continue to use this method, but whereas I used it occasionally in earlier years, I use it rarely at the present time. This is because many of our patients who have chronic mastoiditis have a sclerotic mastoid air cell system and in these patients, a mastoid cavity problem does not result because the cavity is so small but also the operation, even in the most skilled of hands, becomes a dangerous one and can lead to iatrogenic complications. This important contribution, however, continues to have its place, albeit somewhat diminished, in the treatment of chronic mastoiditis.

Dr. Palva describes the history of obliterative techniques for chronic otitis media and mastoiditis. In recent years, more than anyone else, he has pioneered, promoted, and carefully described his method of obliteration. In his paper, he has described some refinements of this technique, for example the use of bone-chips, or bone-pâté, as well as fibrin in trying to shape the medical obliterative segment. I continue to use Palva's flap when obliteration seems indicated. We use this only if mastoid cavities are quite large. This is a very helpful technique, although it is not necessary to use it in all instances, again because mastoid cavities are often sclerotic in chronic mastoiditis. It is my personal opinion that another reason this technique works so well in Dr. Palva's hands is because he is such a meticulous and careful surgeon, and if he were to use another technique I have a feeling that it would work almost as well. My experience with the use of bone-pâté is that it promotes quite a bit of postoperative reaction and may lead to surrounding granulation tissue and cellulitis which requires careful control. When using obliteration and an open-cavity technique, it is important to consider the middle ear/mastoid barrier, and also to consider the mesotympanic space to enhance tympanoplasty, grafting, and ossiculoplasty. Dr. Palva now uses fibrin and other techniques in attempts to accomplish this. I have recently described, and currently perform as a relatively routine matter in our primary mastoidecotmies, the IBM or intact-bridge tympanomastoidectomy. In this instance, I combine the desirable features of both the open and closed cavity methods, while preserving and sculpturing the facial buttress, which provides an excellent mesotympanic space or even enhances it, to promote improved results with ossiculoplasty. I obliterate the enlarged aditus by using a sheet of gel film with either bone-pâté or cartilage, followed by a graft. This method also provides a better middle ear demarcation if one uses an obliterative method as described by Palva.

It is probably appropriate that we end this session with a consideration of surgical approaches to the Eustachian tube. This is because the

Eustachian tube continues to be our chief nemesis, not only in terms of cause or pathogenesis of otitis media including chronic otitis media and mastoiditis, but all the other forms of otitis media as well. It also is our major problem in trying to achieve a good result postoperatively when using various forms of tympanoplasty and ossiculoplasty techniques. This is because no matter what technique is used, if air will not ventilate the middle ear and round window adequately after surgery, we end up with atelectasis, the inability of air to reach the round window, and therefore elimination of the phase-differential between the two windows with preferential sound conduction to the oval window which is essential to obtain and retain a good hearing result.

Dr. Morimitsu describes a technique which he correctly states is applicable only to stenosis of the osseous portion or the protympanum of the Eustachian tube. He does this by removing the bony wall of the semicanal and removing the tensor tympani muscle. I, too, have used a modification of this method. Indeed, I always look to see if there is obstruction of the protympanum in cases of chronic mastoiditis. If there is an anterior flap, somewhat like the one described by Dr. Morimitsu, I find it easy to remove bone or tympanosclerosis and to open up the protympanum, which often includes elevating the medial portion of the anterior bony canal wall. One needs to be careful of the internal carotid artery which lies in the posterior inferior dimension of the protympanum, and in some instances there may be a bulge of this bony covering and in rare instances one might even encounter an aneurysm. The problem, however, with this approach or any other approach to the bony Eustachian tube is that the fundamental problem is not the bony tube, typically, but the fibrocartilaginous tube which opens because of palatal muscles which attach to the soft medial two-thirds of the Eustachian tube. Normally the Eustachian tube is closed and when these palatal muscles contract, then air gains access to the middle ear and to the round window. This is a common and large problem, and to date there is no solution in sight.

Once again, I thank you for the privilege of serving as moderator for this panel, whose participants have been pioneers for the various surgical methods they once again describe and discuss with us during these proceedings.

Surgical approaches in otology

P. van den Broek

Introduction

Antwerp is a town with a great cultural heritage. Like many other older European cities it is situated on the bank of an important river, the Schelde, and has a history going back to the Roman Empire. One of the most well-known artists who spent a major part of his life in Antwerp was Peter Paul Rubens (1577-1640) who is considered to be one of the most important painters of all time. He made over a thousand paintings and decorated many churches. Many musea and churches treasure the witnesses of this great man.

One of his paintings from the collection of the National Gallery in London demonstrates the dilemma of the otologic surgeon. The painting is called "the Judgement of Paris" and was painted in 1639. It represents the dilemma of Paris, the son of the king of Troy, who had to make a choice between Minerva, Venus and Juno. His choice would decide his future — choosing Minerva would mean wisdom and choosing Venus would mean beauty. A perhaps slightly forced comparison with the anterior and posterior approach in otological surgery will result in the same conclusion: the first is wisdom, the second is beauty.

The surgical approaches have a shorter history compared with the paintings of Rubens. The retroaural route to the mastoid originated around the middle of the last century and is generally attributed to William Wilde (1815-1876). In 1853 he published his "practical observations on aural surgery" and he described the retroaural incision for drainage of a mastoid abscess.

The actual opening of the antrum and the mastoid was published in 1873 by Schwartze and Eysell. The retroaural approach was for many years the only approach to the mastoid until Kessel, between 1880 and 1885, published several articles advocating the endaural route to the tympanic membrane and disease arising from it.

In the first half of this century the retroaural route became gradually less popular especially for the treatment of chronic ear disease and cholesteatoma. The endaural radical operation outlined by Thies, who reported on 1500 cases in 1933, became a standard procedure resulting later in major advances to be made in reconstructive ear surgery with the one stage fenestration operation by Lempert and the tympanoplastic procedures by Wullstein and Zöllner.

However, whenever the pendulum swings far to one side it will swing back again. In the sixties and seventies there has been a clear revival of the posterior approaches to the mastoid with techniques promoting the maximum preservation of the structures like the combined approach tympanoplasty (CAT, posterior tympanotomy). The most recent history does not yet allow us to draw conclusions. The dilemma is still there and the surgeons' choice will be governed by anatomical, clinical, pathological, technical and sometimes personal and emotional considerations.

Incisions

The incision of the skin is the first step of any surgical approach. In general, an incision should meet the following requirements:

— it should create a broad access to the surgical field,

— it should allow direct extension to an adjacent anatomical area, if this should prove to be necessary,

— it should not jeopardize the possibility of using adjacent skin as a free or pedicled flap,

— it should be cosmetic as much as possible.

In ear surgery most of these requirements will be met without many problems. The surgical approaches can grossly be divided into three:

— A: posterior, retroaural, transmastoid,

— B: anterior, endaural, and

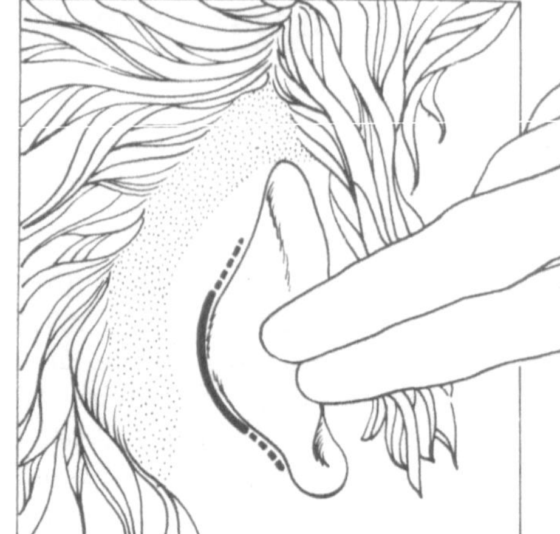

Fig. 1. Retroauricular crease incision

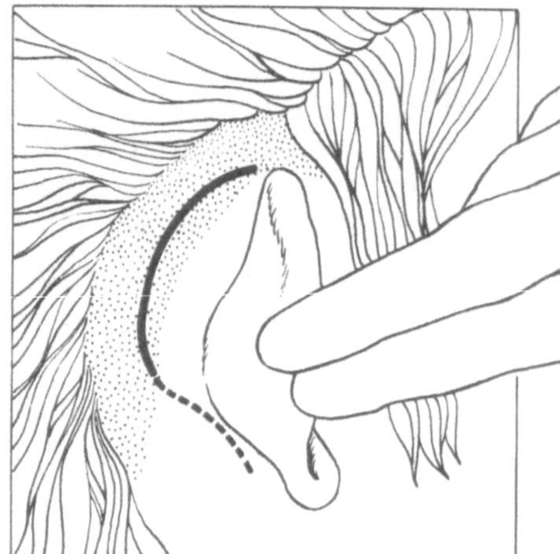

Fig. 2. Extended retroauricular incision for a broad access to the mastoid and middle ear

— C: transmeatal, transcanal.

Every approach can be further divided into a limited, an extended and a modified approach.

Type A — The posterior approach. This approach allows wide access from posterior to the mastoid and the middle ear. If desired, the canal skin can be transected which allows a combined approach. It meets all the requirements outlined before. For the posterior approach three types of incisions may be used.

A1: Retroauricular crease incision (figure 1). This incision is drawn in the retroauricular fold posterior to the concha. It is an excellent incision for limited mastoid operations and for a posterior approach to the external meatus. This can be necessary when the anterior part of the tympanic membrane is obscured by the convexity of the anterior wall of the meatus. It is less suitable for extensive mastoid surgery.

A2: Retroauricular flap incision (figure 2). This incision, which is drawn 2-4 cm behind the auricular fold, can be varied in position. After passing through the skin, the skin is lifted up with the subcutaneous tissues just lateral to the superficial fascial plane. Following the lifting up of the skin, a muscle-periosteal flap based superiorly or anteriorly can be lifted, thus uncovering the mastoid cortex. This incision provides a good access to the entire mastoid area for both limited and extended surgery. The muscle-periosteal flap is used to cover the mastoid defect or can be used in different types of obliterative surgery (Palva et al.).

A3: Extended retroauricular incision (figure 3). When a wider access is needed, the previous incision can be extended in cranial or caudal direction. This is necessary for extensive temporal bone surgery as in temporal bone resection and infratemporal approach for neoplasms (Fisch et al.). In these cases the external meatus is transected in the sagittal plane. The auricle with the most lateral part of the external meatus is retracted anteriorly.

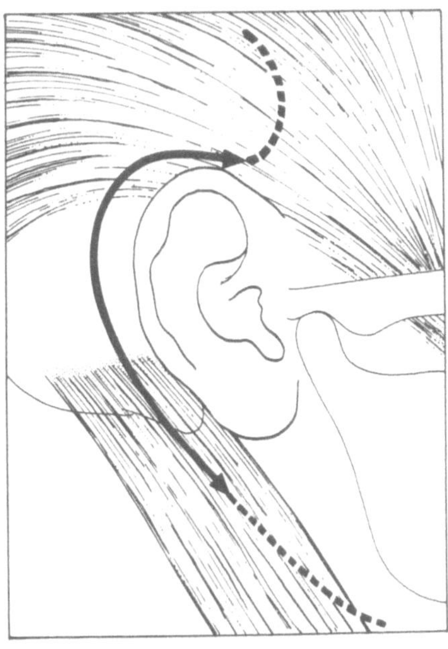

Fig. 3. Wide-field retroauricular incision for extensive surgery of the petrosal bone and infratemporal fossa

Type B — The anterior approach. This approach is often advocated as the ideal to perform surgery on the middle ear and the mastoid as in radical and modified radical operations. It provides the possibility of shaping a cavity as it is seen through the meatus. Access is gained through an endaural incision consisting of an external and endomeatal part. The external part of this incision can be divided into three types:

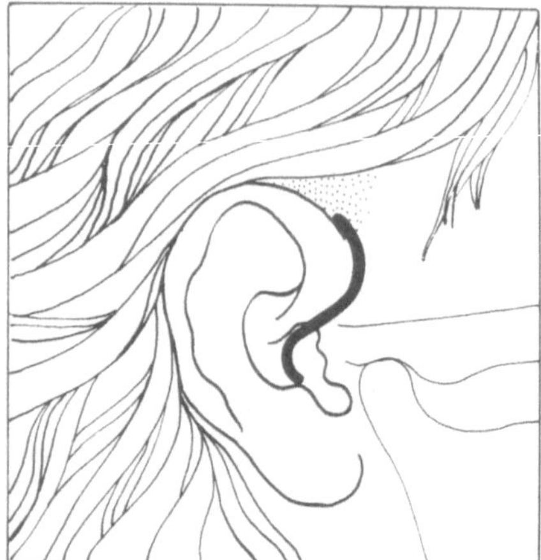

Fig. 4. Regular endaural incision for open cavity surgery

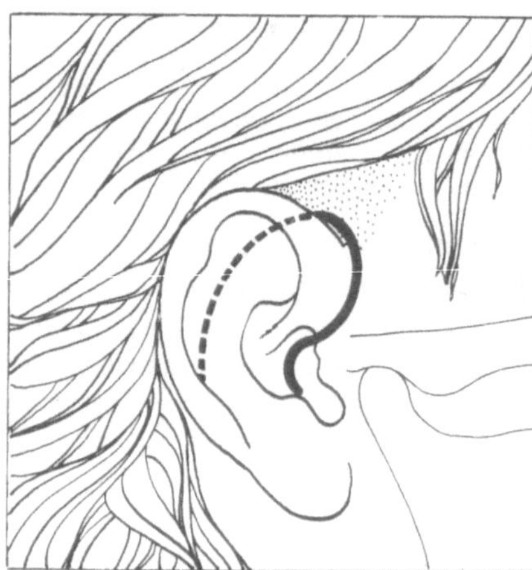

Fig. 5. Extended endaural incision for a wide transmeatal and transmastoid approach

B1: The regular endaural incision (Lempert type, figure 4). The external part of this incision transects the opening in the cartilage between the helix and tragus and it ends along the antero-superior edge of the helix.

B2: The extended endaural incision (Heermann type, figure 5). The incision is taken further over the superior edge of the muscle and ends posteriorly to the ear at the level of the external meatus. It allows a complete detachment of the superior half of the auricle and gives a wide access to the region of the middle ear and the mastoid.

B3: Wide-field endaural incision (Rambo, House type, figure 6). This incision is drawn anteriorly to the helix upwards in a vertical direction. The lower limb will extend either anteriorly to the tragus or join the endaural Lempert incision. Originally used for access to the temporalis muscle for obliterative operations, it has later been used for the middle fossa approach.

Type C — The endomeatal or transcanal approach.
Limited surgery on the tympanic membrane and middle ear can be done through a strictly endomeatal incision. Many incisions have been described. They can be classified as follows:

C1: Simple widening incision of the meatus (figure 7). This incision is prefered by some surgeons for any transmeatal operation instead of a speculum. A slightly better access is obtained but the bleeding from the incision can be troublesome and there can be a small delay in healing.

C2: Medially based tympanomeatal flap incision (figure 8). Incisions to create a medially based

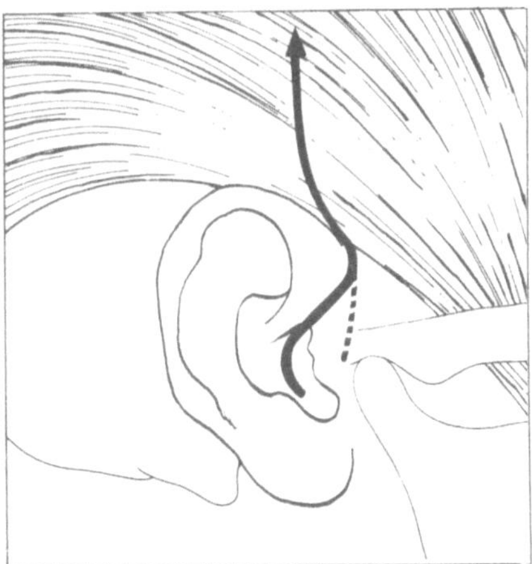

Fig. 6. Wide-field endaural incision for obliterative surgery and middle fossa approach

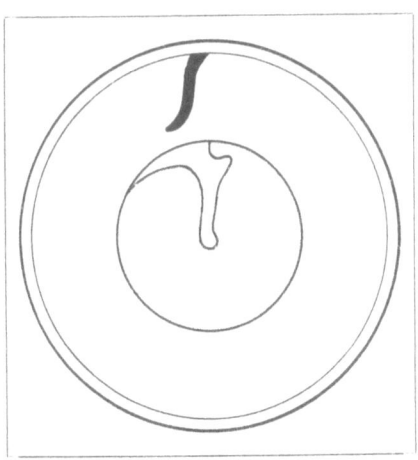

Fig. 7. Simple widening incision of the meatus

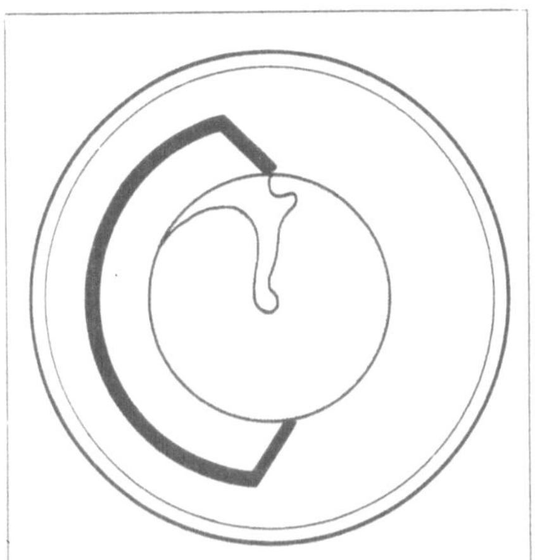

Fig. 8. Medially based tympanomeatal flap incision

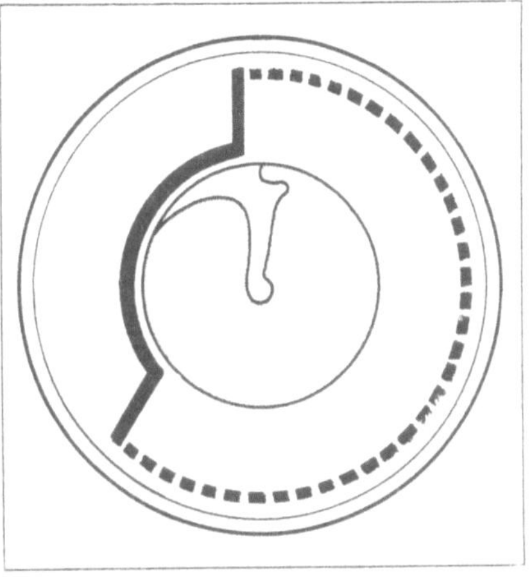

Fig. 9. Endomeatal laterally based incision. Various types

tympanomeatal flap (Rosen type) can be done as for a tympanotomy for otosclerosis. The incision is drawn in the meatus from 12 to 6 o'clock on the posterior side, parallel to the tympanic annulus at a distance between 5 and 8 mm. At 12 and 6 o'clock the incision nearly joins the annulus.

C3: Endomeatal laterally based incision. Various types (figure 9). Incisions to create a laterally based meatal flap. Type C3 is usually an extension of an endoaural incision which has to be completed in the meatus. As preservation of meatal skin is an important part of any ear surgery,

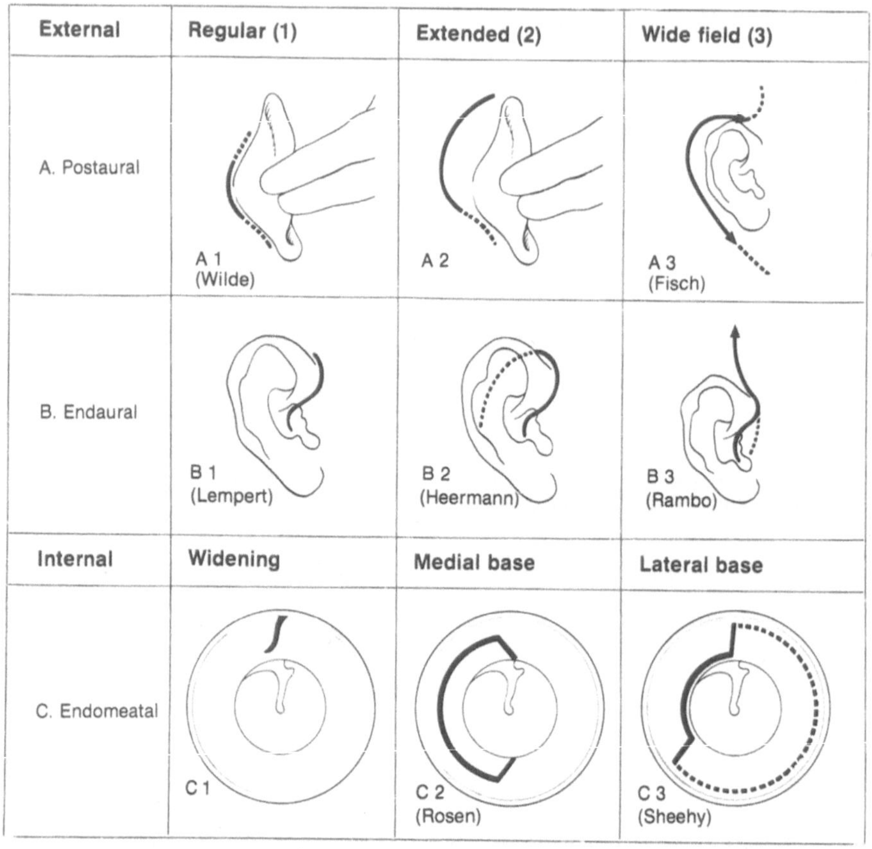

External	Regular (1)	Extended (2)	Wide field (3)
A. Postaural	A 1 (Wilde)	A 2	A 3 (Fisch)
B. Endaural	B 1 (Lempert)	B 2 (Heermann)	B 3 (Rambo)
Internal	**Widening**	**Medial base**	**Lateral base**
C. Endomeatal	C 1	C 2 (Rosen)	C 3 (Sheehy)

Fig. 10. Classification system for incisions in ear surgery

these incisions have to be carefully planned to lose as little skin as possible during the surgery. The flap can be very limited as in the classical Lempert incision but can also be composed of the entire posterior half of the meatal skin. It is impossible to classify all the individual variations described for these endomeatal incisions.

Finally, in an attempt to classify the surgical approaches into a single system which would allow comparison when results are reported, we have summarized the different incisions in a schematic drawing, which allows classifications in a Type A, Type B and Type C approach (figure 10). Each of these is further subdivided into: 1. limited, 2. extended and 3. wide-field, which indicates the extent of the incision used. When a combination of incisions is used as, for instance, in a retroauricular and transmeatal incision, this can be indicated with the classification system presented.

Stapedectomy - Technique and results

J.J. Shea

Anesthesia
The patient is put to sleep with Innovar™ neuroleptanalgesia if small, relaxed, with low blood pressure and generally suited for local anesthesia. Neuroleptanthesia with endotrachael nitrous oxide and endoforane (Forane™) is used if the patient is large, nervous, with elevated blood pressure and generally not suited for local anesthesia. The patient's head is secured to the table with a comfortable head holder, and a speculum holder is used. The middle ear is entered in the usual way taking care not to injure the chorda tympani nerve.

Technique
The technique used depends upon the pathology present. In those ears with localized anterior otosclerosis, the footplate is cut across with a pick and the posterior half of the footplate is removed. The opening is covered with compressed vein from the back of the hand and a platinum teflon cup prosthesis is inserted.

If the otosclerosis is more widespread and invading, the footplate, a small round opening 0,65 mm in diameter, is made with a microdrill and the opening covered with a flap of the lining membrane of the middle ear from the promontory. A platinum teflon cup prosthesis is then inserted.

Twenty milligrams of sugar coated sodium fluoride and 425 mg calcium lactate with vitamin D are given twice daily to all patients with widespread otosclerosis at operation, demineralization of cochlear capsule by polytomography, or rapidly progressive sensorineural hearing loss, for two to four years. This would seem to be of value but I have no firm proof of it.

Repeat operations, which are more common now than before, are more difficult than primary operations, less likely to improve the hearing and more likely to make the patient worse. The patient must be advised of the greater risks of a repeat operation. If possible, the lining membrane of the vestibule should be preserved, if at all possible, and the end of the prosthesis, especially a loop of wire, left in the vestibule beneath the lining membrane of the vestibule if it is not causing the patient any symptoms.

Results
Results with the two groups have been good and generally the same, with no statistical difference between the two, other than more overclosure in the large

fenestra group. Long-term analyses of results present many problems because of the gradual sensorineural hearing loss that is part of the natural history of otosclerosis. For that reason, I chose a two year period five years ago to compare the two techniques as being long enough to be valid but before unrelated sensorineural hearing loss would begin to take place.

One thousand consecutive primary stapedectomy operations performed 5 years ago (1977-1978), when the two techniques described above were being performed just as described, were reviewed. Results after 5 years: (see below).

The only significant difference between the two groups was the larger average dB overclosure in the large fenestra operation. This was probably due to the greater cochlear reserve in ears in which this technique was performed. Generally, the small fenestra operation was done in those ears with more extensive otosclerosis in which the cochlear reserve was less, so it is not surprising the average overclosure was less.

Complications

There have been no perilymph leaks in the large fenestra group because the oval window is covered with vein. There have been no known perilymph fistulas in the small perilymph group because the oval window is covered with a flap of lining membrane of the middle ear from the promontory, and this technique is not used if there is a leak or strong pulse of perilymph when the vestibule is opened. If, when a small opening is made, there is a leak of perilymph, the opening is enlarged to at least half the oval window and a compressed vein used to cover the opening to ensure a good seal.

In this series of 1 000 consecutive primary stapedectomies there were no serious complications during or after operation, no perilymph fistula, no postoperative infection, perforation of the drum, or total sensorineural hearing loss. Further cochlear

	Small Fenestra		Large Fenestra	
	N - 412	%	N - 588	%
Closure AB gap to 10 dB	399	96,8	564	95,9
Overclosure	354	85,9	517	87,9
Average dB gain		9.1 dB		13.9 dB

	Small Fenestra		Large Fenestra	
	N - 412	%	N - 588	%
Further cochlear hearing loss	8	2,0	13	2,2

hearing loss of more than 10 dB of bone conduction and/or decline of more than 10 % for speech discrimination did occur.

In three operations in this series there was a slow perilymph leak when the vestibule was opened, which stopped when the head was elevated, and in each a good result was achieved by removing half the footplate and interposing a vein.

Summary and conclusions
The small fenestra operation is better than the large fenestra operation because it is easier to perform, and less traumatic, and gives equally good results.

The large fenestra operation gives results as good as the small fenestra if the fenestra is small and posterior in the oval window.

I prefer the microdrill to make an opening in the footplate because it is much easier and safer to use than the laser, and gives an opening with living margins, more likely to heal than with the laser in which the margins are vaporized.

I prefer the platinum teflon cup prosthesis to a steel cup piston prosthesis because teflon cup and piston can be altered at operation, if necessary, and the platinum loops give better attachment to the lower incus.

If the incus is so long the lenticular process is not directly over the oval window opening, I use the original teflon piston prosthesis, which gives equally good results as the platinum teflon cup prosthesis.

I have no experience with wire as a prosthesis, except to remove many hundreds of them. Because of the natural spring in wire it is difficult to attach to the incus, and the wire loop at the bottom has a tendency to migrate, become fixed to the margins of the oval window and penetrate the oval window seal.

It would appear that a 0,6 mm diameter prosthesis is optimum, being large enough to get good low tone hearing gain but not too large as to make insertion in a narrow and deep oval window through a thickened footplate impossible.

After one year if the hearing is improved from the first operation, with closure of the AB gap with no decline in comprehension and no dizziness, it is prudent to operate the other ear.

I continue to use sodium fluoride with calcium and vitamin D in most patients with widespread otosclerosis at operation although I have no proof of its value.

Twenty-eight years have passed since the first stapedectomy and reconstruction of the sound conducting mechanism of the middle ear with an artificial prosthesis. The results of this operation, done in various ways throughout the world are good, and have stood the test of time.

About 90 % of ears so operated will have a permanent hearing gain and 1 % will be permanently worse.

Despite the preferences expressed in this report, the results achieved by most competent surgeons throughout the world are remarkably the same, regardless of the technique used, with certain exceptions. Unless a surgeon can equal these results he or she should not perform the stapedectomy operation.

Otitis media - Open techniques

J.A. Rivas

In 1873, more than a century ago, v. Tröltsch proposed a modification of the simple mastoidectomy technique because of the high percentage of recurrence of otorrhea or cholesteatomas. Von Bergman applied the name "radical" to the process of removing the posterio-superior bony wall of the external auditory canal and leaving an open cavity. Almost a hundred years ago, Zaufal described the surgery technique which left the antrum, mastoids, the attic, the middle ear and the canal all exposed. A year later, Stakes described meatoplasty. This radical technique had helped to control the problem of recurring disease because it enables us to completely clean out the mastoid cavity, when necessary, by taking out both the ossicles (except the stapes) and the tympanic remnant (without much attention, however, to hearing function).

In 1910 Bondy became concerned about cases involving perforations with attic cholesteatomas accompanied by an intact pars tensa in patients with good hearing. He proposed a modification

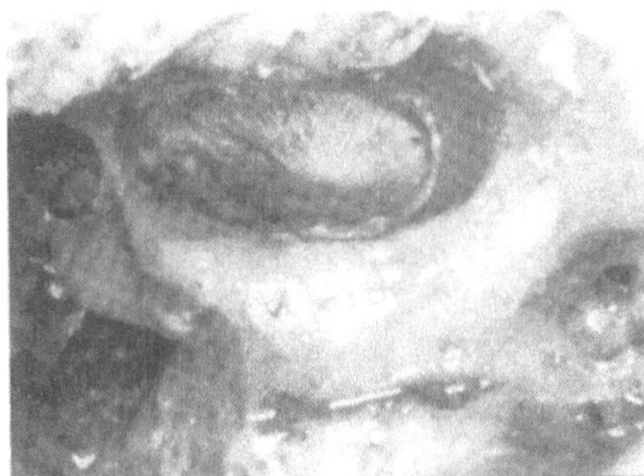

Fig. 1. Modified radical mastoidectomy in which the facial bridge, the ossicles, and the ear drum have been preserved.

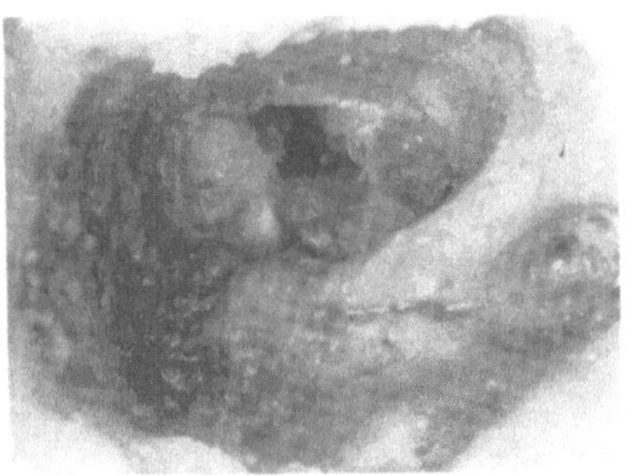

Fig. 2. Radical mastoidectomy in which the facial bridge has been taken out and the ossicles removed.

of the radical operation (figure 1) which would disturb neither the ossicular chain (except at the perforation level of the pars flaccida) nor the intact pars tensa and muscosa of the middle ear. He took down the superior osseous meatal wall and part of the posterior wall, thus effecting the permanent exteriorization of the attic, antrum, and mastoids. With this approach, good hearing was preserved. Bondy's technique, however, was not widely accepted, as ear surgeons continued to be preoccupied more with possible endocranial complications than with preserving or improving hearing. They were mainly interested in obtaining a dry, healthy ear.

Only after Lempert's one-stage fenestration procedure, in 1938, did Bondy's modified radical mastoidectomy become more popular. Its importance was enhanced when Zöllner developed his tympanoplasty techniques in which the sound-conducting apparatus of the middle ear is reconstructed.

Indications for radical mastoidectomy

— Carcinomas in the external auditory canal and middle ear in which most of the temporal bone has to be removed.

— Cholesteatomas with severe sensorineural hearing loss.

Modified radical mastoidectomy and mastoidplasty

Around 1960, when I began my training in ear surgery, I chose the closed technique of conserving the posterio-superior wall of the canal. Later I combined this with a posterior tympanotomy. At first the results were satisfactory, but after one or two years recurrent cholesteatomas appeared. This convinced us to switch to the radical mastoidectomy approach (figure 2) in which the posterio-superior bony wall of the canal is completely excised, the facial ridge is lowered and the bridge is taken out for large and medium sized cholesteatomas located in the middle ear, the facial recess, the attic and/or antrum.

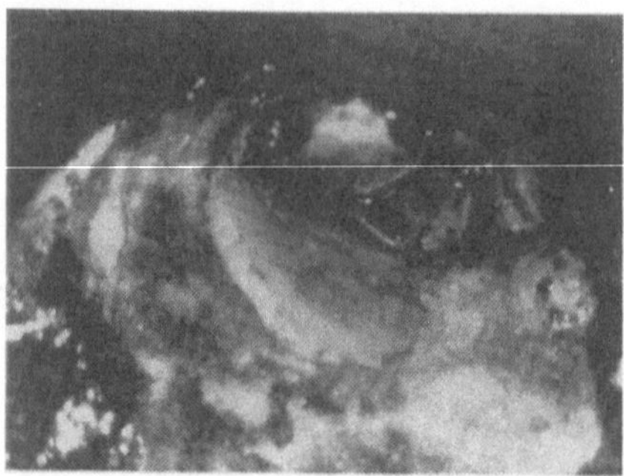

Fig. 3. Mastoidoplasty in which the open cavity has been packed with bone-pâté and cartilage from the concha.

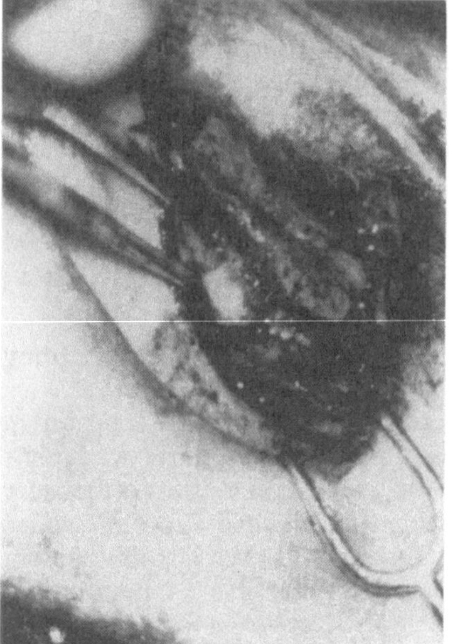

Fig. 4. Meatoplasty. We get a flap of posterior canal skin and cut out a piece of cartilage from the concha.

The operating area is bounded by the following:
— superiorly, the tegmen tympani from the tympanic orifice of the Eustachian tube to the sino-dural angle behind,
— posteriorly, the sigmoid sinus and the sino-dural angle,
— anteriorly, the anterior annulus and the anterior wall of the canal, which is straightened out in order to bring into view the tympanic orifice of the Eustachian tube.

The floor of the mastoid cavity and the external auditory canal should be kept at the same level so as to insure good drainage. The posterior bony wall of the canal is lowered as far as the vertical portion of the facial nerve; it is drilled down until moderate bleeding occurs, continually observing the landmarks of the lateral semicircular canal and the posterior annulus. The medial landmarks are the labyrinth, the facial nerve, the promontory, and the ossicular chain.

In a one-stage surgical procedure, we perform a mastoidplasty (figure 3), using healthy bone drilled out during the mastoidectomy, cartilage from the concha to fill up the attic, and a piece of Palva muscle flap to cover the bone. (The flap is covered with skin from the canal and concha excised during the endoaural and concha incision). In the mastoidectomy we use a postauricular incision.

We prefer to use a single surgical procedure for large and medium sized cholesteatomas involving partial or total destruction of the posterio-superior wall without relating it to the cochlear reserve because our primary objective is to excise the tumor in a one-stage operation. The patient, however, is warned, that if results are not satisfactory, a second-stage operation will follow. We also use it in surgical check-ups for recurrent cholesteatomas.

Meatoplasty (figure 4)
In open mastoidectomy, we make an incision in the canal superiorly and inferiorly to get a flap of posterior skin, lengthening the incision from above to the concha. Once we arrive at the base of the helix, we cut out a piece of cartilage from the concha, taking advantage of its natural curve. We take out the leftover skin from the concha to use it as free flap to cover the resulting open cavity in the external auditory canal. The posterior flap of skin is used to cover the Palva muscle flap from the musculoplasty, thus giving us a canal that is twice as big as the original. We pack the canal with Gelfoam and sponge.

At present we are using the closed technique in small attic cholesteatomas lateral to the malleus and incus, in cases showing an undamaged external attic wall, or when the lesion is minimal and can be repaired with cartilage or autologous or homologous bone. In any case, a posterior tympanotomy is performed, if necessary. We also use the closed technique in those rare cases in which a suspected cholesteatoma is not found, in osteitis, and chronic osteomyelitis of the temporal bone.

Contra-indications in open technique cases
— In chronic simple otitis media perforations accompanied by mucoid otorrhea with central perforations (without cholesteatoma) that could result in spontaneous closing of the perforation.
— In acute otitis media accompanied by mastoiditis.
— In chronic tubercular otitis media.
— In chronic allergic otitis media.

Anesthesia
We always use general anesthesia when performing mastoidectomies (and our patients prefer it) on children and young people as well as adults with controlled hypotension. This gives us an operating area relatively free of bleeding. Patients are discharged on the second or third day after surgery.

Postoperative care
We use analgesics; however, if there are signs of infection, cultures and antibiograms are made, followed by immediate administration of antibiotics, antibiotic powder, sulfas, and fungustatic agents.

The outer dressing is changed on the first day of postoperative treatment and the patient is discharged; in some cases, on the second day following surgery. The first postoperative treatment in the office is scheduled for the

Comparison of results obtained with open and closed technique
As you can see on the charts, we have compared our hearing results from both open and closed techniques.

	OPEN TECHNIQUE			CLOSED TECHNIQUE		
dB	NUMBER OF CASES	%		NUMBER OF CASES	%	
Hearing gain						
0	16	34,78	58,67	13	15,85	71,93
1-10	15	32,60		37	45,12	
11-20	9	19,56		18	21,95	
21-30	2	4,34		2	2,43	
31-40	1	2,17		2	2,43	
Hearing loss						
1-10	2	4,34	6,51	3	3,65	12,17
11-20	1	2,17		5	6,09	
21-30	0	—		2	2,43	
31-40	0	—		0	0	
TOTAL	46	100		82	100	

The percentages of recurrent cholesteatoma in the two techniques are as follows:

RECURRENT CHOLESTEATOMA				
NUMBER OF CASES	TECHNIQUE	RECURRENCE	%	FOLLOW-UP
46	Open	2	4,34	12-24 months
61	Closed	5	8,19	6-48 months
TOTAL CASES		7		

fourth day. On the eighth day we remove the sponges, leaving the Gelfoam. If epidermization is not progressing, the area is covered with a skin graft two weeks later. As the epidermization in the surgical cavity progresses, the number of postoperative visits is reduced to once every six months for a period of five years.

Otitis media - Closed techniques

ABSTRACT

C.W. Jansen

Closed techniques in chronic middle ear surgery follow the principle of closed aeration of the middle ear, including the mastoid. In contrast to acute mastoiditis where antrostomy is also done to provide re-aeration, preservation and improvement of tubal function in cholesteatoma needs a special technique, which was introduced in 1958 by the author.

Different kinds of techniques which more or less follow the same principles have been originated later on.

Partial or total removal of the posterior bony canal wall and reinstallation is done instead of preservation of the posterior bony wall.

The postoperative evaluation of middle ear surgery needs an exact explanation of each technical procedure to ensure a correct follow-up of cases and comparison of results.

On the other hand, one has to realize that many factors have to be taken into account. For example computerization, and also the way of publication, will bring up new problems which cannot be solved just by simplification.

Chronic otitis media - Obliterative techniques

T. Palva

Early obliteration dates back to Mosher[1] in 1911, who employed subcutaneous full thickness post-auricular tissues down to the sterno-mastoid muscle to occlude the antrum and epitympanum. He used a superior pedicle which leaves the obliteration material insufficiently supplied by arteries and nerves. Tongues of temporalis muscle have also been brought to mastoid cavity for obliteration but these grafts frequently suffer from insufficient blood and nerve supply and generally contain an insufficient bulk.[2]

Starting from Popper's idea[3] (1935) to line the mastoid cavity with thin periosteum, in the 1950's, I started to employ his basic form of incision with a meatally based pedicle but included all subcutaneous tissues in flaps of various sizes not to line but to obliterate the mastoid cavity.[4] Technical improvements in the obliteration procedure were made in the early 1970's to avoid possible late cavitation of the ear canal in large cavities. Cortical bone-pâté is collected and pressed tight for bony obliteration of Trautmann's triangle and of the main part of the posterior cavity. Building up a new posterior annulus at its original level is facilitated by using bone-pâté and periosteum containing mastoid tip bone chips, now together with fibrin glue. Similarly, this material can be cemented posteriorly to the soft ear canal to give it real new bone support. Biopsy specimens removed on occasional revisions many years later provide evidence of vital, firm new bone in the obliterated areas.

Other methods for obliteration have included abdominal fat as free grafts, similar to those used for frontal sinus obliteration, bone from the iliac crest, fresh cartilage from the concha or homograft denatured nasal cartilage. Also artificial materials have come up from time to time, starting from methyl methacrylate and including various types of plastic materials. These materials act as foreign bodies, create a giant cell reaction, become exposed, infected and must be removed.

Technique of obliteration

The prerequisite for open surgery with tympanoplasty and obliteration is that the surgeon can do competent bone work in the mastoid and epitympanum. One must be able to skeletize all three semicircular canals, and if need arises follow infected and granulating cell tracks until healthy bone appears. The surgeon must also follow the temporal dural laminal inward bend down to geniculate ganglion area and have the lamina directly visible at all areas. This direct vision must extend to the anterior epitympanic cell close to the Eustachian tube. All diseased tissues are removed from the two triangles, one formed by the tensor tympani muscle with the facial nerve to its ganglion, and by the facial nerve with the ampullar end of the superior semicircular canal, temporal bone lamina forming the short side of both these triangles. It goes without saying that diseased tissues should also be removed from the meso- and hypotympanum, and from the Eustachian tube orifice. However, these latter areas are all anterior to the obliteration itself and disease, if left there, will make itself quickly visible by inspection through the ear canal.

In Shrapnell's membrane cholesteatoma not involving the mesotympanum, the surgery I recommend entails preservation of the soft ear canal as an intact tube, detaching it from the annulus and then removing the posterior bony wall. Stapes can be made more prominent by cutting of long process of the incus and reconstruction on the lenticular process can be made with a malleus head. The defect in the Shrapnell's membrane is finally patched from the medial side. The soft ear canal can either be packed with vaseline gauze or with 2 or 3 expandable tampons. The posterior tympanic membrane fibrous annulus will be in contact with the new bone-pâté/bone-chips annulus and the cavity will be filled with the flap and additional bone-pâté.

In the ears with extensive disease of the middle ear cleft, with no pars tensa, the ear canal skin can be cut in two halves, forming large swing doors.[5] These can be lifted forward with the ear canal skin and the tympanic cleft cleaned meticulously. One must often drill deep between the cochlea and the jugular bulb as well as remove all diseased mucosa from the facial and tympanic sinus. Before reconstruction there are only bare bony surfaces including the Eustachian tube orifice and the window niches.

I do surgery also in these ears in one stage and either cover the promontory bone with thin silastic sheeting or thin lyophilized dura. If the other ear has normal hearing, as fortunately is the case in 85 % of patients, staging of the surgery is not necessary. If the middle ear becomes ventilated, hearing will be reasonably good. If not, the patient will have the same hearing level as before surgery but the ear will be safe and dry and the use of a hearing aid is possible. Staging may be used if improvement in hearing levels is the primary hope on the patient's list.

Results

I have recently analysed two series of ears, operated on between 1974 and 1983. Group I consisted of 126 ears with cholesteatoma, the primary surgery having been done by myself. Group II consisted of 154 referred cases in which primary surgery had been made elsewhere and the surgery done by myself was a revision after an earlier combined approach tympanoplasty (CAT), open cavity method or obliteration surgery. All cases have been followed at the outpatient department by myself annually but also at other times patients have a free access to consultation if the ear is not symptom free. The observation period ranges from 1 to 11 years with an average follow-up time of 5,1 years.

After preoperative treatment, ears in Group I were dry in 39 % of patients and showed Staphylococci in 33 %. The number of Pseudomonas or Proteus infection was relatively low (8 % and 6 % respectively). In Group II, infected ears were clearly more frequent (78 %) despite energetic treatment and the frequency of Pseudomonas infection (21 %)

Table 1. Results of preoperative bacterial cultures				
	Group I		Group II	
	N	%	N	%
Staphylococci	41	33	54	35
Pseudomonas	10	8	32	21
Proteus	8	6	2	1
Miscellaneous	18	14	32	21
Ear dry	49	39	34	22
Total	**126**	**100**	**154**	**100**

Table 2. General data on open surgery with obliteration				
	Group I		Group II	
	N	%	N	%
Total	126	100	154	100
Preoperative data:				
The opposite ear deaf	8	6	2	1
Facial paralysis	—	—	1	1
Operated ear deaf	2	2	6	4
Peroperative data:				
Carcinoma	—	—	1	1
Labyrinthine fistula	14	11	18	12
Bare carotid artery	1	1	1	1
Dural and brain herniation	—	—	1	1
Cholesteatoma lateral to ossicles	4	3	—	—
Rigid footplate	—	—	1	1
Complications:				
Temporary facial nerve palsy	3	2	—	—
Sensorineural loss (35 dB)	1	1	—	—
Accidental opening of vestibule	1	1	1	1
Deaf ear	1	1	—	—
Postoperative revisions:				
Residual cholesteatoma	1	1	1	1
Retraction pocket	1	1	2	2
Meatoplasty	4	3	3	2
Removal of Proplast	2	2	2	1
Removal of tympanic cholesterol cyst	1	1	—	—
Eosinophilic granuloma	1	1		
Tuberculosis	—	—	1	1
Tympanoplasty	3	2	1	1
Removal of tubal prosthesis	2	2	1	1

clearly higher than in Group I (table 1).

The peroperative (table 2) data disclosed labyrinthine fistulae in 11 % of patients in Group I and 12 % in Group II and thus the figures as such do not differ. It is worth noting, however, that Group II developed fistulae except in one case, during the interval between the last surgery and the revision performed by myself. Two ears with large, bare carotid artery in the middle ear, one large brain herniation and one carcinoma were unexpected additional findings. In Group II surgery as a rule was more demanding and more extensive. The advancement of disease was also manifested by 6 deaf ears (4 %) before surgery. Squamous epithelium grew in most crevices of the tympanum and in 83 ears (54 %) all soft tissues were removed from the tympanic cleft, including the tubal orifice.

Postoperatively (table 2), there were 2 ears with paresis and one with total paralysis of the facial nerve, all in Group I. The first two recovered in 2 weeks and 2 months, respectively. In the third, the abnormally high-placed nerve was totally cut with the drill, grafted and made a good recovery in 6 months. The frequency of temporary paralysis, putting both groups together, was thus 0,8 %.

The only deaf ear in both groups (0,4 %) resulted from the removal of cholesteatoma covering extensive labyrinthine fistulae in the horizontal and superior canals. Two accidental openings of the vestibule resulted in no damage to the inner ear.

Recurrence of cholesteatoma was seen in the form of one residual and one retraction pocket in Group I (1,6 %). The former was operated in 1977 when a biopsy indicated that all hypotympanic squamous epithelium had probably not been removed. The ear was watched and in 2 years a cholesteatoma regrowth was already noticeable and the revision was done one year later. The retraction pocket developed in cholesteatoma-like formation 2 years after surgery but because of good hearing the patient could be brought to accept revision surgery only 2 years later. His hearing has remained good over the observed 7-year period.

In Group II one ear with an epitympanic residual cholesteatoma was revised 2 years later. In 2 ears, retraction pockets were treated conservatively for several years but were then revised. Counting all 5 ears of recurrent cholesteatoma together from both groups, gives a frequency of 1,8%.

Meatoplasty as a secondary procedure was done under local anesthesia in 7 ears (2,5 %). In all ears it prevented further accumulation of epithelium and wax and gave a small healed cavity as an end result.

A reperforation developed in 2 ears (1,6 %) in Group I and in 4 ears (2,6 %) in Group II. Ninety-four (75 %) of ears in Group I and 113 (73 %) in Group II have been dry during the whole observation period and none is draining continuously. One instance of drainage has been noticed in 29 ears (10 %) of all cases and 2 to 3 times in 24 ears (8,6 %). In 7 ears (2,5 %) there has been drainage more than three times during the postoperative time and two were really longstanding. In one of them, even revision surgery was done without result but finally, tuberculosis could be proved in both cases. An antituberculus medication was given for both patients and since then these two ears have remained dry.

In most ears the cause for drainage was found to be myringitic changes in the ear drum, or external ear canal irritation. These were quickly brought to an end with 20 % silver nitrate surface treatment supplemented by 3 % boric acid in 70 % alcohol ear drops for 3 weeks.

In this connection the results of hearing are given only as average levels for the two groups (table 3). These figures are somewhat better postoperatively, but as all ears are included, the spread is large and the differences are not significant. A detailed analysis related to tympanic pathology will be reported separately.

Table 3. Hearing results (Average for 0,5, 1 and 2 kHz)

Preoperative	**Group I**	**Group II**
Air	45,4	52,9
Bone	17,7	18,8
A-B gap	27,7	34,2
Hearing level 40 dB or less	59 ears	39 ears
Postoperative		
Air	41,6	44,7
Bone	16,8	17,8
A-B gap	25,3	26,9
Hearing level 40 dB or less	69 ears	62 ears

Discussion

Eradication of cholesteatomatous disease is the primary aim of surgery in chronic ears, followed by reconstruction of the middle ear mechanisms for hearing improvement or preservation. My policy for 25 years has been to advocate open surgery which is combined with tympanic cavity and ear canal reconstruction and mastoid obliteration. The 126 primary and 154 revision ear surgeries performed and followed up by myself testify that residual cholesteatoma after thorough surgery is a rarity (0,7 %) and retraction pockets (1,1 %) have nearly disappeared. However, when all ears in this series are followed up for a period of 10 years, the figures are probably slightly higher but in all likelihood the total of ears with recurrent cholesteatoma remains less than 5 %.

It is equally clear that if one takes figures of any Institute that has surgeons of different levels of training, the figures for recurrent cholesteatoma will be higher. In a recent series of 178 ears with obliteration surgery re-examined at an average 13,9 years later, the rate of recurrent cholesteatoma was found to be 8,1 %. Considering that the surgery was performed by two general otolaryngologists in a non-university hospital, the method itself must be regarded sound and applicable at all levels.

Most of the surgeons with international reputation who have

used CAT have reported unacceptably high figures for cholesteatoma recurrence. I fail to see how this method could be recommended for cholesteatoma involving the antrum and mastoid. Neither is there any cause to revert to open cavities as a certain number of large cavities will always break down. As a matter of fact, in my revision group several ears with complications like dura-brain herniation or dural infectious processes were found in connection with open cavities. Similarly, the development of fistulae between the previous surgery and the present revision occurred mostly in the open cavity ears.

The failure of an earlier obliteration surgery to give a dry or cholesteatoma free ear could practically always be traced to the technique. The earlier surgeons had not used bone-pâté and bone chips for medial cavity obliteration and the musculo-periosteal flap had sometimes been so short that it did not reach even the antrum area. In larger cavities this provided space for retraction, and when meatoplasty had not been performed, a cholesteatomatous retraction pocket developed.

In chronic ear surgery there can be no compromise to good training and thorough knowledge of temporal bone anatomy. For an occasional ear surgeon, open surgery is the only alternative. Even if one were not confident in ear canal and middle ear restoration, one should at least be capable of obliteration of the posterior and medial part of the cavity with bone-pâté and let the musculo-periosteal flap come down anteriorly to it. This, combined with a large meatoplasty would result in a healthy small cavity. With increasing experience, one can proceed to normal ear canal and middle ear restoration.

Acknowledgements: This work was aided by a grant from Signe & Ane Gyllenberg Foundation.

References:

1. MOSHER H.P. A method of filling the excavated mastoid with a flap from the back of the auricle. *Laryngoscope* 21: 1158-1163, 1911.
2. GUILFORD R.R. Obliteration of the cavity and reconstruction of the auditory canal in temporal bone surgery. *Trans. Am. Acad. Ophthalmol. Otolaryngol.* 65: 114-122, 1961.
3. POPPER O. Periosteal flap grafts in mastoid operations. *S. Afr. Med. J.* 9: 77-78, 1935.
4. PALVA T. Reconstruction of ear canal in surgery for chronic ear. *Arch. Otolaryngol.* 75: 329-334, 1962.
5. PALVA T. Obliteration of the mastoid cavity and reconstruction of the canal wall. In: Gibb A.G., Smith M.F.W., eds. Otology. Butterworths international medical reviews, Otolaryngology 1, London, Butterworth & Co. 19-29, 1982.
6. LINDROOS R. Long-term results of surgery for chronic otitis media. M.D. Thesis, University of Helsinki, 1-75, 1984.

Musculotubal canal approach for stenotic Eustachian tube

T. Morimitsu, T. Nagai, M. Nagai, K. Enatsu, M. Ide

Introduction

Malfunction of the Eustachian tube results in persistent middle ear effusion, recurrent otitis media, tympanic perforation, middle ear atelectasis, adhesive otitis and cholesteatoma causing severe hearing loss. In cases with inadequate tubal function, therefore, it is impossible to reconstruct the non-perforated ear drum or dry ear, even though the tympanoplastic surgical procedures have been done fairly well.

Although it is beyond the scope of this paper to discuss the functions of the Eustachian tube, its patency and drainage by its ciliary epithelium are fundamental. Clinically complete closure of the tube is not so frequent but it is also desirable to develop a surgical technique to reconstruct the normally functioning tube. In this paper, a surgical approach for the stenotic osseous tube will be reported combined with discussion on literature.

Review of literature

Stenosis at the cartilaginous segment has been repaired by many kinds of shunt or bypass operation: tympano-maxillary shunt by Drettner & Ekval (1969)[1], tympano-frontal shunt by Goode & Glasscock (1975)[2], tympano-nasopharyngeal shunt by Misurya (1975)[3], and experimental study on tympano-oropharyngeal shunt by Lapidot et al. (1977)[4].

When tubal stenosis was not complete, Zöllner (1963)[5] inserted radioactive materials, silk thread, and more lately polyethylene tubes, via the nasopharynx to the nasal opening. The inlay was left in place for two weeks to three months depending upon the extent of obstruction. Although his results were fairly good, he admitted that it was sometimes impossible to reopen the stenosed tube.

Wright & Wright (1977)[6] constructed an Eustachian tube prosthesis and reported a success rate of 79 %.

Parkin et al. (1983)[7] examined various kinds of Eustachian tube stentings and concluded that small polyethylene stents were most successful.

Surgical techniques to treat the stenosis or closure at the osseous portion have been reported by some authors.

Wullstein (1963)[8] treated total obstruction of the osseous portion of the tube during tympanoplasty by blind drilling with a burr and implanted amnion, obtaining a fair result, however he admitted that he was not likely to try this procedure again in the future. Moreover, the risk of damaging the carotid artery cannot be neglected.

Kumazawa (1965)[9] transplanted the maxillary mucous membrane on the surgically enlarged tubal surface after his "Tubotympanobrückenplastik".

House et al. (1969)[10] opened the stenotic osseous tube with the middle cranial fossa approach in 6 cases with good results.

Glasscock (1973)[11] stated that the middle cranial fossa Eustachian tuboplasty is a practical procedure for dealing with bony or fibrous closure of the osseous segment of the tube and it allows the surgeon to reconstruct the tube and stimulate regrowth of normal mucous membrane from the cartilaginous tube. He reported the results of 9 cases.

Holmquist (1973)[12] reported a case in which a small metal piece, lodged in the bony part of the tube, was successfully removed with a combined postauricular transcanal approach. And he suggested that his surgical approach might be used to correct blockage and malfunction of the tube.

Misurya (1975)[13] operated on two cases of severely blocked osseous Eustachian tubes with his combined transcanal pre-auricular approach. In his method, the anterolateral wall of the osseous external ear canal is resected with Gilgi's saw and replaced after the enlargement of the tubal isthmus.

Morimitsu et al. (1976)[14] reported the musculotubal canal approach for the surgical correction of the stenosed osseous tube which will be reported in this paper.

Surgical technique of musculotubal canal approach

The principle of this approach is to enlarge twice the tubal lumen by removing the musculotubal canal septum after extraction of the tensor tympani muscle as follows:

— Elevation of the anterior wall skin of the external ear canal and exposure of the chorda tympani and the anterior tympanic ligament.

— The tympanic ostium of the Eustachian tube is enlarged with a diamond burr and the cochleariform process is exposed.

— The semicanal of the tensor tympani muscle is opened and the muscle fibers are extracted thoroughly, and then the musculotubal canal septum is removed, keeping the mucous membrane intact (illustration 1).

— In the deepest part of the muscular semicanal, the cartilaginous tube is exposed and resected, opening the lumen of the

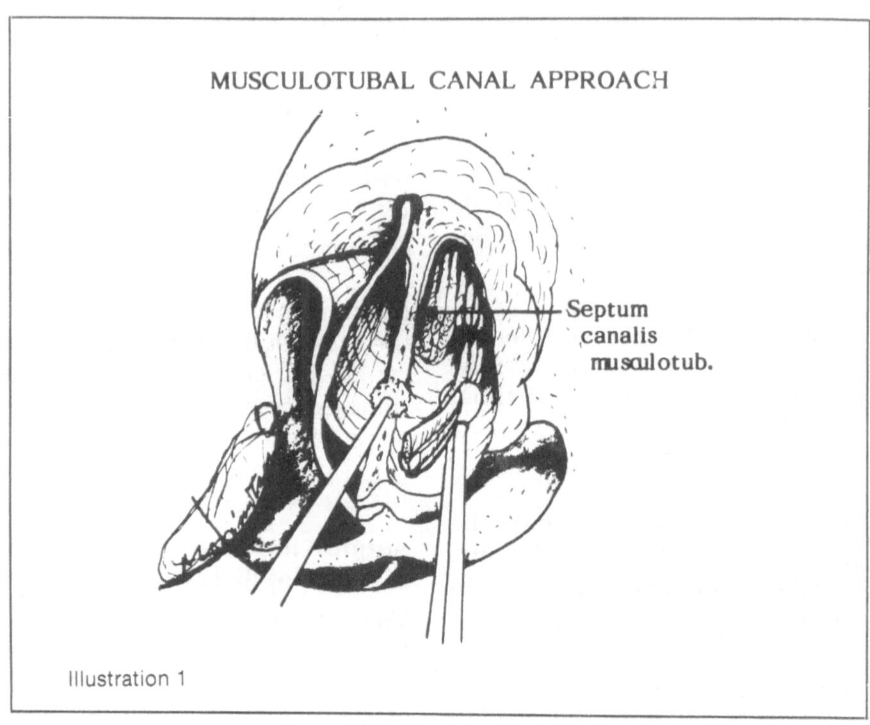

Illustration 1

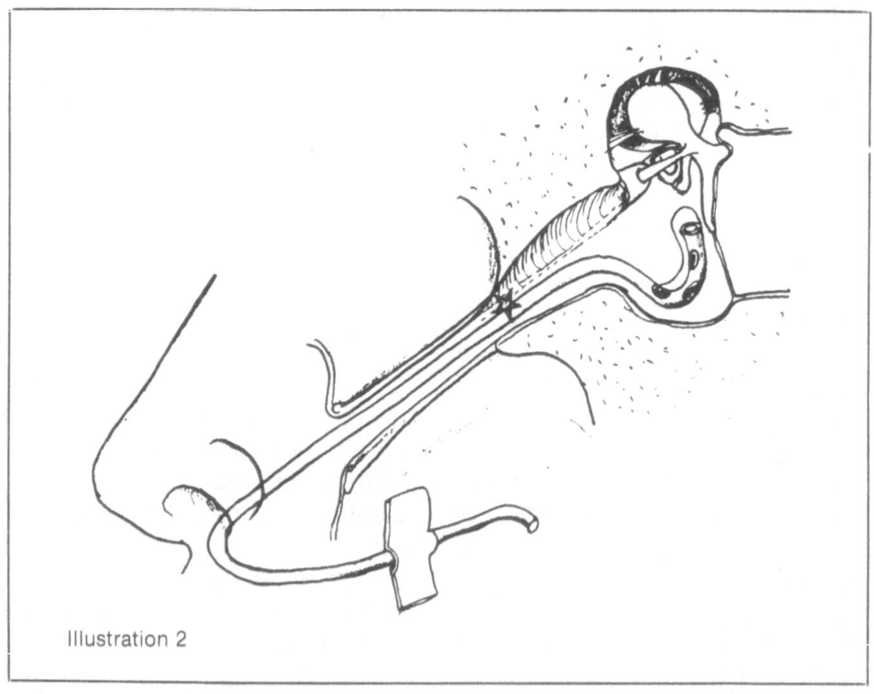

Illustration 2

cartilaginous segment of the tube.

— After the total removal of the septum, the mucous membrane of the tube is cut and opened, covering the muscular semicanal cavity.

— A polyethylene tube is inserted through the enlarged isthmus and covering the canal surface with ciliated mucous membrane is expected (illustration 2).

— After surgery, inflation or infusion of a steroid solution is carried out daily through the inserted tube until it slips out spontaneously.

In this technique, the anatomical orientation to avoid the risk of damage to the carotid artery is very easy and the preservation of the ciliated epithel, which is absolutely necessary for normal tubal function, is also assured.

Selection of cases and clinical results

From 1976 to 1984, 1600 tympanoplasties were done and 12 of these cases were indicated for tuboplasty by musculotubal canal approach because of stenosis at the osseous Eustachian tube.

Diagnosis of tubal stenosis is performed as follows:

— Inflation with an Eustachian catheter, listening to the inflating sound with an otoscope or observing the tympanic cavity under a surgical microscope.

— Bouginage with various sizes of bougies and measuring the depth of the stenosis. If the depth is about 25 mm long, the stenosis is located at the tubal isthmus.

— Observation of the nasopharyngeal tubal ostium with a nasopharyngoscope during swallowing, inflation and bouginage.

— Bouginage from the tympanic ostium during the tympanoplasty, determined finally for tuboplasty.

Eight of 12 cases had gone through surgery previously scratching radically the tubal mucous membrane and filling bone chips which was a method widely used in Japan in pretympanoplastic era. Another 2 cases had undergone radical conservative surgery and the remaining 2 cases had been submitted to tympanoplastic procedure. All of the patients earnestly wished for dry ears at least and good hearing if possible.

In 3 cases the stenosed tube could not be reopened because the stenosis spread to the cartilaginous portion.

In 7 of the 9 cases in which the surgical procedure could be done completely, the tube became patent and the intact ear drum could be reconstructed. Four of these cases showed significantly improved hearing.

But in 2 cases, tubal stenosis relapsed soon after removal of the polyethylene tube. One of them was operated on again with a good result but the other case was abandoned as the patient did not want further surgical treatment.

Surgical technique to correct the stenotic osseous Eustachian tube is not yet established. Even with our technique, the cases indicated for this method are very limited. And it will be very difficult to restore satisfactory functioning of the tube when the mucous membrane is damaged severely and the cartilaginous portion is damaged also. However, the authors believe that the effort to establish a surgical technique for tuboplasty should be pursued since there are patients with tubal stenosis.

References:

1. DRETTNER B, EKVALL L. Chronic obstruction of Eustachian tube treated with tympano-maxillary shunt. *Acta Otolaryngol (Suppl)* 263:2932, 1969.
2. GOODE R.L., GLASSCOCK M. The tympano-frontal shunt: A procedure for the treatment of chronic Eustachian tube insufficiency. *Laryngoscope* 85:100-112, 1975.
3. MISURYA V.K. Tympano-nasopharyngeal shunt operation. A new method of middle ear ventilation. *J. Laryngol. Otol.* 89:189-197, 1975.
4. LAPIDOT A., TERREE D., REZVANI F. et al. Eustachian tube bypass: Experimental evidence for total Eustachian substitution. *O.R.L.* 86:498-505, 1977.
5. ZÖLLNER F. Therapy of the Eustachian tube. *Arch. Otolaryngol.* 78:394-399, 1963.
6. WRIGHT J.W. Jr., WRIGHT J.W. 3d. Preliminary results with use of an Eustachian tube prosthesis. *Laryngoscope* 87:207-214, 1977.
7. PARKING J.L., JOHNSON L.P., STRINGHAM J.C. Transtympanic Eustachian tuboplasty and tolerance of stenting materials. *Otolaryngol. Head & Neck Surg.* 91:407-411, 1983.
8. WULLSTEIN H. Eustachian tube in tympanoplasty. *Arch. Otolaryngol.* 71:408-411, 1963.
9. KUMAZAWA T. Über Tubotympanobrükkenplastik. *Proct. Otologia Kyoto* 58:216-224, 1965.
10. HOUSE W.F., GLASSCOCK M.E. 3d, MILES J. Eustachian tuboplasty. *Laryngoscope* 79:1765-1782, 1969.
11. GLASSCOCK M.E. 3d. Middle cranial fossa Eustachian tuboplasty. *Arch. Oto-Laryngol.* 97:15-16, 1973.
12. HOLMQUIST J. Eustachian tube surgery. *J. Laryngol. Otol.* 87:1029-1032, 1973.
13. MISURYA V.K. Eustachian tuboplasty. *J. Laryngol. Otol.* 89:807-813, 1975.
14. MORIMITSU T., MATSUMOTO I., SHIBATA K. et al. Musculotubal canal technique. A method of Eustachian tuboplast. *Otolaryngol. Tokyo* 48:973-978, 1976.

SYMPOSIUM I
Eradication of the pathology

Chairman: D. Austin

Eradication of pathology

D. Austin

Many factors must be considered in a standardized system of reporting the eradication of pathology. The more important items include:

- The type of pathology
  - — Reversible
  - — Non-reversible
    - □ Cholesteatoma
    - □ Tympanosclerosis
    - □ Osteomylelitis
- The anatomical region involved
- The method of eradication
  - — Sharp dissection
  - — Blunt dissection
  - — Burring
- The surgical risks of eradication
- The risk of non-eradication
- The surgical plan
  - — Closed
  - — Open

Many other factors may be conceived as entering into a complete system describing the eradication of pathology. A system to be useful, however, must be acceptably simple and short. It must also be capable of modification as surgical methods change to be long-lived. Finally, the system must be able to be adapted to the computer because of the increasing complexity of data base management in our age of rapid widespread communication.

Management of the mastoid - The UDT-system; a new classification in ear surgery

E.H.M.A. Marres

The strategic location of the middle ear cleft and mastoid air cells makes every infection of the middle ear and mastoid capable of creating intracranial complications or complications of the middle ear cleft and of the mastoid, the facial nerve, the labyrinth and sigmoid sinus. With the advent of antibiotics the majority of patients with an acute otitis media are controlled by medical treatment. Only a few cases do not respond to this therapy and require surgery. Surgery is indicated when the acute symptoms have not been controlled by antibiotics and otorrhoea continues for 4 to 8 weeks after the onset of the disease or when the following complications are present, when the case is first seen:

— intracranial complications,
— subperiosteal or subcutaneous abscess in the postauricular region,
— Bezold's abscess,
— labyrinthitis.

In such cases a proper knowledge of the anatomy of the middle ear cleft and the temporal bone is necessary. The same applies to the knowledge of the function of the middle ear and the character of the disease especially in cases of chronic otitis media.

Additionally, these multifaceted problems can be handled by a wide variety of surgical approaches. Personal experience and philosophy until now have been the guidelines on deciding which of the several surgical procedures to use to solve a patient's chronic otitis media problem. It is clear, that the choice of surgical approach depends on the operation which is to be carried out and on the region of the temporal bone which has been infected. However, the terms epitympanotomy or atticotomy, antrotomy, mastoidectomy, attico-antrotomy or epitympanomastoidectomy, posterior tympanotomy or combined approach tympanoplasty, modified radical and radical mastoidectomy, hold different meanings for different surgeons in the surgical management of the temporal bone. Therefore, a more accurate anatomical description in relation with these surgical terms is necessary.

Surgical management of the patient with chronic otitits media rests on two basic principles:

— management of the attic and mastoid,
— management of the middle ear cleft.

Management of the attic and mastoid

The surgical approach of the attic and mastoid depends on the deci-

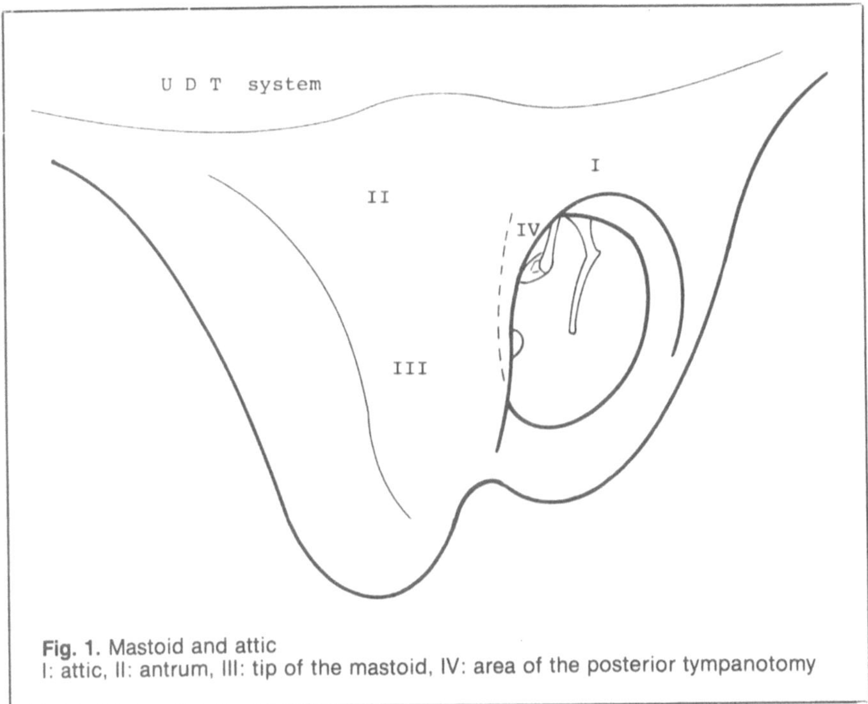

Fig. 1. Mastoid and attic
I: attic, II: antrum, III: tip of the mastoid, IV: area of the posterior tympanotomy

sion to preserve or to remove the superior and posterior bony wall of the ear canal. It is not my intention to discuss the indications of the canal wall up or down techniques, but I would like to try to give a more accurate classification of the various terms in use for the surgical approaches of the attic and mastoid.

A good classification should be understandable and simple for everybody. It is necessary to divide the surgical region of the attic and mastoid into four different areas (figure 1), namely the attic (I), the antrum (II), the tip of the mastoid (III) and the area of the posterior tympanotomy (IV). It is also necessary to indicate whether we preserve or remove the superior posterior wall of the ear canal. In this manner we have a good, accurate and understandable classification method usable in all cases where surgical management of the attic or mastoid or both is necessary.

If we use the canal wall up technique we indicate this with the letter U and the canal wall down technique with the letter D in combination with the Roman numerals I, II, III and IV corresponding to the areas of the mastoid. This classification has the advantage, that it is comparable with the classification of Wullstein and Zöllner relative to tympanoplasty in type I to IV. The U I

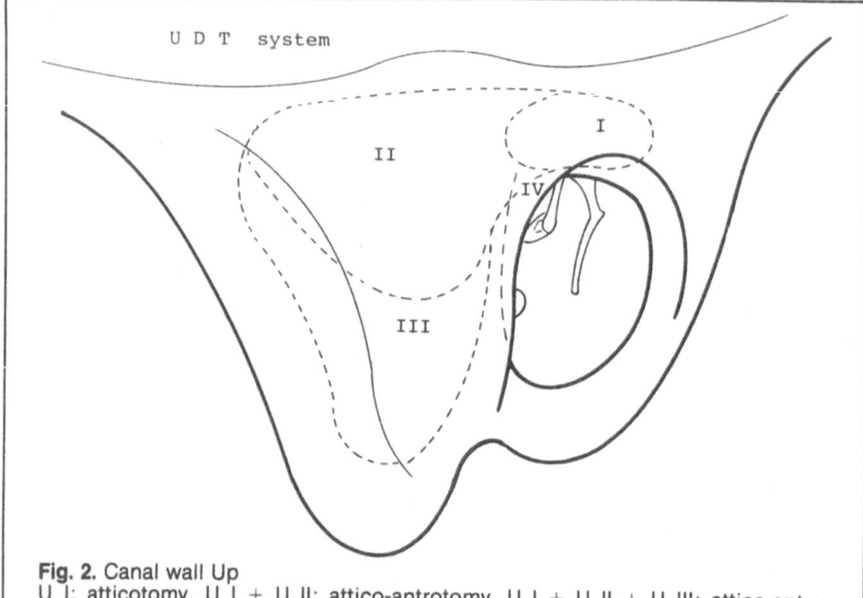

Fig. 2. Canal wall Up
U I: atticotomy, U I + U II: attico-antrotomy, U I + U II + U III: attico-antro-mastoidectomy, U I + U II + U III + U IV: posterior tympanotomy

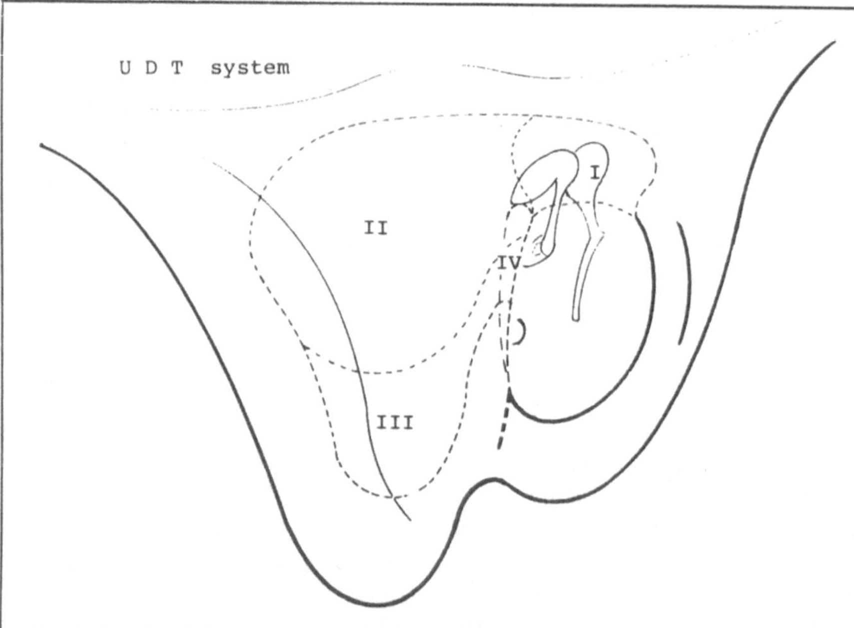

Fig. 3. Canal wall Down
D I: atticotomy, D I + D II: attico-antrotomy, D I + D II + D III: modified radical mastoidectomy, D I + D II + D III + D IV: radical mastoidectomy

to IV and D I to IV operations are marked out in the figures 2 and 3.

Management of the middle ear cleft

Classification of tympanoplasties in types I to IV is accepted by every ear surgeon and needs no modification.

Conclusion

With the classification of surgery of the mastoid into U I to IV and D I to IV in combination with the usual classification of tympanoplasties into T I to IV, we can determine every surgical treatment of the mastoid and middle ear reconstruction. If we accept this new UDT classification, confusion in the various terms relative to mastoid surgery and middle ear reconstruction will no longer exist.

The epitympanum and ossicular chain

S.R. Wullstein

The inner architectural design of the epitympanum is the best evidence of the complexity of its function and its readiness for the patho-physiological reactions. Because of the way it responds to external solicitations, it is a "key area" in middle ear pathology.

The anatomical topographical landmarks are of particular interest in discussing how to eradicate the pathology and how to reconstruct the structures. They are:

— the ventral part of the epitympanum e.g. the anterior region in front of the malleus - the recessus protympanicus and the recessus supratubalis, separated each from the other by the tensor tympani fold;

— the lateral part of the epitympanum between the lateral surface of the ossicular masses and the inner side of the lateral epitympanic wall.

The borderline between the epitympanum and meso-hypotympanum is lined up by a narrowing, the second "bottleneck" in the middle ear ventilation (the first one is the Eustachian tube), the so-called tympanic diaphragm, the name introduced by the French anatomists Chatelier and Lemoine in 1948. It is situated nearly horizontally and parallel to the rotation axis of the ossicles. It follows the profile line of the tensor tympani canal with the processus cochleariformis as well as the course of the horizontal part of facial nerve. It is formed anteriorly by the tensor tympani fold, dorsally by the lateral incudal fold. The tympanic diaphragm has two openings - the anterior and posterior tympanic isthmi.

The tensor tympani fold stretches caudally between the processus cochleriformis with the tensor tympani tendon and the canal of the tensor tympani muscle, cranially to the crista anterior which is the bony ridge where the petrous and squamous part of this region sutures together. The tensor tympani fold belongs to the obligate folds of the middle ear. It plays an important rôle in two functional units:
A. the mechanics and acoustics, as well as in,
B. the physiological ventilation and clearance of the middle ear system.

A. During the process of vibration of the ossicular chain and the tympanic membrane the movements of the tensor tympani fold have been observed (Marquet) to correspond to the vibration of the ossicles and to the amount of air displaced in the epitympanum so long as the sound perception continues and the tensor tympani muscle does not fatigue.

B. The tensor tympani fold deflects the air coming from the Eustachian tube during swallowing or active insufflation. It leads this air inflow inferiorly through the anterior meso-hypotympanal canel via the inferior ventilation pathway around the promontory hump - as a cap - into the region of the round window niche and the sinus tympani.

It is impossible for the airflow to enter the epitympanum directly from the Eustachian tube via the recessus supratubalis. The airflow can only reach the epitympanic space through the tympanic isthmi in the tympanic diaphragm passing the two ventilation pathways - inferior and superior - described in the earliest days of tympanoplasty by H.L. Wullstein.

The position of the tensor tympani fold is a result of the development of the pneumatic spaces of the middle ear, e.g. of the bony formation and the preformation of the air-filled spaces as well as of the necessary inner air pressure. Therefore, according to the interrelationship and correspondence of these three factors during the postnatal development of the pneumatic spaces, the position of the tensor tympani fold arises either more oblique or more horizontal. In the case of a very deeply developed recessus protympanicus the tensor tympani fold will be positioned more horizontally. The recessus supratubalis remains very flat or vice versa.

If the widening of the tympanic tubal orifice cranially to the bony canal of the tensor tympani muscle is strongly developed then the tensor tympani fold is pushed more cranially during the developmental stage; its position remains more oblique. This situation results in a very flat recessus protympanicus with nearly no air-filled space in front of the malleus head very often causing localized osteitic fixation of the head of the malleus to the tegmen of the tympanum.

The fact that the tensor tympani fold separates the two recessi is also very important for the pathology of the chronic middle ear diseases especially for the cholesteatoma cases. The direction of the further growth into the depth of the pyramid via recessus supratubalis leads to the development of the dangerous tubal cholesteatoma or via the recessus protympanicus to the development of a silent paralabyrinthine cholesteatoma from the "anterior point of danger".

Furthermore, the only possible way of ventilating Prussak's space as well as for air filling of the lateral epitympanic air cushions is the posterior tympanic isthmus. Prussak's space is lined laterally by the Shrapnell membrane, medially by the neck of the malleus, cranially by the first level of the lateral malleolar folds and has as its bottom the anterior and posterior folds of v. Tröltsch. These two folds cannot be renamed nowadays as Prussak's folds because every change from the well-known classical nomenclature makes only more confusions. The same is true for the terms of recessus protympanicus and recessus supratubalis. They are based on the very early description done by A. Hammar in 1902, later by Pernkopf and others. The modern term - the sinus epitympani - creates only more confusion.

As already noted, the lateral incudo-malleolar folds are situated in two levels. In this way - as a lightweight structure - they build two floors of air cushions, the superior and inferior ones. We call these air-filled spaces the lateral epitympanic air cushions. The first description of these membranes dates back to 1878 by A. Politzer. Our studies on comparative anatomy have shown that these formations of folds as epitympanic air cushions exist in the primates also. The hypothesis is that these lateral epitympanic air cushions play an important and protective rôle as a damping system for absorption of the overloading energy and help to adapt very quickly the whole vibrating system of the middle ear for the next information which follows (S.R. Wullstein). The holographic pictures with the different vibration patterns done by v.Bally clearly demonstrate that the pars flaccida together with Prussak's space and all lateral epitympanic air cushions represent a functional unit contrary to the vibration patterns of the dense pars tensa.

The patho-morphological substrate in the early stages of the middle ear inflammation should be looked for in the reactions of the mucosal lining and its folds.

Nearly all acute bacterial infections develop per continuitatem via the Eustachian tube. The most anterior part of the epitympanum is very well provided in blood supply by the vessels coming from the branches of the external carotid artery as well as from the branches of the internal carotid artery. They anastomosize, according to Hansen, in the bony region around the Fissura Glaseri and the bottom of the recessus protympanicus. There is a triangle known as an "anterior point of danger" for the silent and deep development of the paralabyrinthine cholesteatoma (H.L. Wullstein), situated directly over the ganglion geniculi in front of the anterior crus of the anterior semicircular canal. This is also the region of increased metabolic processes in the bony substance without any sign of inflammation, only as a result of the non-interrupted biomechanics and biokinetics during the whole life (permanent rotation, torsion, declination and inclination of the pyramids in the base of the skull - A. Serzer and J. Krmpotic and others). The increased metabolism leads to morphological changes in the bony substance described by G. Kelemen as a "pagetoid-like" bony deformation.

The first reaction of inflammation coming from the Eustachian tube is hyperaemia, tissue oedema, exudation, cellular infiltration in the supplying region of the anterior tympanic artery e.g. the region of the tensor tympani fold with the recessus protympanicus and recessus supratubalis. Inflammation overlaps very quickly to the neighbouring soft tissues, to the mucosal lining and mucosal folds of the lateral epitympanic air cushions. This tissue reaction can be recognized from the external view otoscopically or microscopically by the hyperaemia, oedema and fluid behind the pars flaccida and in the region of the posterior quadrant of the pars tensa, also in the surrounding region of the canal skin in the so-called vascular bundle from the superior external canal wall.

The next step is the blockade of the tympanic diaphragm with complete interruption of ventilation and mucociliary clearance. At that stage the Eustachian tube can be free from any sign of infection. But as long as interruption of ventilation and clearance in the region of the tympanic diaphragm continues to exist the pathological process in the epitympanum and in the retrotympanic spaces cannot but result in different patho-morphological features as well as cholesteatoma, adhesions, fibrosis, tympanosclerosis, ostitic ossicula fixation etc.

The protympanum

P. Savary

The protympanum is essentially the vestibule of the Eustachian tube. Schwabart was the first author to introduce this term to designate the vestibule of the Eustachian tube. Its posterior margin is the projection on the promontory of the anterior margin of the sulcus. Its anterior margin is the actual wall of the middle ear, the carotid canal and the aperture of the Eustachian tube.

According to many authors, this vestibule may include the osseous part of the Eustachian tube. It is bordered on the top by the anterior attic, more specifically by the sus-tuberian fosset[1] from which it is separated by a very thin osseous layer. A little further on, it is bordered by the canal of muscle of the malleus. Clinically, the vestibule may be partially visible, because its external margin comes directly from the exterior part of the Eustachian tube and very often is in direct continuity with the external auditive canal and its anterior margin.

The exhaustive radiological study by Ars from Brussels and Claus from Antwerp (1980)[2] with X-rays and tomographies taken in Guillen's unilateral transorbitary position, has permitted to measure carefully the different surfaces and dimensions.

The Mucosa

Comparing the research done on the mucosa, we find that Akaan-Penttilä,[3] from Finland and many other authors have found that this part of the anatomy had a respiratory ciliary and pseudo-stratified mucosa, decreasing from the Eustachian tube towards the antrum. Others, like Daniel,[4,5] Diamant,[6,7] Ingelstedt[8] and Tos[9] insisted that the high incidence of natural otitis media in the rat, might be related, among other causes, to its horizontal Eustachian tube. According to these same authors, it is well established that humans with large mastoid cavities, with more horizontal Eustachian tube and greater goblet cells density are more subject to otitis. Daniel, Brinn et al.,[4] from North Carolina brought forward the hypothesis that the seromucosa glands may secrete immunoglobulins, as do the human salivary glands, in the light of Sadé's[10] hypothesis that a lack of ventilation in the middle ear is the most important factor in the chronicity of middle ear otitis. This assertion is also based on Elner's observations of the rôle of gas exchange in the normal human middle ear. Now let the researchers (unfortunately too few) work in peace on pure middle ear pathology.

How to eradicate lesions
Let us remember that we, surgeons, must quite frequently invent new eradication means, since each ear is a personal challenge. In the preparation of this paper, I was not able to find any common denominator for the adequate eradication of all the lesions, even after 22 years of practice in cophosurgery.

☐ *Access to the protympanum*
Our method of intervention, by closed technique, does not include the double incision called "vascular strip", on the contrary, we complete the detachment of the external auditive canal up to the sulcus. It is very important to scrape the anterior spine of the canal which is the anterior petrosquamous suture. We immediately touch the anterior margin of the middle ear.

☐ *The drilling of the mastoidian cavity*
This implies that we open the facial recessus widely to facilitate the access to the anterior part of the middle ear.

☐ *Tympanic membrane remnants*
It is essential to clean all the tympanic membrane remnants, including the ones in the anterior part. Several times we have found tympanosclerosis and cholesteatomatous cysts in these remnants. We must always remember that a seemingly partially affected tympanic membrane is actually often totally affected.

☐ *Drilling of the anterior margin*
This is necessary only when the wall is bulging and hinders the anterior sulcus. In any other circumstance, it is useless and not recommended.

☐ *Shall we drill the anterior sulcus?*
The answer is definitely, no. Should the eradication of the lesions be so difficult as to necessitate the drilling of the anterior sulcus, chances are that the lesion recurs and that the grafts lead to failure by lack of support.

☐ *Instruments*
We must remember that this mucosa is far more delicate than that of the middle ear and vicious scarring could obliterate the Eustachian tube and transform a demonstrative technique into a total functional failure.

It is often useful and sometimes necessary to favour its opening toward the upper part in order to facilitate the attical ventilation. Finally, we must avoid burring its anterior margin which is directly in touch with the carotid canal. The visibility of this region must be supported by a total mobility of the operation table, of the microscope and the surgeon.

The lesions
☐ *The mucous clots*
They must be taken off carefully with an aspirator. It may either be passive, accumulated or se-

creted. In this particular case, the functional prognosis is bad. Nasal hygiene is highly recommended after the operation.

☐ *The fibrous tissue*

Associated to tympanosclerosis, it often takes over from the mucosa. It must be cleaned off carefully. The middle-term prognosis is rather bad, since, in most of the cases, it is associated to the more or less generalized tympanosclerosis. However, in the case of pure tympanosclerosis, the envelope is soft and can be removed rather easily.

☐ *The cholesteatoma*

In Canada - and it is probably a phenomenon common to all the technically-advanced countries - there seems to have been a decrease in the number of cholesteatomas of the middle ear in recent years. We attribute this to the caring of the Eustachian tube dysfunctions by myringotomy and intubation. Nevertheless, cholesteatoma still exists and is either encapsulated in its sack or invading. When encapsulated, it may be carefully cleansed, while taking particular care of the mucosa. On the contrary, if it is invading and intraosseous, particularly in this anterior region of the ear, I perform a radical mastoidectomy, without immediate reconstruction and when it is clean, about six months later, I reconstruct the middle ear and the posterior wall by means of a tympano-ossicular homograft.

☐ *Natural osseous- and surgical fibrous obliteration*

In previous times, the surgical fibrous obliteration was part of the classical mastoidectomy technique. It was done in order to avoid tubal otorrhoeas coming from large cavities of total mastoidectomy. In these cases, it is impossible to ensure adequate and durable ventilation of the middle ear and therefore, any attempt to rebuild will only lead to failure.

References:

1. ANDREA M. La Region Anterior de la Caja del Timpano y de la Fosita Supratubarica. *Anales O.R.L. Iber. Amer.* VIII, 3: 245-256, 1981.
2. ARS M. The Tympanic Cavity: Tomographic Anatomy. *Ann. Otolaryngol.* 6: 311-315, 1981.
3. AKAAN-PENTTILÄ. Middle Ear Mucosa, *Acta Otolaryngol.* Stockholm, 93: 251-259, 1982.
4. DANIEL H.J., BRINN J.E. FALGHUM ROBERTS BARRET KATHRYUR. Comparative Anatomy of Eustachian Tube and Middle Ear Cavity in Animal Models for Otitis Media. *Ann. Otol. Rhinol. Laryngol.*, 9: 82-89, 1982.
5. DANIEL H.J., CARMINE F.H., COOK R.A. Otitis Media in Two Strains of Laboratory Rats. *J. Aud. Res., 11: 276-278, 1971.*
6. *DIAMANT M. Otitis and Pneumatisation of the Mastoid Bone. Acta Otolaryngol.* (Stockholm), 28 suppl. 41, 1940.
7. DIAMANT M. Otitis and the Size of the Air Cell System. *Acta Otolaryngol.* (Stockholm), 21, 543, 1940.
8. INGELSTEDT S. Chronic Adhesive Otitis. *Acta Otolaryngol.* (Stockholm), supp. 188, 1963.
9. TOS M., BAK-PEDERSON K. Goblet Cells Population in the Pathological Middle Ear and Eustachian Tube of Children and Adults. *Ann. Otol. Rhinol. Laryngol.* 86: 209-218, 1977.
10. SADE J. The Biopathology of Secretory Otitis Media. *Ann. Otol. Rhinol. Laryngol.* 83, suppl. 11: 59-70, 1974.

Management of the hypotympanum

R. Charachon

In middle ear surgery, the hypotympanum does not usually offer the same difficulties as in glomus tumour surgery. Nevertheless, it is the starting point of the anterior hypolabyrinthine cell tract. Osteitis, epidermization and cholesteatoma may present a challenge in close contact with internal carotid artery, cochlea, jugular bulb and facial nerve.

The hypotympanum is a recess between the tympanal bone and petrous bone with usually many pneumatized cells which may entrap epithelial cysts. Anteriorly, it is close to the internal carotid artery and posteriorly close to the jugular bulb (figure 1). Besides normal variations, anomalies may be found: rarely total malposition of the internal carotid artery, more often a very high jugular bulb reaching the round window or even the oval window. Lack of bone may be found on the internal carotid artery and more often on the jugular bulb. Above the hypotympanum and behind the facial nerve is the cochlea.

The depth of the hypotympanum depends on the level of the jugular bulb. In sclerotic temporal bone, the hypotympanum may be absent or very shallow and smooth. On the contrary, in 30 % of cases, according to L. Girard (figure 2), in well pneumatized temporal bone, the hypotympanum is large and the anterior hypolabyrinthine cell tract is well developed. This tract joins, medially to the facial nerve, the posterior hypolabyrinthine tract underneath the posterior semicircular canal. This junction occurs at the border between the posterior end of the hypotympanum and the inferior retrotympanum. We propose to call it the weak point of the retrotympanum.

Lesions and their management
Management of lesions invading the hypotympanum must be very careful. Landmarks must be exactly located, i.e. first of all the facial nerve along its mastoid part according to the procedure, very deep posterior tympanotomy in closed technique or total lowering of the posterior wall in open technique.

Osteitis may involve hypotympanum cells. A diamond burr may remove it. But in the case of petrositis or external malignant otitis, osteitis involves all the cell tracts. Instead of using the Ramadier approach, we propose opening the posterior hypolabyrinthine cells between the sigmoid sinus and the facial nerve, under-

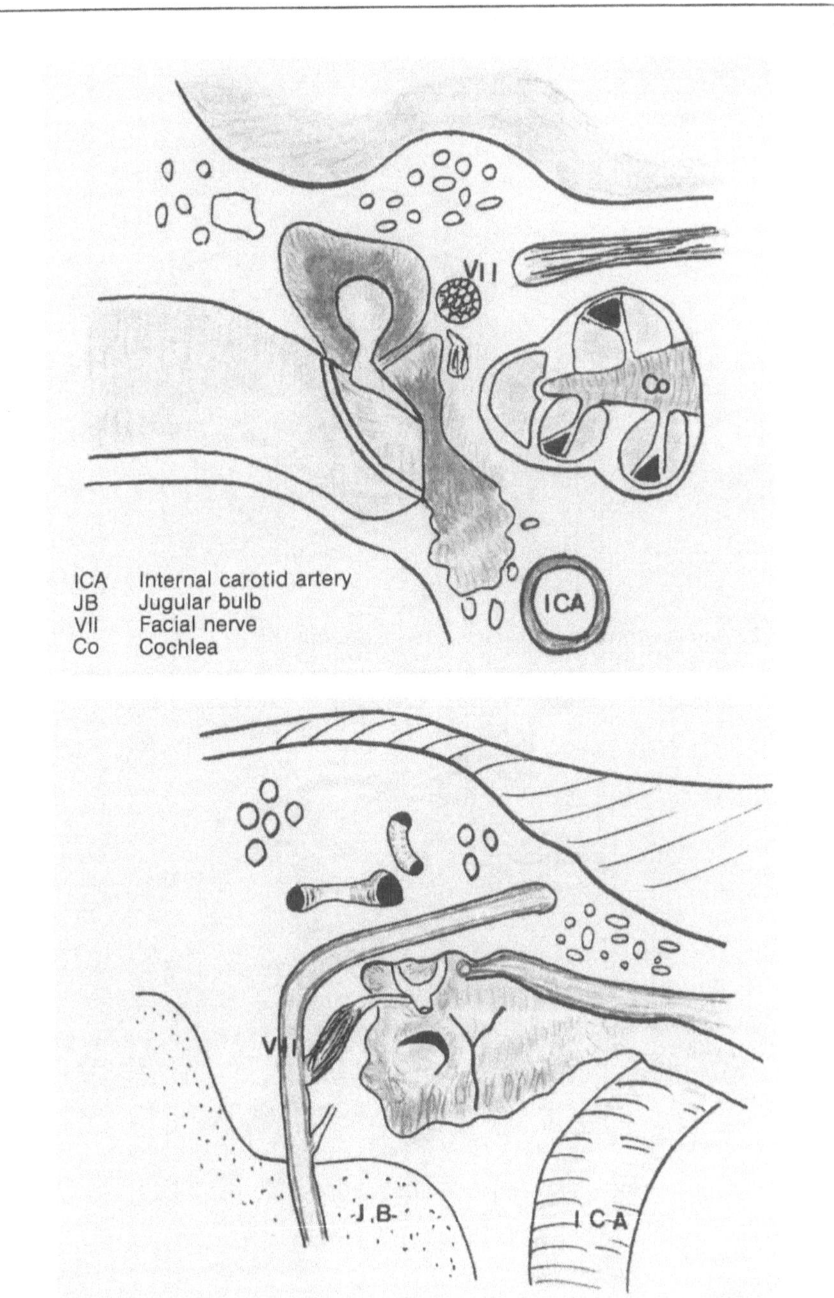

Fig. 1. The hypotympanum has usually many pneumatized cells. It is anteriorly close to the internal carotid artery, and posteriorly close to the jugular bulb. Above the hypotympanum is the cochlea and behind it is the facial nerve.

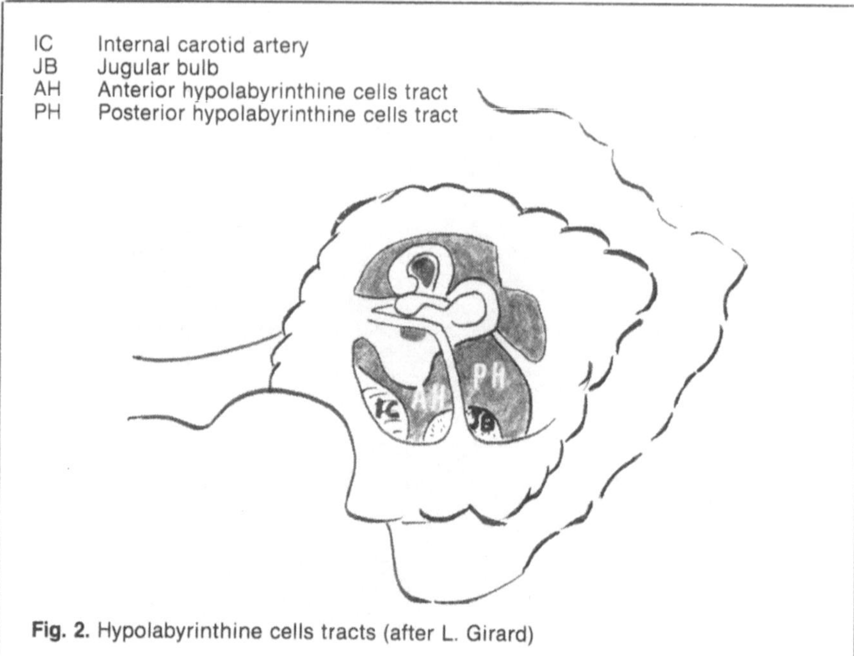

Fig. 2. Hypolabyrinthine cells tracts (after L. Girard)

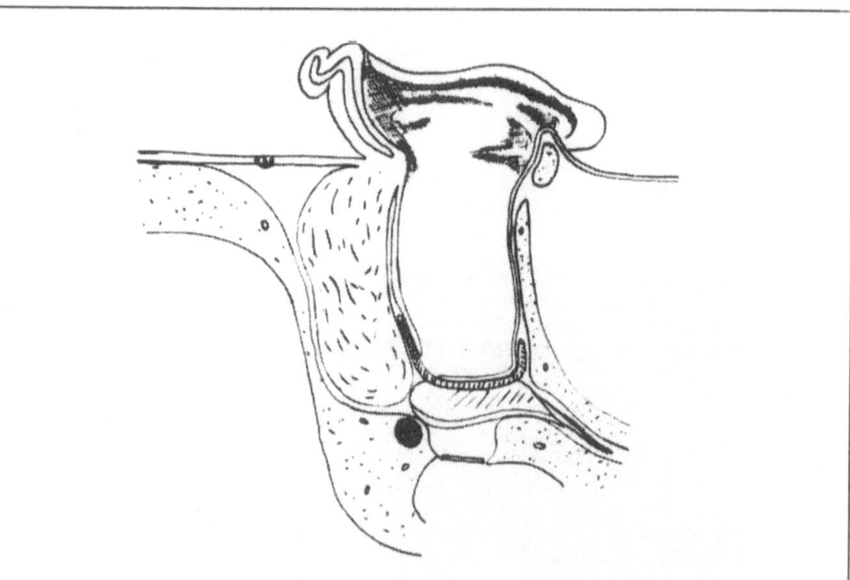

Fig. 3. Epidermization of the hypotympanum reaching the protympanum and the Eustachian tube.
A thick silastic sheeting with a long horn is placed in the mesotympanum and the Eustachian tube during obliteration procedure.

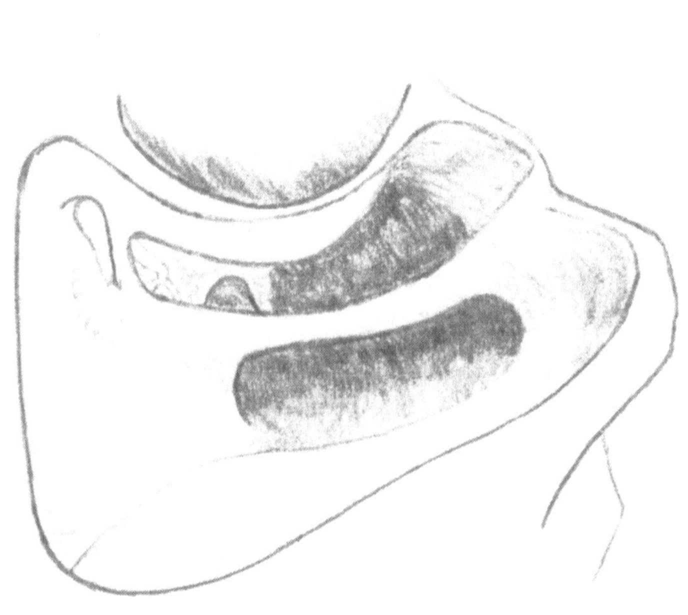

Fig. 4. Opening of the posterior hypolabyrinthine cells tract between sigmoid, sinus and facial nerve underneath the posterior semicircular canal during ICWT. This procedure allows control of a hypotympanum cholesteatoma invading the weak point of the retrotympanum medially to the facial nerve.

neath the posterior semicircular canal, to reach the petrous apex.

Epidermization of a smooth hypotympanum may be easy to remove but it may progress towards the protympanum and the Eustachian tube (figure 3). If the mucous membrane of the Eustachian tube is replaced by squamous epithelium, open technique is advisable. Opening of the Eustachian tube is necessary, taking care of the internal carotid artery. All the mucosa must be removed. Then a silastic sheeting with a long horn is placed for guiding mucosa regrowth and it is left in place for at least 18 months.

If the hypotympanum is rich in pneumatized cells, epidermization invades them and a **cholesteatoma** appears spreading out from cell to cell. All the cells have to be removed with a diamond burr taking care of the cochlea above, the internal carotid artery anteriorly, the jugular bulb below and the facial nerve posteriorly. It is necessary to locate exactly the facial nerve either by a large tympanotomy or by removing the posterior bony canal, according to pneumatization of the mastoid. In such cases, we found twice a cochlear fistula. Even if its endostal layer is intact, prognosis is poor.

According to our experience, cholesteatoma is very often situated posteriorly and involves the weak point of the retrotympanum, medially to the facial nerve. It is necessary to skeletonize the mastoid part of the facial nerve and to open the posterior hypolabyrinthine cells between the sigmoid sinus and facial nerve, underneath the posterior semicircular canal. This may be done in pneumatized cases as high as the sinus tympani (figure 4).

If the hypotympanum cholesteatoma is very large, growing downward along the internal carotid artery and jugular vein, a part of the tympanal ridge must be removed after locating the facial nerve. Open technique with or without posterior obliteration is usually necessary.

Sometimes, the hypotympanum cholesteatoma becomes an intrapetrous one: a trans-otic approach with re-routing of the second and third portions of the facial nerve, is the only way to remove it.

Management of the retrotympanum

M.C.H. Gersdorff, J.-P. Maisin

Foreword

☐ I would like to begin by thanking very sincerely Professor Marquet for his friendly invitation. I am also indebted to Prof. Guerrier (Montpellier, France), Dr. Proctor (Detroit, USA), Prof. Carachon (Grenoble, France), Dr. Deguine (Lille, France), Prof. Portmann (Bordeaux, France), Dr. Sanna (Parma, Italy), Dr. Sheehy (Los Angeles, USA) and Prof. Zini (Parma, Italy) for their collaboration in preparing my lecture.

☐ The posterior region of the tympanic cavity, the retrotympanum, is probably the most complicated area to study from both the anatomical and the surgical point of view. Before considering surgical techniques for removal of diseased tissue from the retrotympanum, it is helpful to recall its specific anatomy.

☐ The retrotympanum is derived from the second branchial arch. The ossification of Reichert's cartilage will result in the formation of Proctor's styloid complex, composed of three eminences: the pyramidal, styloid and chordal eminences.

☐ Arising from the eminences with between them, the promon-

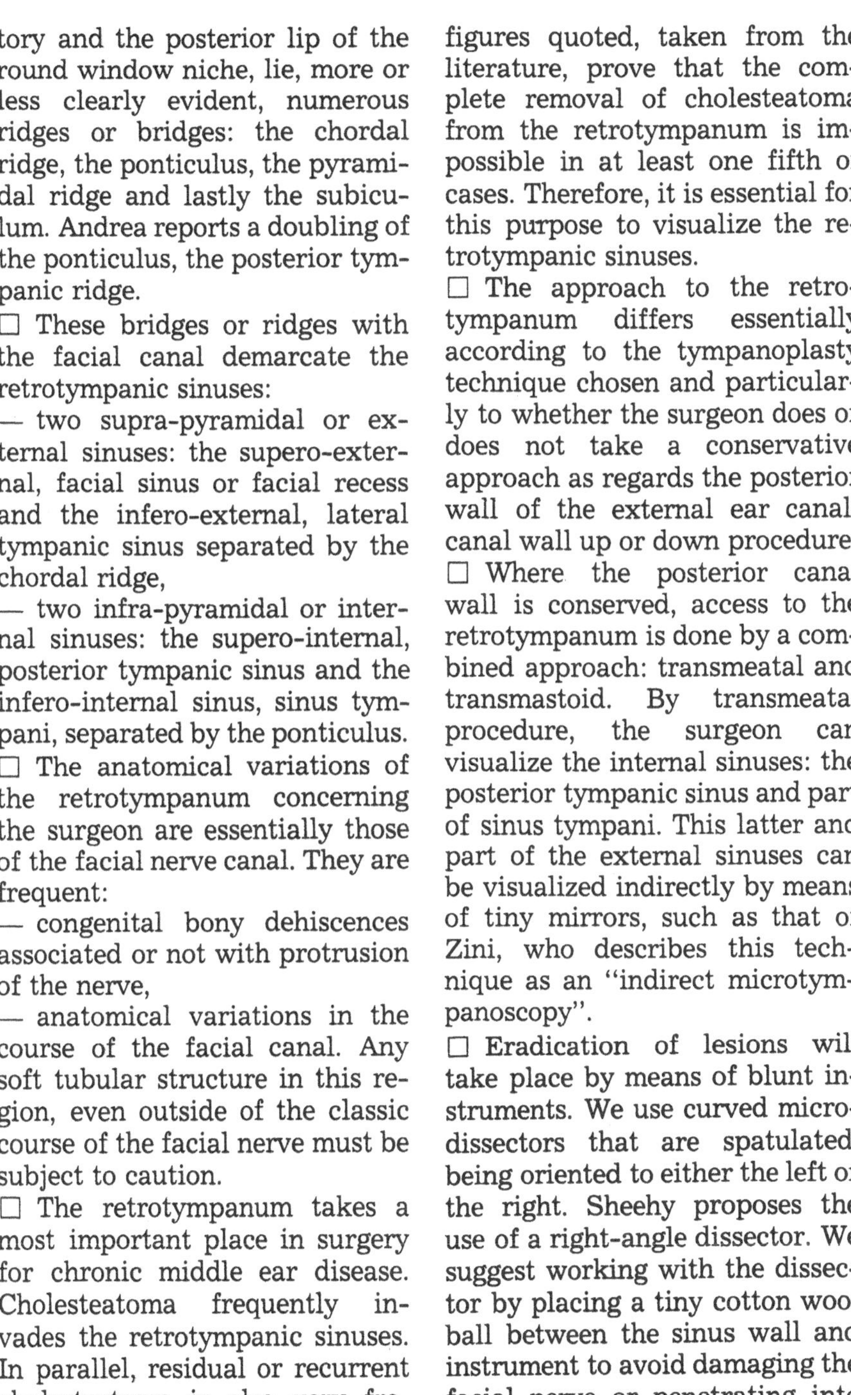

tory and the posterior lip of the round window niche, lie, more or less clearly evident, numerous ridges or bridges: the chordal ridge, the ponticulus, the pyramidal ridge and lastly the subiculum. Andrea reports a doubling of the ponticulus, the posterior tympanic ridge.

□ These bridges or ridges with the facial canal demarcate the retrotympanic sinuses:

— two supra-pyramidal or external sinuses: the supero-external, facial sinus or facial recess and the infero-external, lateral tympanic sinus separated by the chordal ridge,

— two infra-pyramidal or internal sinuses: the supero-internal, posterior tympanic sinus and the infero-internal sinus, sinus tympani, separated by the ponticulus.

□ The anatomical variations of the retrotympanum concerning the surgeon are essentially those of the facial nerve canal. They are frequent:

— congenital bony dehiscences associated or not with protrusion of the nerve,

— anatomical variations in the course of the facial canal. Any soft tubular structure in this region, even outside of the classic course of the facial nerve must be subject to caution.

□ The retrotympanum takes a most important place in surgery for chronic middle ear disease. Cholesteatoma frequently invades the retrotympanic sinuses. In parallel, residual or recurrent cholesteatoma is also very frequently seen in this region. The figures quoted, taken from the literature, prove that the complete removal of cholesteatoma from the retrotympanum is impossible in at least one fifth of cases. Therefore, it is essential for this purpose to visualize the retrotympanic sinuses.

□ The approach to the retrotympanum differs essentially according to the tympanoplasty technique chosen and particularly to whether the surgeon does or does not take a conservative approach as regards the posterior wall of the external ear canal: canal wall up or down procedure.

□ Where the posterior canal wall is conserved, access to the retrotympanum is done by a combined approach: transmeatal and transmastoid. By transmeatal procedure, the surgeon can visualize the internal sinuses: the posterior tympanic sinus and part of sinus tympani. This latter and part of the external sinuses can be visualized indirectly by means of tiny mirrors, such as that of Zini, who describes this technique as an "indirect microtympanoscopy".

□ Eradication of lesions will take place by means of blunt instruments. We use curved microdissectors that are spatulated, being oriented to either the left or the right. Sheehy proposes the use of a right-angle dissector. We suggest working with the dissector by placing a tiny cotton wool ball between the sinus wall and instrument to avoid damaging the facial nerve or penetrating into the labyrinth.

□ The retrotympanum can be approached from behind by posterior and inferior tympanotomy. Proposed by Jansen, this technique effects the opening into the external sinuses of the retrotympanum, first the cells of the facial sinus and then the lateral tympanic sinus. This technique allows a very satisfactory overall view. However, the internal sinuses and more particularly the sinus tympani, are only partly visible directly. Indirect micro-tympanoscopy with a mirror increases vision without however always ensuring that it is complete.

□ In the case of persistent cholesteatoma of the posterior wall of the sinus tympani, only the inter-sinuso-facial approach enables eradication to be complete. Following the description by House and Glasscock for glomic tumors, Charachon has adopted this approach for total removal of cholesteatoma. It consists of reaching the inner and lower region of the retrotympanum by passing under the facial nerve between the lateral sigmoid sinus and the posterior semicircular canal.

□ The main danger of such an approach is accidental opening of the posterior semi-circular canal. This danger may cause the majority of surgeons to hesitate and to transform an operation initially planned as "canal wall up" into a "canal wall down" procedure.

□ By definition, a radical mastoidectomy comprises the opening and then the elimination of the retrotympanic external sinuses with their lesions. The wide opening made to the middle ear facilitates vision of the internal sinuses but the sinus tympani however does not necessarily become completely visible. Rotation of the operating table generally makes it possible. If not, the removal of the lesions has to be done with great prudence using tiny cotton wool balls and curved blunt micro-dissectors.

□ Complete removal of infection from the retrotympanum would appear to be possible whichever surgical technique is chosen. The surgeon must constantly bear in mind - particularly where the posterior meatal wall is to be retained - the risks of residual disease or recurrences of cholesteatoma in this region, while not failing to respect the precious neighbouring structures: labyrinth and facial nerve.

*

* *

The posterior region of the tympanic cavity, the retrotympanum, is probably the most complicated area to study from either the anatomical point of view or that of surgery.

"The posterior tympanum is the most complicated area in the middle ear and yet it must be fully understood in order to control disease and to enable restoration of some function in the middle ear" (Proctor, 1971).

Access to the retrotympanum is difficult for the anatomical reasons set forth in the paper "Anatomy of the retrotympanum" (Scientific exhibitions, p. 310). Whatever surgical approach is followed[1], it is essential to achieve good visualization of the region. The retrotympanum does indeed take a most important place in surgery for chronic middle ear disease, whatever the nature of the inflammatory tissue: mucosal pathology, epidermization or cholesteatoma.[2,3,4]

Cholesteatoma frequently invades the retrotympanic sinuses. If one considers the retrotympanum as including the oval and round windows, cholesteatoma occurs in this region in 79 % of the ears we operate upon[5] and in 63 % of cases treated by Ogala and Palva.[6] In parallel, residual or recurrent cholesteatoma is also very frequently seen in this region. In the case of closed technique surgery, 19 % and 42 % of residual and/or recurrent disease have been encountered in the work respectively by Chuard (and Deguine)[7] and by ourselves.[8]
With the open technique also there are frequent recurrences of cholesteatoma (20 % of residual or recurrent cholesteatoma, 20 % of which in the region of the stapes according to the findings by Charachon et al.[9] - open technique with Palva-type obliteration).

Therefore, one can understand how important it is to achieve as complete as possible a removal of all inflammatory pathological matter from the retrotympanum and for this purpose to visualize all the retrotympanic sinuses (figures 1, 2).

Is this possible without damaging the facial nerve or the labyrinth? The figures quoted, taken from the literature referred to in this work, prove that a perfect vision and the removal of lesions in the retrotympanum are impossible in at least 1/5 of cases, no matter which means of approach is practised (canal wall up or down). Let us see, in the light of the experience of renowned surgeons and also that of our own, how this aim may be attained.

*

* *

The approach to the retrotympanum differs essentially according to the tympanoplasty technique chosen, and particularly to whether the surgeon does or does not take a conservative approach as regards the posterior wall of the external ear canal (canal wall up or down). Even with the closed technique, when visualization of the retrotympanum is inadequate, some surgeons,[10] do not hesitate to recommend that the posterior wall of the external ear canal be temporarily removed and then restored to place at the end of the operation: "Should it prove impossible to remove such disease completely, the posterior

Fig. 1. Sinuses of the retrotympanum

	External or supra-pyramidal sinuses	**Internal** or infra-pyramidal sinuses
Superior	Facial sinus	Posterior tympanic sinus
Inferior	Lateral tympanic sinus	Sinus tympani

meatal wall must be temporarily removed to give better access to the depths of the recesses (temporary conversion of a closed cavity into an open cavity)".

Rather than speaking of open or closed technique, we shall therefore first of all describe the retrotympanum according to whether or not there is conservation of the posterior canal wall: canal wall up or down.

Canal wall up
Where the posterior canal wall is conserved, access is obtained to the retrotympanum via a combined approach: transmeatal and transmastoid.

Transmeatal procedure
By this route the surgeon can visualize the internal sinuses: the posterior tympanic sinus and part of the sinus tympanic. The latter, and part of the external sinuses, can be visualized indirectly by means of tiny mirrors, such as that of Zini, who describes this technique as an "indirect microtympanoscopy".

Eradication of lesions, with direct or indirect vision, will take place by means of blunt instruments. We use curved micro-dissectors that are spatulate, with two angulations and of two lengths, being oriented to either the left or the right, i.e. four instruments marketed by Met-Fischer under the name of "micro-dissectors". Sheehy,[11] proposes the use of a right-angle dissector.

We suggest working with the dissector by placing a tiny cotton wool ball between the sinus wall and the instrument to avoid damaging the facial nerve or penetrating into the labyrinth, which may have become exposed because of the pathology. Fragments of epidermis cling particularly well to cotton wool. The procedure permits the exeresis to be effected meticulously, and as completely as possible followed by verification with the use of a Zini mirror should there have been incomplete direct vision.

Transmastoid procedure
The retrotympanum can be approached from behind forwards by posterior and inferior tympanotomy and by the intersi-

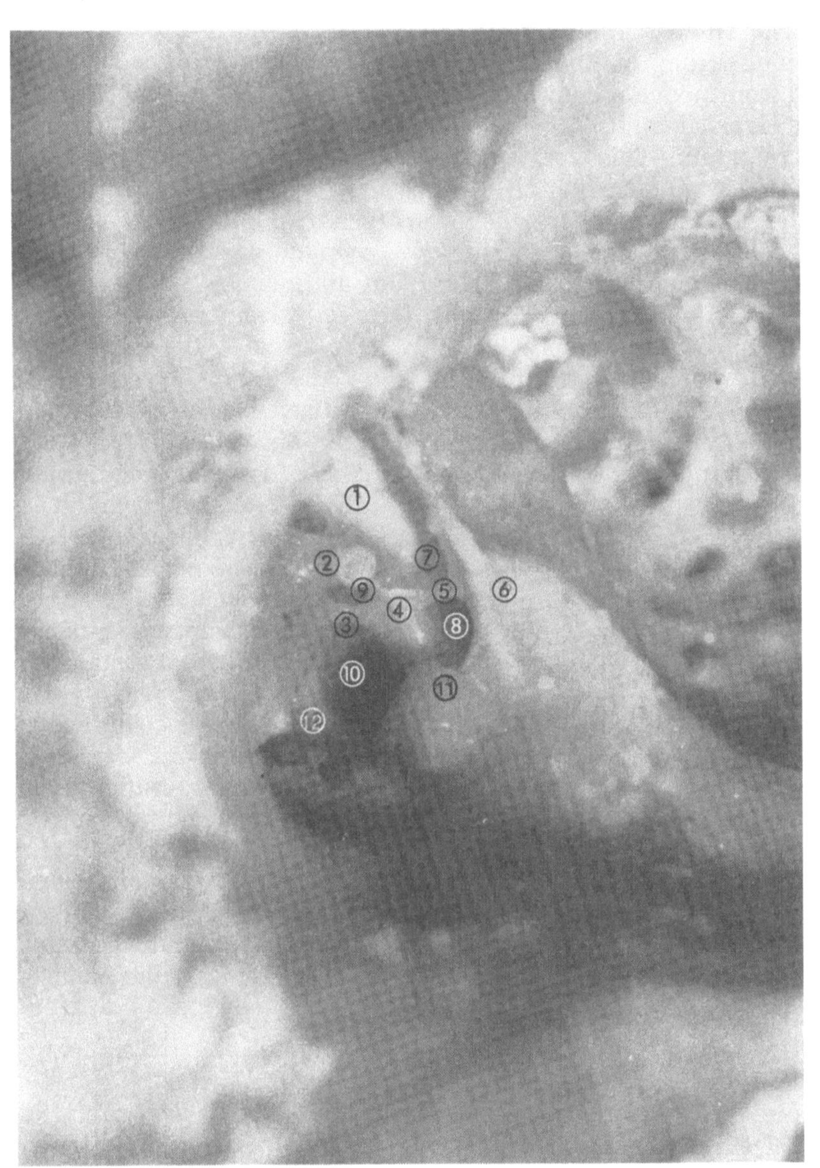

Fig. 2. Anatomy of the retrotympanum

1 = facial nerve
2 = stapes
3 = ponticulus
4 = pyramidal eminence
5 = chordal ridge
6 = chordal eminence
7 = facial sinus
8 = lateral tympanic sinus
9 = posterior tympanic sinus
10 = sinus tympani
11 = styloid eminence
12 = subiculum

nuso-facial route. *Posterior and inferior tympanotomy* effects the opening from behind forwards and from above downwards into the external sinuses of the retrotympanum. This work, carried out first with a cutting drill then with a diamond drill, attains first the cells of the facial sinus and then the lateral tympanic sinus. This technique proposed by Jansen[12] has been developed by the majority of the otologists in favour of a closed-technique tympanoplasty (combined approach), for instance Portmann[10] and Sheehy[11].

A correct posterior and inferior tympanotomy must scrupulously respect the neighbouring structures: the fossa incudis and the short process of the incus (where the incus is maintained in place), the tympanic sulcus (inner edge of the external auditory meatus), the lateral semicircular canal and the facial canal.

Correctly carried out, this approach completely opens up the external sinuses of the retrotympanum and allows a very satisfactory overall view to be had of the retrotympanum, the stapes and the windows. The internal sinuses, and more particularly the sinus tympani, are however only partly visible directly. Despite the posterior tympanotomy, indirect microtympanoscopy with a mirror increases vision without however always ensuring that it is complete.[13]. The exeresis technique requires two-handed work, with a small sucker used at the same time as a microdissector or microhook. The small sucker is used via the transmastoid, the microdissector or hook by the transmeatal route. The inter-sinuso-facial approach only can enable complete eradication in the case of an incomplete vision, even indirectly, and of persistent cholesteatoma of the posterior wall of the sinus tympani. This approach has been described by House and Glasscock[14] for the removal of tympano-jugular glomic tumors. The same technique was adopted by Portmann.[15] Charachon and Junien-Lavillauroy[16] and Charachon and Roux[17] describe the advantage of using this approach for total eradication of some cholesteatomas by closed technique. This surgical approach consists of reaching, via the transmastoid route, the inner and lower region of the retrotympanum and the infra-labyrinthic region of the temporal bone by passing under the facial nerve between the lateral sinus and the posterior semicircular canal.

In surgical position, the surgical approach takes place therefore between the lateral sinus to the rear, the facial nerve in front, the posterior labyrinth above the sigmoid sinus and the jugular bulb below. This approach is associated with posterior and inferior tympanotomy.

The main danger of such an approach is accidental opening of

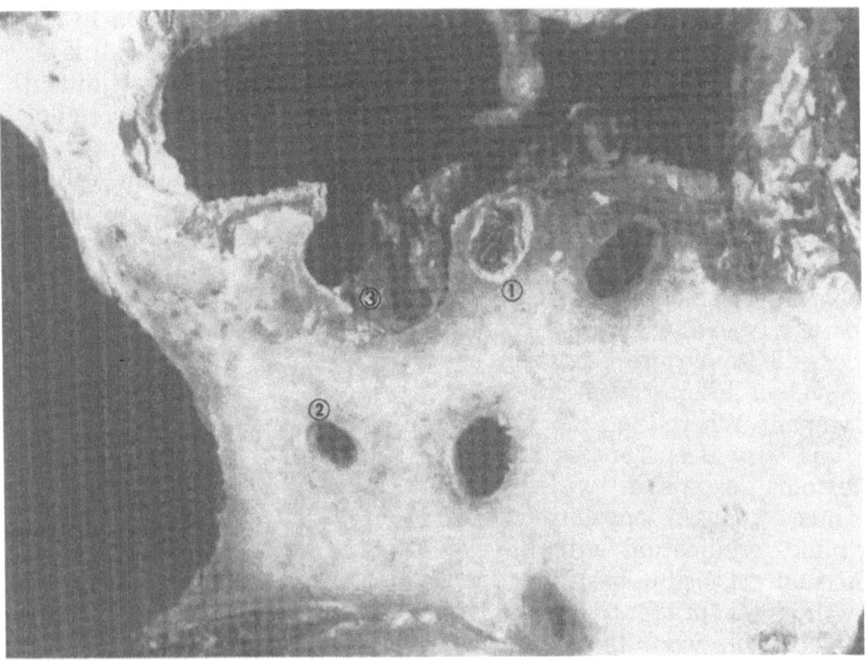

Fig. 3. Anatomical relationships between the posterior semicircular canal (2) the sinus tympani (3) and the facial nerve (1).

the posterior semicircular canal (figure 3). It should be practised with prudence, and by an experienced surgeon who is familiar with the anatomy of the region. The interest of the approach lies in that it is the only one to enable complete and direct vision into the depth of the sinus tympani. The dangers may, justifiably, cause the majority of surgeons to hesitate and to transform an operation initially planned as "canal wall up" into "canal wall down", or else - as Portmann [10] proposes - to perform a provisional excision of the posterior meatal wall, effecting the temporary conversion of a closed cavity into an open one.

Canal wall down

With radical mastoidectomy, the posterior wall of the external ear canal is drilled, and the bony structures overlying the proximal part of the facial canal mastoid segment are completely lowered. To be correct, the procedure should extend as far as the epitympanum above and to the sulcus tympani below.[11,10] Respect for the external semicircular canal and the facial canal is mandatory. By definition, this operation comprises the opening and then the elimination of the retrotympanic external sinuses with their lesions (facial sinus and lateral tympanic sinus).

The wide opening made to the middle ear facilitates vision of the internal sinuses but the sinus tympani however does not necessarily become completely visible. It can be cleared of lesions by the transmeatal procedure described above. In cases of "canal wall down" technique, rotation of the operating table (and with it the patient's head) generally makes it possible to ensure complete removal of lesions from the sinus tympani. Where the sinus tympani is very deep, and/or cholesteatoma extension widens the sinus tympani posteriorly, a "blind" eradication, without even an indirect vision, has to be done with great prudence, using the tiny cotton wool balls that we have found to be of aid in avoiding injury to the facial nerve or to the possibly denuded posterior labyrinth.

Exceptionally, the inter-sinuso-facial approach might be indicated with the "canal wall down" technique. In our experience it has never yet been necessary, except for two cases of "natural" inter-sinuso-facial opening effected by the cholesteatoma itself.

Complete removal of infections from the retrotympanum would therefore appear to be possible whichever surgical technique is chosen (canal wall up or down). Recognition should nevertheless be given to the difficulty of the techniques described and the meticulous skill required of the surgeon, who must constantly bear in mind, particularly where the posterior meatal wall is to be retained, the risks of residual disease or recurrence of cholesteatoma in this region (at least 1/5 of them) while not failing to respect the precious neighbouring structures: labyrinth and facial nerve.

Conclusion

The surgical anatomy of the retrotympanum, or styloid complex, comprises four sinuses, subdivided into the external (facial and lateral tympanic) and the internal (posterior tympanic and sinus tympani).

These sinuses are frequently the site of mucosal lesions, epidermal affections or cholesteatoma, the removal of which varies according to the surgical technique chosen; canal wall up or down.

In the case of canal wall up, the internal sinuses can be reached by transmeatal approach with direct visualization, and/or indirect vision by means of Zini mirrors.

By transmastoid approach the surgeon attains the external sinuses by posterior and inferior tympanotomy, and, if necessary for the sinus tympani, by the inter-sinuso-facial route. In the case of canal wall down, the external sinuses and their lesions are eliminated on performance of radical mastoidectomy. The internal sinuses are approached with direct or indirect visualization.

References:

1. GUERRIER Y., ANDREA M., PACO J. Les repaires anatomiques du cholestéatome dans la caisse du tympan. *Ann. Oto-laryng.* (Paris), 97, 15-28, 1980.
2. ZINI C., SHEEHY J.L., SANNA M. Microsurgery of cholesteatoma of the middle ear. *Libreria Gnedini*, Milano, 1983.
3. SHEEHY J.L., ROBINSON J.V. Cholesteatoma surgery at the otologic medical group: residual and recurrent disease. *Am. J. Otology*, 3, 209-215, 1982.
4. SHEEHY J.L., BRACKMANN D.E., GRAHAM M.D. Cholesteatoma surgery: residual and recurrent disease. A review of 1024 cases. *Ann. Otol-Rhinol-Laryngol.* 86, 451-473, 1977.
5. GERSDORFF M., HAMOIR M. La chirurgie du cholestéatome. *Cahiers O.R.L.*, 17, 561-584, 1982.
6. OJALA K., PALVA A. Late results of obliterative cholesteatoma surgery. *Arch. Otolaryngol.*, 108, 1-3, 1982.
7. CHUARD P. Le cholestéatome de l'oreille moyenne. Thèse, Université de Lille, France, 1982.
8. GERSDORFF M., HAMOIR M. Cholesteatoma surgery of the middle ear: reflection on recurrences. *Arch. Otorhinolaryngol.* 237, 77-82, 1982.
9. CHARACHON R., ROUX O., EYRAUD S. Le cholestéatome de l'oreille moyenne. *Ann. Otolaryng.* (Paris) 97, 65-78, 1980.
10. PORTMANN M. The ear and temporal bone. Masson Publishing U.S.A., 1979.
11. SHEEHY J. Surgery of chronic otitis media. In Otolaryngology vol. 1, Chapter 20, Harper and Row, Publishers, Inc. 1977.
12. JANSEN C. The combined approach for tympanoplasty. *J. Laryngol. Otol.*, 82, 779-789, 1968.
13. DONALDSON J.A., ANSON B.J., WARPEHA R.L., RENSINK M.J. The surgical anatomy of the sinus tympani. *Arch. Otolaryng.* 91, 219-227, 1970.
14. HOUSE W.F., GLASSCOCK M.E. Glomus tympanicum tumors. *Arch. Otolaryng.* 87, 550-554, 1968.
15. PORTMANN M. Quelques cas de tumeurs glomiques envahissantes de l'os temporal. *J.F. O.R.L.*, 20, 25-28, 1971.
16. CHARACHON R., JUNIEN-LAVILLAUROY C. Intérêt de la voie inter-sinuso-faciale sous-labyrinthique. *Ann. Oto-laryng.* (Paris) 92, 445-449, 1975.
17. CHARACHON R., ROUX O. La suppression du cholestéatome du sinus tympani et de la gouttière postérieure de la caisse. *J.F. O.R.L.*, 30, 191-194, 1981.

Management of the oval and round windows

M.E. Wigand

In spite of numerous attempts to document both middle ear pathology and its surgical management for the purpose of electronic data processing (e.g. Schmitt, Shea, Strauss) only little attention was paid to the recording of oval and round window abnormalities. Schmitt provided space for six pathological features of the oval and round windows, while documentation of surgical measures was confined to the oval niche, dealing predominantly with the handling of squamous epithelium or mucosa grafting. Strauß, who has outlined a model for the recording and electronic processing of data resulting from middle ear surgery, takes notice only of the width of the oval window, but does not mention the round window. In the documentation sheets of Gerhardt and Mercke no particular space is reserved for the description of window pathology, nor for the performed window surgery. Though there exist instructive descriptions of graded changes in middle ear malformations, otitis media or otosclerosis (Gristwood, Guerrier et al., Shea) no overhead system exists for the uniform documentation of different lesions.

Every new approach has to take into account the still ongoing development of middle ear surgery. Since earlier systems have lost their interest by the evolution of more recent concepts of pathology and newer surgical techniques, the avoidance of too specified catalogues, therefore, seems mandatory. With this in mind, an open end system was designed for the recording of findings and their management within the oval and round window niches. It is based on three statements referring to

— the etiology,
— the morphology of pathological abnormalities, and
— the surgical management.

The type of disease (etiology) may be recorded elsewhere, because it concerns all parts of the middle ear. Morphology and surgical management, however, have to be described separately for each window.

The mode of description should be easily understandable. Instead of numerical codes speaking signatures could be used. Modern personal computers have shown the practicability of clear text documentation. At the same time, a graded system of overlapping keywords and of more specific signatures could enhance an immediate provisory description and leave space for a later definite specification. All efforts should be made to design a system of documentation simple enough to be accepted by the busy and tired surgeon after some hours of work. A personal interview with the computer certainly could enhance a valuable recording of all significant features of middle ear operations. The following examples shall give an idea of what was intended.

Etiology

The etiology of a middle ear lesion deeply influences the prognosis. Postoperative evaluation, matter of fact, has to reconsider the nature of a pathological process. Clinical terms of the diagnosis change over the years. Their submission to the basic phenomena of general pathology therefore seems useful. The respective keywords would be sufficient to roughly identify the interesting case reports. Their sub-grouping could be realized by the signatures, which may be added or not added, according to the personal circumstances. Their completion may be carried out later, for instance, after a pathohistological examination of specimens. Such an open system of graded precision offers several advantages, all of which cannot be discussed here (table 1).

Table 1. Etiology of pathological abnormalities

Clinical terms	Keywords	Signatures
Atresia auris Dislocation, atrophy	Dysplasia	Dyspl. Min Dyspl. I, II, III Dyspl. N. VII Dyspl. A. Staped Dyspl. Jug. bulb. etc.
Injury, fracture etc.	Trauma	Trauma direct Trauma indirect Trauma al. body
Otosclerosis v. Recklinghausen etc.	System. disease	Syst. otosclerosis Syst. other
Otitis media Tympanosclerosis Cholesteatoma etc.	Inflammation	Infl. simpl. Infl. purul. Infl. granul. Infl. fibros. Infl. calcin. Infl. cholest., etc.
Fibroma, neuroma Glomustumor, carcinoma	Neoplasia	Neo. benign Neo. malign.

The main feature of this system is the replacement of different diagnoses by the combined recording of the localization and the pathology of a lesion.

Morphology

Similar reasons foster the idea of a system of graded precision with regard to the documentation of formal abnormalities. For the postoperative evaluation of microsurgical interventions the quantification of both the extent and the intensity of a window lesion is of particular importance. We have also to consider that different changes may be combined and overlap. An open descriptive formula is, therefore, recommended, offering free space for labelling the findings by screening keywords (compulsory) and by grading signatures (voluntary). Reading the sheet would stimulate the surgeon to give a fast but complete report on his own observations at the oval and round windows (table 2).

For example: the existence and position of the inner ear windows in congenital atresia are of utmost importance for the functional result. Abnormal distance between both windows or their vertical rotation may definitely influence the audiological gain of a tympanoplasty even with good mobility of the windows. The grade of occlusion of the oval window by the

Table 2. Morphology of pathological abnormalities of the oval and round windows

Formal observations	Keywords	Signature
Absent or displaced windows, rotation of window axis	Abnormal position	Posn. absent Posn. displ. Posn. rotat.
Overlying masses, the hidden window	Occlusion	Occl. part. revers. Occl. tot. revers. Occl. part. irrevers. Occl. tot. irrevers.
Narrow and atretic windows, obliteration of niches	Obstruction	Obst. part. soft Obst. tot. soft Obst. part. hard Obst. tot. hard Obst. oblit. niche
Perilymph fistula, erosion of labyrinthine capsula	Pathological aperture	Apert. platin. erosion Apert. small perf. Apert. total perf. Apert. extend. perf. Apert. alien. loco
Immobility of window, stapedial reflex, round window reflex	Dysfunction	Funct. reflex posit. Funct. easy mob. Funct. dub. mob. Funct. obvs. fix Funct. aplasia

Table 3: Management of middle ear window lesions

Clinical terms	Keywords	Signatures
Blunt or sharp dissection Drilling, infracture (hook) etc.	Manipulation	Manip. blunt Manip. sharp Manip. drill Manip. hook Manip. coagul. Manip. laser
Platinotomy, platinectomy enlarged window formation	Fenestration	Fen. small Fen. large Fen. abnormal
Closure of fistula or rupture Reconstruction of window	Closure	Clos. glue Clos. gelfoam Clos. fascia Clos. fat Clos. bone Clos. others
Interposition to footplate Piston techniques Vestibulopexy Differential window exposure Atopic fenestration etc.	Sound	Sound no Sound to chain Sound to drum Sound shadow Sound others

overhanging facial nerve may prohibit the establishment of a columella. The degree of oval niche obliteration implies dangers for the inner ear, their recording is, therefore, of great value, as Gristwood has shown us.

Our open system of documentation by speaking signatures is still provisory and incomplete. **Its principle, however allows its continuous improvement by addition or omission of special attributes to basic phenomena.**

Management
Finally, recording of the management of oval and round window lesions may also be abbreviated by a few basic principles such as opening, closure and reconstruction of a sound conductor. Table 3 canalizes the different clinical terms into the physical phenomena (keywords) which might be specified by specific attributes (signatures). The proposed list of speaking signatures is still preliminary and incomplete. Discussion and recommendations for change or additional paragraphs are hoped for.

The applied technique of surgical dissection of a window may have far-reaching consequences and should, therefore, be mentioned. Whether the opening of the oval window was performed by a hook or drill or laser is worthwhile recording such as the technique of window closure. Blunt dissection of mucosal folds or soft adhesions will not stimulate fresh scar formation, while sharp removal of mucosa and granulation injures the epithelium and causes ulceration, which always makes the functional prognosis doubtful. Bone removal may stimulate apophytic bone formation. Removal of squamous epithelium from the windows is difficult and dangerous especially with footplate erosion or from a hidden round window. Also the extent of fenestration has far-reaching consequences for the postoperative evaluation. There is particular need for an international nomenclature of this subject as of the type of the reconstructed sound conductor. Contemporary literature lacks reports on comparable systems of documentation. Even the "standard classification" (D.M. Lierle 1965) does not refer to the oval and round windows.

Conclusion
In conclusion, the above mentioned ideas on a system of documentation of the management of pathology within the oval and round niches cannot be more than a first attempt to outlay a flexible matrix for the postsurgical electronic data processing. Its principle consists of recording both the surgical findings and the surgical therapy using keywords and speaking signatures instead of diagnoses and code numbers. Open-end lists are preferred to limited word rows, in order to be able to realign the sets of items with future developments. The next step toward realization

would be a review of the proposed system by more electronic data processing - experienced people who could also integrate the corrected lists into a complete system of middle ear documentation.

Literature:

GERHARDT H.-J., Department of Oto-Rhino-Laryngology, Humboldt-University, Berlin (GDR), Personal communication 1984.

GRISTWOOD R.E. A note on progression of the otosclerotic focus. *Clin. Otolaryngol.* 7, 257-260, 1982.

GRISTWOOD R.E. Stapes Footplate Pathology in Otosclerosis and the Progression of the Otosclerotic Focus in South-Australia, Politzer-Society-Conference on Surgery of the Temporal Bone, Montreux, 1983.

LIERLE D.M. Standard Classification for Surgery of Chronic Ear Infection. *Arch. Otolaryngol.* (Chicago) 81, 204-205, 1965.

GUERRIER Y., ANDREA M., PACO J. Les repaires anatomiques du cholestéatome dans la caisse du tympan. *Ann. Oto-Laryng. (Paris) 97, 15-28, 1980.*

MERCKE U., Departement of Oto-Rhino-Laryngology, University of Lund, Sweden. Personal Communication 1984.

SCHMITT H.G. Ein Vorschlag zur Dokumentation und Statistik der Ohroperationen. *Medizinische Dokumentation* 4, Heft 2, 1960.

SHEA, J. J. JBM Port-A-Punch Card System for Otosclerosis Surgery. *Laryngoscope* (St. Louis) 74, 245, 1964.

STRAUSS P., WÖHRL K., DAU J., LIPPERT H. Ein Modell für verschiedene Grossrechnertypen zur Erfassung, Speicherung und Auswertung von Daten bei Ohroperationen. *Laryngol. Rhinol. Otol.* 56, 878-884, 1977.

Management of labyrinthine fistulae

M. Sanna

Introduction

The labyrinthine fistula is the most common complication of cholesteatoma. Most commonly, its location is in the lateral semicircular canal. The fistula may be subtotal with only partial exposure of the perilymphatic space, or total, with complete exposure. A fistula may be found in any of the semicircular canals (monofocal and plurifocal fistulas). A fistula may occur in the oval window or in the promontory (cochlear fistula). Generally, labyrinthine fistulas develop very slowly.

History

As far as we know, Politzer[1] was the first to advocate, in 1909, a conservative approach and stressed the importance of leaving the cholesteatoma matrix undisturbed, in order to preserve the cochlear and vestibular functions. Nylen[2] was the first, in 1923, to envisage surgery by removing the matrix and leaving the fistula uncovered.

The 50's and 60's were characterized by considerable progress in the field of surgical techniques. As a result of such developments, the notion of matrix removal emerged, the fistula being covered by various materials such as skin, mucous membrane, fascia, vein or bone (Timm,[3] Utech,[4] Eckel[5]). In the same period a large number of authors, however, agreed that such an operation was absolutely contra-indicated when a labyrinthine fistula was present. Similar, and at times, greater problems arose when closed tympanoplasty was introduced. Indeed, no agreement has been reached yet, as to how the fistula should be managed, and authors still have conflicting opinions on this subject.

Management of the fistula
Once the presence of a fistula has been detected, and its size approximately determined, the surgeon is faced with two problems:
— what technique should be adopted, i.e. the open or closed technique,
— how the matrix should be handled, i.e. removing it or leaving it undisturbed.

Surgical technique
If small fistulas pose no problems, the opinions of various authors are conflicting when the fistula is large. For some authors (Wullstein,[6] Palva et al.,[7] Abramson et al.,[8] Gacek,[9] Freeman,[10] Wayoff et al.[11]) this is one of the conditions that preclude any procedure other than a radical or modified radical mastoidectomy. Others, however (Law et al.,[12] Sheehy,[13] Smyth,[14] Sanna et al.[15]), believe that even a large fistula can be managed by a closed technique.

Management of the Matrix
On the subject of management of the matrix, opinions are extremely conflicting. The dimension of this disagreement between different authors is clearly demonstrated by the antithetic points of view expressed in different papers.

— Wullstein (1968)[6] proposes a two-stage procedure and removes the matrix during the second stage.
— Ritter (1970)[16] believes that the tissue overlying the fistula should be left in place on the basis of an increased incidence of hearing loss in cases in which the membrane was removed.
— Palva et al. (1971)[7] come to the opposite conclusions and suggest removing the matrix in all cases.
— Sheehy and Crabtree (1973)[17] first proposed a staged procedure in closed tympanoplasty, leaving the matrix at the first stage.
— Tos (1975)[18] removes the matrix and then closes the fistula.
— Law et al. (1975)[12] claim that the surgical procedure should be staged, leaving the matrix at the first stage and removing it at the second stage of a closed technique.
— McCabe (1978) removes the matrix in all cases.
— Freeman (1979) prefers leaving the matrix over the fistula.
— Wayoff et al. (1979)[11] recommend removing the matrix even though a risk to the inner ear is involved.

— Fisch (1980) prefers to remove the skin even in fistulas larger than 2 mm.
— Sanna et al. (1980-1982)[19] prefer to stage the operation.
— Finally, there are yet other authors, including Gacek (1974)[9] and Sheehy (1978),[13] who believe that the matrix should either be removed or left "in situ", depending on the different cases. More specifically, when a closed technique is adopted, the matrix should be removed at the first stage if the fistula is small, but left in place initially and removed at the second stage if the fistula is large. When the procedure is an open technique, the matrix shall always be left undisturbed.

We (1980-82) agree with this last group of authors. We left the matrix in place in the cases in which we adopted an open technique. We prefer to perform a closed tympanoplasty with the matrix being left over the fistula initially and removed at the planned second stage.

As we have seen, there still exists a controversy over how to handle the matrix over the labyrinthine fistulas, and these conflicting opinions have not yet been settled.

Management of extensive and/or multiple fistulas

There is a considerable risk to the inner ear in a patient with an extensive or multiple fistula, regardless of the method of management or the surgical technique followed. In these cases, prognosis is very poor. Sheehy[13] reports a 56 % total loss of hearing; Pfaltz[20] claims that there is no chance of preserving the function of the ear.

Cochlear fistula

Special mention should be made of the cochlear fistula cases, this being the type of fistula that is most often responsible for dead ears preoperatively as well as postoperatively, as a result of an attempt of removing the matrix (Palva et al., 1971; Gacek, 1971; Law et al., 1975; Amyth, 1980). Our experience with the cochlear fistula, limited as it may be, proves that even this type of fistula can be managed using a closed tympanoplasty and removing the matrix at the second stage. This manœuvre, however, is much more delicate in these types of fistulas than in fistulas involving the lateral semicircular canal.

Personal experience

Between January 1971 and De-

Table 1. Labyrinthine fistula - 116 cases in 859 cholesteatomas (13,5 %)

	No.	%
Lateral semicircular canal	92	79,3
Multiple	13	11,2
Oval window	5	4,3
Cochlea	6	5,2

Table 2. Size of the fistula - 116 cases

	No.	%
Small (0.5-1 mm)	11	9,5
Medium (1-2 mm)	19	16,4
Large (>2 mm)	86	74,1

Table 3. Operative procedure in cholesteatoma cases - comparison of fistula with non-fistula cases

	Fistula cases	Non-fistula cases	Total cases
Closed tympanoplasty	61 (52,6 %)	612 (82,4 %)	673 (78,3 %)
Open tympanoplasty	18 (15,5 %)	33 (4,4 %)	51 (5,9 %)
Classical or modified radical mastoidectomy	37 (31,9 %)	98 (13,2 %)	135 (15,8 %)
TOTAL	116	743	859

Table 4. Labyrinthine fistula - evolution of the techniques - 116 cases

Operative procedure	1971-1979	1980-1983	TOTAL
Closed tympanoplasty	17 (38,6 %)	44 (61,7 %)	61 (52,6 %)
Open tympanoplasty	7 (16,0 %)	11 (15,2 %)	18 (15,5 %)
Classical or modified radical mastoidectomy	20 (45,4 %)	17 (23,7 %)	37 (34,9 %)
TOTAL	44	72	116

Table 5. Closed tympanoplasty - management of cholesteatoma matrix with respect to size of fistula - 61 cases

Size of fistula	Number of cases	Matrix "in situ"	Matrix removed
Small	9 (14,7 %)	2 (7,1 %)	7 (21,2 %)
Medium	18 (29,5 %)	2 (7,1 %)	16 (48,5%)
Large	34 (55,8 %)	24 (85,8 %)	10 (30,3 %)
TOTAL	61	28	33 *

* In 25 cases the fistula was covered (with fascia in 24 %; with fascia and bone dust in 76 %), the remaining 8 cases (small fistulas) were not covered.

Table 6. Management of large fistulas - 86 cases

Operative procedure	No.	Matrix "in situ"	Matrix removed
Closed tympanoplasty	34	24 (70,6 %)	10 (29,4 %)
Open tympanoplasty	16	14 (87,5 %)	2 (12,5 %)
Classical or modified radical mastoidectomy	36	33 (91,7 %)	3 (8,3 %) (2 labyrinthectomies)
TOTAL	86	71 (82,6 %)	15 (17,4 %)

cember 1983, we operated on 116 cases of labyrinthine fistulas out of a total of 859 cases of chronic otitis media with cholesteatoma. Tables 1 and 2 show the location and size of the fistulas, respectively. Table 3 reports the surgical techniques used in the two groups (the fistula group and the non-fistula group). Our attitude to the management of the labyrinthine fistula has changed over the years (table 4).

Table 5 shows the management of the matrix with respect to the size

Table 7. Labyrinthine fistula - closed tympanoplasty (planned second stage) - matrix "in situ" - 28 cases		
Fate of the matrix	No.	%
Matrix not found	19	67,8 [Bony closure 11 (58 %)]
Residual cholesteatoma	9	32,1 [Bony closure 1 (11 %)]

of the fistula, and table 6 the management of large fistulas.

Table 7 shows the evolution of the matrix in 28 cases in which it had been left "in situ" in a staged closed tympanoplasty. All 28 cases were reviewed. To our great surprise, in 19 of these cases no trace of the matrix could be found and the region of the fistula was covered by newly formed mucous membrane in all 28 cases; in 12 cases the bony closure of the fistula had occurred. In the 9 cases where we found a residual cholesteatoma, mucous membrane had newly formed over the fistula and this enabled us to remove the cholesteatoma without having to open into the membranous canal.

Results

The review of our results will take into consideration the postoperative bone conduction - about 50 % of cases have a 5-year follow-up. We divided the results into two separate groups and looked at the results obtained with open techniques and with closed tympanoplasty. Table 8 reports the results obtained in 55 cases operated on with an open technique.

Table 9 reports the results of 61 cases managed by combined approach tympanoplasty, divided into two groups: in one group, we consider 28 cases in which the matrix had been left "in situ"; in the other group, we have 33 cases in which the matrix had been removed at the first stage.

Discussion

Currently, the major problems that the surgeon has to solve are:

— Should the matrix covering the fistula be removed or should it not?

— When should the matrix be removed?

Table 8. Labyrinthine fistula - results in open procedures - 55 cases			
	Open tympanoplasty 18 cases	Classical or modified radical mastoidectomy 37 (29) cases*	Total 55 (47) cases*
B.C. unchanged	17 (94,4 %)	23 (79,4 %)	40 (85,1 %)
B.C. deteriorated (between 20 and 30 dB or more)	—	3 (10,3 %)	3 (6,4 %)
Dead ear	1 (5,6 %)	3 (10,3 %) (labyrinthectomy in 2 cases)	4 (8,5 %)

* 8 cases with preoperative total hearing loss are not considered in the results.

Table 9. Labyrinthine fistula - results in closed tympanoplasty - 61 cases

	Matrix "in situ" 28 cases	Matrix removed 33 (32) cases*	Total 61 (60) cases*
B.C. unchanged	26 (92,8 %)	29 (90,6 %)	55 (91,7 %)
B.C. deteriorated (between 20 and 30 dB or more)	2 (7,2 %) (1 case with cochlear fistula)	2 (6,2 %)	4 (6,7 %)
Dead ear	—	1 (3,2 %)	1 (1,6 %)

* 1 case with preoperative total hearing loss was not considered in the results.

— What technique should be adopted?

From our results, we can claim that when an extensive fistula is present, it is better to leave the matrix "in situ" when an open technique is adopted. When a closed technique has been chosen, the matrix can be safely removed in most of the cases with a small fistula, but is is safer to leave the matrix at the first stage with large fistulas.

The open technique is recommended in multiple fistulas and in the only hearing ear.

The risk to the inner ear is less if the matrix is left over the fistula in any type of technique, and this risk is lesser still if a closed technique is adopted and the operation is staged.

Conclusions

In all cholesteatoma cases, the presence of a labyrinthine fistula should always be suspected, and not until it has been detected or excluded with certainty should one go in for any manœuvres to remove the matrix at the level of the lateral canal. Once the presence of the fistula has been detected and its probable size assessed, the cholesteatoma matrix can be removed from all other areas of the fistula, which must be left undisturbed until complete removal of the disease. At this point a decision has to be made as to the procedure to be adopted. There are many factors affecting the choice of the surgical procedure, such as the opposite ear, size of the fistula and cochlear function. As to whether the matrix should be left in place or not, opinions differ considerably.

The technical ability of the surgeon to carefully remove the cholesteatoma matrix without disrupting the membranous labyrinth **is very important.** Experience, no doubt, is important in developing this ability. Anyway, it is much safer and more prudent to leave the matrix which covers a labyrinthine fistula, especially if it is a large one, and to adopt a staged strategy.

The location and size of the fistula are very important in deciding whether or not the matrix should be removed. If the fistula involves the cochlea, the risk of hearing loss is greater.

When the fistula is 2 mm or larger, or an extensive fistula is present, the matrix must be left undisturbed in the first stage and eventually removed at the second look. If we are operating on the only hearing ear, removal of the matrix is absolutely not indicated and an open technique is recommended.

In our hands, a stage closed tympanoplasty is the best way of handling the labyrinthine fistulas, leaving the matrix undisturbed at the first stage and removing it during the second stage.

In 2/3 of our cases, the matrix had disappeared at the second stage. In the remaining 1/3 there was a residual cholesteatoma, usually in the form of a small cyst. There were no cases of massive recurrence of cholesteatoma. In 12 out of 28 cases, the fistula was closed by new bony formation.

Using this technique, better functional results are obtained and the risk of inducing total hearing loss is almost completely eliminated.

References:

1. POLITZER A. A text-book of the Diseaes of the Ear. 5th Ed. Lea and Feldger, Philadelphia, 1909.
2. NYLEN C.O. The labyrinthine fistula symptoms. *Acta Otolaryngol.* Suppl.: 111, 1923.
3. TIMM C. Zur Behandlung der chronischen Otitis Media mit Labyrinthfistel. *Z. Laryn. Rhinol.* 31: 481-483, 1952.
4. UTECH H.: Ein Beitrag zur Therapie der Labyrinthfisteln. *HNO* (Berlin) 7: 349-350, 1959.
5. ECKEL W. Beiträge zum Problem der Labyrinthfisteln. *HNO* 8: 1-11, 1959.
6. WULLSTEIN H. Operationen zur Verbesserung des Gehöres. Thieme, Stuttgart, 311, 1968.
7. PALVA T., KARJA J., PALVA A. Opening of the labyrinth during chronic ear surgery. *Arch. Otolaryngol.* 93: 75-78, 1971.
8. ABRAMSON M., MARKER L.A., McCABE B.F. Labyrinthine fistula complicating chronic suppurative otitis media. *Arch. Otolaryngol.* 100: 141-142, 1974.
9. GACEK R.R. The surgical management of labyrinthine fistulae in chronic otitis media with cholesteatoma. *Ann. Otolaryngol.* Suppl.: 10, 1974.
10. FREEMAN P. Fistula of the lateral semicircular canal. *Clin. Otolaryngol.* 3: 315-321, 1978.
11. WAYOFF M., FRIOT J.M., CHOBAUT S.C., SIMON C. Les fistules du canal semi-circulaire externe. *Oto-Neuro-Opht.* 51: 3-12, 1979.
12. LAW K.P., SMYTH G.D.L., KERR A.G. Fistulae of the labyrinth treated by staged combined approach tympanoplasty. *J. Laryngol. Otol.* 471-478, 1975.
13. SHEEHY J.L. Mangement of labyrinthine fistula. *Clin. Otolaryng.* 3: 405-414, 1978.
14. SMYTH G.D.L. Cholesteatomatous fistula of the labyrinth in chronic ear disease. Churchill Livingstone Publ., 189-195, 1980.
15. SANNA M., SCANDELLARI R., JEMMI G. Il trattamento della fistola labirintica nella chirurgia del colesteatoma. *Atti 67º Congr. Soc. Ital. ORL,* 97. Publ. Minerva Medica, Milano, 1980.
16. RITTER F.N.: Chronic suppurative otitis media and the pathological labyrinthine fistula. *Laryngoscope* 80: 1025-1035, 1970.
17. SHEEHY J.L., CRABTREE J. Tympanoplasty: staging the operation. *Laryngoscope* 83: 1594-1621, 1973.
18. TOS M. Treatment of labyrinthine fistulae by a closed technique. *ORL* 37: 41-47, 1975.
19. SANNA M., SCANDELLARI R., DELOGU P., ZINI C. Il trattamento della fistola labirintica nelle timpanoplastiche chiuse. *Atti 69º Congr. Soc. Ital. ORL.* 163. Publ. Verducci, Roma, 1982.
20. PFALTZ C.R., Complications of otitis media. *ORL* 44: 301-309, 1982.

Eradication of the pathology from nervous structures during middle ear surgery

K.L. Pulec

Techniques for the successful removal of pathology from nervous structures during middle ear surgery are available. The development of neuro-otological techniques and the routine use of intact canal wall tympanoplasty for the treatment of chronic otitis media has made the open technique used in the past to manage disease purposefully left behind, unnecessary and undesirable. Knowledge and routine use of these techniques makes it possible to obtain total removal of cholesteatoma and benign neoplasms without causing injury to nerves and brain.

The most common type of pathology which involves nerves, dura and brain encountered in middle ear surgery is related to infection. Cholesterol granuloma, edematous mucosa and polypoid granulation tissue need not be totally extirpated. Only gross removal to establish proper drainage is required. The presence of this tissue, however, can distort landmarks and increase the risk of injury to nerves and brain for that reason. In addition, edematous mucosa and granulation tissue is often combined with the basement membrane of squamous epithelium and cholesteatoma within the middle ear and mastoid and makes the dissection more hazardous. It is mandatory that all basement membrane of the living portion of squamous epithelium within the middle ear and mastoid be totally removed. Most well-trained, experienced surgeons report no residual disease within the mastoid and approximately four percent residual disease within the tympanum usually in the area of the round or oval windows where dissection is purposely less aggressive to avoid risk of sensorineural injury in the infected ear. This residual disease, when left on purpose or unknowingly, can safely be removed by a transcanal tympanomeatal flap approach during a planned second-stage reconstruction of hearing or if a mass becomes evident behind the intact tympanic membrane. Other benign conditions which occur in the tympanum and must be removed from neural tissue are, in decreasing frequency, glomus body tumor, neuroma, meningioma, hemangioma, ceruminous gland adenoma, and histiocytosis X. In the case of histiocytosis X, less than total removal is often successful.

Technique

Three techniques may be used. In the majority of cases, the capsule of benign neoplasms and the basement membrane of cholesteatoma can be dissected from the mucous membrane which lines the middle ear and covers the nerve sheath and dura. In the majority of cases, the tumor mass merely occupies the middle ear space or mastoid air cell space and is easily lifted from the mucous membrane. It is important that the surgeon always approach important structures in areas of virgin anatomy where there is no disease. Bone is then removed to the margin of the disease and the disease can then be removed from the nerve sheath or dura with no question about the exact position of the important structure. For example, in the case of cholesteatoma filling the upper half of the mastoid and antrum, the approach involves first the removal of bone 4 or 5 mm inferior to the lower margin of the cholesteatoma sac to expose the facial nerve sheath. The dissection of bone from the facial nerve sheath is then carried toward the disease so that the facial nerve sheath is carefully protected from injury. It is not only a matter of safety, but the prompt identification of any important structure and hence, its preservation, usually greatly shortens the time required for the surgical procedure.

A second technique involves removal of a portion of the nerve sheath or dura by sharply dissecting away the surface layers of the nerve sheath or dura to ensure complete removal of pathology. This technique is especially useful in secondary surgery where a firm adhesion is found between the cholesteatoma, the basement membrane or the capsule of a neoplasm. When such a situation is encountered, the bulk of the disease is removed, and the area in question is usually left as an island of residual disease. When the questionable area has been thoroughly exposed and properly identified, a circumferential incision through clearly normal facial nerve sheath or dura through approximately one half of the thickness of the entire layer is made with a sharp, small scalpel similar to a #15 Bard-Parker blade. The surface layers to be removed with the disease are grasped by a cup forceps and kept under tension as the knife edge is used in a slicing sharp dissection to split the layers of tissue. With practice, this skill can be mastered so that the facial nerve sheath, middle-fossa dura or posterior-fossa dura can be split to remove a surface layer and still leave a thin, but protective deep layer.

A third technique involves complete removal of nerve sheath to expose the naked facial nerve fibers or arachnoid and brain. Benign disease will easily be removed from brain or the nerve fibers, in almost every case, with the exception of the rare neglected infiltrating glomus body tumor. In the case of removal of facial nerve sheath to extirpate all pathology, the method of exposure of the nerve sheath and incision is similar to that used for facial nerve decompression with the exception that a segment of the sheath is excised. Once the dissection has been started, the area to be removed is grasped with a cup forceps and kept under tension while the incisions are extended with a sharp knife or Bellucci scissors. The use of proper surgical technique will result in normal facial and other cranial nerve function following this dissection. No covering is required following removal of the sheath from the nerve fibers. The use of Silastic film to prevent adhesions between exposed facial fibers and the raw medial surface of a tympanic membrane graft is desirable.

Repair with fascia in areas where the dura has been excised from the middle or posterior fossa is usually needed. Fascia, perichondrium, periosteum or other mesodermal autograft or homograft tissue is placed under the edges of the bone or under the edges of the remaining dura and held in place if necessary by some firm support to prevent cerebrospinal fluid otorhinorrhea. In the case of dural exposure through the tegmen tympani, no firm support is required for small bony exposures. Whenever the bony opening is 1 cm or greater in diameter, it is necessary to place a firm support of SupraMid between the dura and the interior of the skull to prevent later herniation of brain into the mastoid. In most cases, this can be accomplished by cutting the SupraMid in an oval shape so that it can be placed through the opening into the middle fossa and then positioned so that it will not fall through the hole. In the case of an intact canal wall technique, no covering is necessary over the mastoid side of the SupraMid. Should the surgeon already be confronted with a radical mastoid cavity, he can obliterate it with bone paste which can be packed right against the SupraMid. Should he wish to leave the cavity, the SupraMid must be covered by fascia within the cavity.

Case Report

A 52-year old white attorney was seen in consultation on 10/20/76 with the diagnosis of left congenital cholesteatoma. He gave a history of drainage from the left ear during childhood and left hearing loss since the age of 11. At the age of 19 he had a left ear infection and a myringotomy was performed. Two years later, he developed vertigo which lasted for one week. With the exception of left hearing loss, he had no difficulty until June 1976 when he first noticed brief episodes of left facial spasm. The spells occurred 3 times, lasting one minute each in the period of one week. On 9/28/76, the referring surgeon had performed an exploratory mastoidectomy and had found extensive cholesteatoma. One week before my examination, he developed unrelenting, severe, left hemi-facial spasm.

Physical examination revealed a dry central perforation on the left and evidence of a recently healed endaural incision. The face had normal motion with periodic left-sided spasms. Audiogram showed normal hearing on the right for pure tones and speech. The left ear had a conductive hearing loss of 64 dB with 88 % speech discrimination. Polytomography demonstrated an extensive lytic process involving the left petrous apex. A polytome Pantopaque study demonstrated that the cholesteatoma extended 2 mm into the left internal auditory canal at its superior edge. Neurosurgical evaluation revealed no defects other than the VIIth and VIIIth nerves on the left side. On 11/18/76 under a general anesthetic, a left postauricular incision was made. A complete mastoidectomy and labyrinthectomy was performed. A dry, white, tightly packed congenital cholesteatoma was found to be filling the entire petrous apex. The cholesteatoma was attached to the facial nerve along the entire medial surface of the tympanic portion and to the posterior edge of the labyrinthine portion. The cholesteatoma had eroded the bone and completely surrounded the dura of the internal auditory canal. By removing the bone from the entire circumference of the facial nerve from a point 5 mm proximal to the stylomastoid foramen to the internal auditory canal, it was possible to remove the cholesteatoma completely. It was necessary to move the facial nerve from side to side in order to dissect the basement membrane from the entire circumference of the nerve sheath. The cholesteatoma could not safely be dissected from the middle fossa nor the posterior fossa, and for that reason, the dura was split and the superficial layers removed with the cholesteatoma in several large areas. The internal auditory canal was opened and the VIIIth nerve was severed within the canal. Fascia graft was placed under the tympanic membrane to close the perforation. Gelfoam was packed lightly into the perforation in the internal auditory canal dura. Abdominal fat removed through a separate low transverse abdominal incision was packed into the entire petrous apex and mastoid to close the cerebrospinal fluid leak and to obliterate the large surgical defect. The wound was closed in layers with interrupted chromic catgut and running silk sutures. The patient's postoperative course was uneventful with the exception of a 10 % left facial weakness. He had no spasms of the face. He was discharged on the sixth postoperative day. He returned to work 4 weeks after surgery and had at that time a 5 % left facial weakness (figure 1). At 4 months, the wounds were well healed, the face was normal and he had no tinnitus, vertigo or facial spasm. Follow-up examination on 1/31/78 revealed normal facial function (figure 2) and no complaints. He remains well and free from any recurrent symptoms 7 years postoperatively.

Comment

This case illustrates most of the technical problems which can confront the otologic surgeon in the management of congenital cholesteatoma. In order to accomplish total removal of all basement membrane of squamous epithelium to prevent any recurrent problems, it was necessary to expose the facial nerve sheath from the spinal fluid of the internal auditory canal throughout its course almost to the stylomastoid foramen and it was necessary to dissect the basement membrane from the facial nerve sheath and at times, part of the sheath was removed where there was any question that basement membrane might still be present. The bone of the petrous apex was eroded by the disease and it was necessary to dissect the cholesteatoma and split the dura over both the middle cranial fossa and posterior cranial fossa. The dura of the internal auditory canal had to be partially excised to ensure complete removal of disease. This added the problem of cerebrospinal fluid leak. Closure must be carefully performed so that excessive pressure is not placed upon the fragile facial nerve passing through the dural openings. Closure and obliteration of the entire apex and mastoid with abdominal fat similar to that used in the closure after the removal of acoustic neuroma is an effective method.

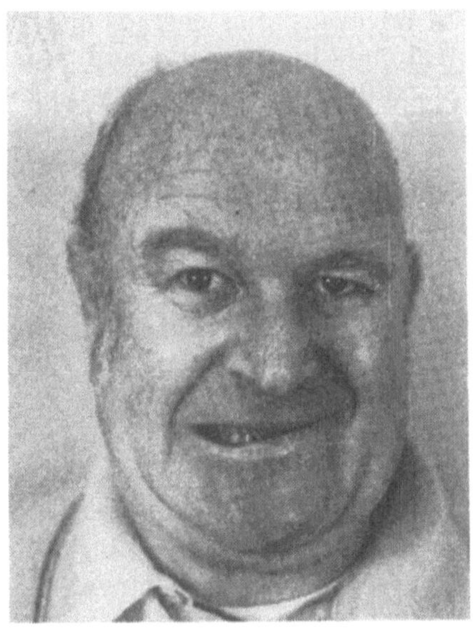

Fig. 1: One month postoperative congenital cholesteatoma removal. 5 % left facial weakness.

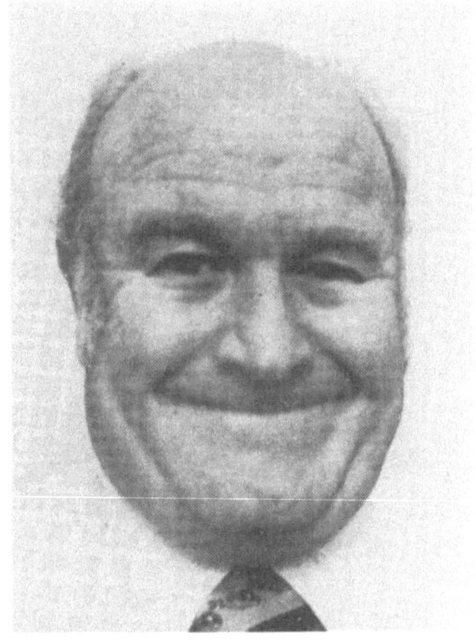

Fig. 2: Fifteen months postoperative removal left congenital cholesteatoma. Normal facial function.

In an occasional case of cholesteatoma, the surgeon will occasionally find it necessary to incorporate the middle cranial fossa approach. This addition is necessary when the cholesteatoma extends beyond the epitympanum and extends along the floor of the middle cranial fossa. When the disease extends medially to the geniculate ganglion and the superior semicircular canal, it is usually impossible to safely obtain total removal by the tympanic or mastoid approach. In such a case, it is desirable to perform a small tempero-craniectomy and use a self-retaining dural retractor. With the exposure afforded by this approach, cholesteatoma and the basement membrane of the squamous epithelium can safely and directly be dissected from the labyrinth, facial nerve, cochlea and any fistula present, and the carotid artery and Eustachian tube.

Three techniques for the removal of pathology from nervous structures during middle ear surgery have been described. Procedures to expose pathology in any part of the temporal bone and ways to repair defects in the dura have been discussed. Routine use of these methods is imperative for success in middle ear surgery.

This lecture was sponsored by Ear International, 1245 Wilshire Boulevard, Suite 509, Los Angeles, California 90017, USA.

SYMPOSIUM II
Reconstructive surgery

Chairman: E.H. Huizing

Biocompatible implant material

J.J. Grote

Since the beginning of reconstructive middle ear surgery there has always been an interest in implant materials. The use of alloplastic implant materials in the middle ear was disappointing because of extrusion.[1,2] However, it is worthwhile to realize that the most successful middle ear reconstruction, in otosclerosis patients, is performed with alloplastic implants.[3]

For good postoperative evaluation of the results with alloplastic implants two types of criteria are important: material criteria and surgical criteria. Because of the difference in surgical aims it is obvious that orthopedic surgeons need different implant materials than otologists. But also in the reconstruction of a middle ear the demands for the canal wall will be different from those for a chain reconstruction.

The material criteria concerns the biocompatibility of a material which can be discussed in two ways.[4] The reaction of the implant on the body with local and general reactions, also called the cytotoxicity of the implant material, and the influence of the body on the prosthesis which eventually can lead to degradation and loss of function. This is the biofunctionality of the implant. Biocompatibility is the first prerequisite for a useful implant material and this has to be tested extensively in vitro, in animal experiments and in clinical studies, with long postoperative periods.

The capacities of an implant material are dependent on its surface activity. To indicate the interaction of the surface of an implant material and the body we can regard an implant material as bio-inert, biotolerant or bio-active. A foreign body will always be encapsulated by a fibrous capsule with a different amount of reactive cells, especially foreign body giant cells. An implant material is bio-inert if no reaction of the surface to the body occurs and the encapsulation is only a small fibrous capsule without further reaction. A biotolerant material will have a good capsule around the implant material without signs of cellular activity as giant cells, whereas a bio-active material will give a real bonding with the surrounding tissue on the surface and will in this way be integrated.

In the past, implant materials had a solid structure but, during the last decade several investigators developed porous materials, which enabled the host tissue to grow into the pores of the implant, giving a good integration in the body. It was found that macropores of 100 micron were ideal for the ingrowth of fibrous tissue and especially of bone tissue, whereas micropores of several microns seemed to be essential, especially in porous ceramic implant materials for remodelling and integration.[5]

For a good postoperative evaluation of different implants in reconstructive middle ear surgery we must have sufficient insight into the biocompatibility and reactivity of the implant material. Therefore, the following information concerning new implant materials is necessary:

— *Generic names.* Not only the generic names of the material used, but also of the additives which might be part of the implant material are necessary. These generic names can give us the information on cytotoxicity and biofunctionality.

— *Structure.* With structure has to be mentioned not only the composition of the material with regard to the density and to the crystallographic structure in case of ceramic, but also the porosity indicating the macropores and the micropores which will be of influence on the integration capacity and the remodelling capacity.

For 10 years we have studied different types of implant materials,[6,7] in the last 7 years we have been using calcium phosphate in the form of hydroxyapatite. Hydroxyapatite resembles the anorganic basis of normal living bone tissue. We have tested this implant material in vitro, in animal experiments and in clinical studies for several years.[8,9,10] This ceramic can be made in dense and porous form with macropores of 100 microns and micropores of several microns, which are essential for the remodelling process.

To illustrate the different problems which can be found in the description of implant materials, the need for an exact description of calcium phosphate ceramics will be discussed. Calcium phosphate is present in the body in different forms. The main forms are hydroxyapatite and B whitlockite which is also called tri-calcium phosphate. In the human body tri-calcium phosphate is soluble and therefore not present in crystallographic form. The sintering technique however, can give a tri-calcium phosphate ceramic.[11] For a good understanding it is necessary to indicate which type of calcium phosphate is used as the difference between these bone-like implant materials is their biodegradability. Apatite ceramics in dense form are not degradable and B whitlockite or tri-calciumphosphate ceramics are biodegradable under certain circumstances. This biodegradation is dependent on the crystallography, the stoichiometry, which is the calcium/phosphor ratio, and the porosity, especially the microporosity.[12] We use hydroxyapatite in dense form and in macro-microporous form. The dense form is bioreactive, but will not be remodelled in living bone tissue. Hydroxyapatite is the main substance of living bone tissue matrix. The more the material is like the host's, the better it is for the implant.

Apart from the material criteria, the surgical criteria are also important for a successful use. Therefore, a good terminology for the different types of prostheses is necessary. Austin[13] made a very detailed survey of the situations which can be found in middle ear reconstruction. Essential is the presence or absence of the malleus handle and the stapes superstructure. He indicates two types of prostheses: the columella type and the assembly. A columella is a connection which has direct contact with the drum membrane. There are two possibilities: a short columella which is the connection between the stapes superstructure and the drum membrane in case of a missing malleus, and a long columella which is the connection between the footplate and the drum membrane. Columella's always had the highest extrusion rate because of their contact with the drum membrane. There still is the idea that better implant materials will prevent extrusion and the interposition of cartilage seems to diminish extrusion rate. However, direct contact of a columella against the drum membrane is not ideal, not even in cases of good integration in the prosthesis. The drum membrane will fold over the prostheses and eventually will extrude them. Therefore, assembly prostheses will have better integration possibilities in the middle ear.

To simplify the nomenclature of these different prostheses, I suggest the following terminology which is based on the missing part which has to be replaced:

part which has to be replaced:
— **stapes prosthesis,** as we all use in otosclerosis surgery;
— **stapes/incus prosthesis,** in case of a missing stapes superstructure and incus, but if the malleus is present. The prosthesis forms an assembly between the stapes footplate and malleus handle, a good design for such a prosthesis with regard to the transmission function is not yet available;
— **incus prosthesis,** which is replacing the missing incus, between stapes head and malleus neck;
— **drum membrane prosthesis,** in case the drum membrane and malleus are absent or either a total drum membrane perforation needs an alloplastic implant;
— **canal wall prosthesis,** in which the posterior and superior canal wall is missing;
— **total middle ear prosthesis,** in case of an empty middle ear and a missing posterior canal wall.

I will give some examples of hydroxyapatite prostheses, which I have been using for several years now.[10] Some of them have proven their reliability in a sufficiently long postoperative period and other prostheses are still in an experimental phase. Because of the problems with the drum membrane and the extrusion rate of columellas, I have chosen the assembly approach. The incus prosthesis is made of dense hydroxyapatite and connects the head of the stapes with the handle of the malleus. Its shape is such that there is no connection with the bony annulus or the facial ridge and it is easy to use in middle ear reconstruction. Another example is the stapes/incus prosthesis, which is a connection between the malleus handle and mobile footplate. The prosthesis can be placed in the centre of the mobile footplate and is made of dense hydroxyapatite with a good connection between the footplate and handle of the malleus.

The canal walls prosthesis is made of porous hydroxyapatite giving a good ingrowth of living bone tissue and will be remodelled in living bone. If the soft tissues are handled in a correct way it gives a nice new ear canal. Drum membrane and malleus prostheses and total alloplastic middle ear prostheses are still in an experimental phase.

Conclusion

Postoperative evaluation of alloplastic implant prostheses can only be compared if biomaterial criteria with generic names of the materials, including the additives, and the composition, including porosity, will be mentioned, in order to have some more insight into the biocompatibility and reactivity of the material. Description of the type of prosthesis, according to the suggested terminology, is also essential for judging the results. A good description of biomaterial criteria and surgical criteria can lead to improvement of these implants which will be necessary for the development of middle ear reconstructions.

References:

1. GUILDFORD F.R. Use of prosthesis in conduction mechanism. *Arch. Otolaryngol.* 80: 80-86, 1964.
2. PORTMANN M. Management of ossicular chain defects. *J. Laryngol. Otol.* 81: 1309-1323, 1967.
3. SHEA J.J. A technique for stapes surgery in obliterative otosclerosis. *Otolaryngol. Clin. North Am.* 1: 199-215, 1969.
4. HOMSY Ch. A. Biocompatibility in selection of materials for implantation. *J. Biomed. Mater. Res.* 4: 341-356, 1970.
5. HOMSY Ch. A. On alloplasts for otology. In: Biomaterials in Otology ed. J.J. Grote, Publisher Martinus Nijhoff, Boston 1984.
6. KUYPERS W., GROTE J.J. The use of Proplast in experimental ear surgery. *Clin. Otolaryngol.* 2: 5-15, 1977.
7. GROTE J.J., KUYPERS W., DE GROOT K. Use of sintered hydroxyapatite in middle ear surgery. ORL, *J. Otorhinolaryngol. Relat. Spec.* 43: 248-254, 1981.
8. GROTE J.J., KUYPERS W. The use of biomaterials in reconstructive middle ear surgery. Chapter 67 in: Biomaterials in reconstructive surgery, Ed. Rubin L.R. Publisher C.V. Mosby: 1983.
9. V. BLITTERSWIJK C.A., GROTE J.J., KUYPERS W. Hydroxyapatite in the infected middle ear, 93-104 in: Biomaterials in Otology ed. J.J. Grote. Publisher Martinus Nijhoff, Boston 1984.
10 GROTE J.J. Tympanoplasty with calcium phosphate. *Arch. Otolaryngol.* 110: 197-199, 1984.
11. DE GROOT K. Degradable ceramics in D.F. Williams (ed.). Biocompatibility of clinical implant materials, vol. 1, CRC Press, Boca Raton Fla. 199-224, 1981.
12. KLEIN C.P.A.T., VAN DER LUBBE H.B.M., DRIESSEN A.A., DE GROOT K., VAN DEN HOOFF A. Biodegradation behaviour of various calcium phosphate materials in subcutaneous tissue, in ceramics, in surgery, Ed. P. Vincenini, Elsevier, Amsterdam, 105-116, 1983.
13. AUSTIN D.F. A decade of Tympanoplasty: Progress or regress? *Laryngoscope* 92: 527-530, 1982.

Autogeneic and allogeneic grafting materials

W.M.S. Ironside

During the past twenty years, there has been an increasing use of human materials to replace structures of the ear, malformed developmentally, affected by chronic disease or surgically sacrificed. Unfortunately, there has been a lack of consistency in the terms used to describe these grafts, but to delve into the origins of words applied to grafts confuses rather than helps. In the end one has to settle for what has been accepted already.

There are a variety of ways in which grafts can be classified but the ones of interest are:

☐ *By the relationships between donor and recipient:*
— autograft when donor and recipient are the same organism,
— isograft when donor and recipient are twins,
— allograft when donor and recipient are different genotypes,
— xenograft when donor and recipient are of different species.

In the past there was a tendency to refer to the grafts from donor to a different genotype recipient as a homograft which has pertinence in grafts within the human species but not within other species. But 'allo'graft derived from the Greek 'allos' meaning "different" holds good when grafting in any species.

More recently there has been a move to qualify further the graft by indicating that it is the "gene" which is important in this classification. But here there does not seem to be agreement for at least two forms have acceptance. Allogenous is used by Kuijpers and Veldman 1980[1] and others and allogeneic by Lindenmann, 1971[2].

Having discussed the problems with the word specialists at the Oxford University Press Offices, they suggested, after consideration, that "allogeneic" was the correct adjective.

☐ *Classification of grafts by site:*
— orthotopic - donor tissue to same site,
— heterotopic - donor tissue to different site.

Fortunately there is no disagreement about these terms. During the past two decades or more otologists have used increasingly:

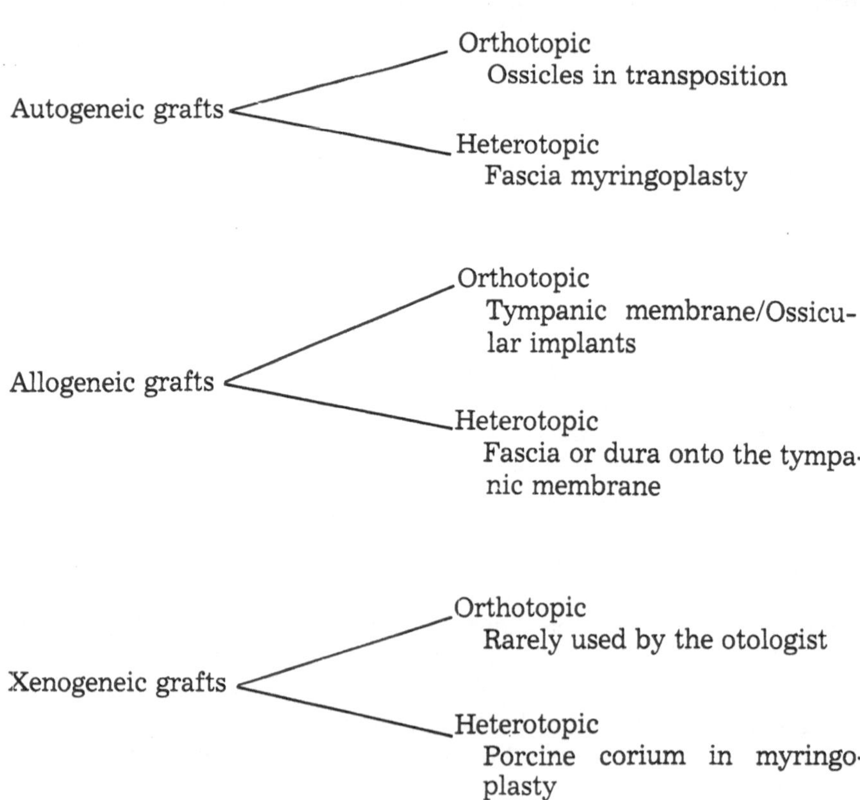

It is accepted that the autogeneic grafts, given an adequate blood supply, and in the absence of infection, will be incorporated into its new position and will be gradually replaced by host tissues so that restoration of function achieved by grafting will be permanent. But with allogeneic and xenogeneic grafts the process is prolonged (Kingma & Hamde 1964).[3]

The reason for this difference lies in the necessity to attempt to destroy the antigenicity of the non-autogeneic graft, and while this may or may not be achieved completely (Veldman et al. 1978).[4] the tissues are altered, changing in some instances their handling characteristics, slowing up the revascularisation of the graft and delaying the replacement of the graft by host tissue — in extreme circumstances the graft remains totally avascular and unchanging.

The common methods of preservation of non-autogenetic grafts appear to affect the grafts differently, as a consequence the reaction of the host to these grafts differ.

Freeze-drying. While this method of preservation is convenient in regard to packaging and the grafts have an indefinite shelf life, it has been shown by Steffert (1967) that the antigenicity of the grafts is not completely eliminated by the process. There is initially, after implantation, an apparent acceptance on the part of the host and then during the second week there is evidence of mild rejection which gradually settles; the graft then proceeds through the various stages of integration or replacement by host tissues. Unfortunately, during the rejection period, fibrosis tends to occur in the graft and surrounding tissue. While this may indeed be helpful and a distinct advantage when allogeneic bone is used to restore the posterior meatal wall, or when placed in the mastoid cavity to support such a posterior wall, it would be unwelcome in the middle ear.

Furthermore, freeze-drying has a physical effect upon soft tissues such as the tympanic membrane. This results in considerable shrinkage of the tissues which is not completely restored by immersion in fluid and by electron microscopy one can see spaces formed presumably by ice formation. This shrinkage and disruption of soft tissues is of particular disadvantage when trying to replace a tympanic membrane which must be matched in dimensions as far as possible.

Alcohol. The first tympanic ossicular block graft to be inserted was prepared in alcohol by Glasscock and House, (1968)[5]. Animal experiments by Van den Broek and Kuijpers (1974)[6] have revealed that alcohol is effective in eliminating antigenic reaction in the rats middle ears and osteogenesis occurs. Many surgeons over the past years have successfully used alcohol stored allogeneic ossicles. Since alcohol is an excellent antiseptic agent, sterility of these grafts is ensured. On the other hand, fluid is progressively extracted from soft tissues stored in alcohol, so that the tissues shrink and become rubbery hard; storage and delivery present a problem from a fire hazard aspect. For these reasons alcohol is reserved only for the preservation of ossicles and these collected in a surgeon's department.

Tanning. Another method of preserving grafts is by immersion in an aldehyde solution only (Perkins 1970)[7] or as a first step. The major effect of this treatment with formaldehyde or gluteraldehyde is on the collagen which develops intermolecular and intramolecular cross linkages resulting in a resistance to proteolytic digestion (Tavis et al. 1975)[8] and a greater stability of the graft (Cox et al. 1973)[9]; the mechanisms of cross linking are still poorly understood (Woodroof 1978).

It is known that a greater number of, and more stable crosslinks are formed with gluteraldehyde than with formaldehyde (Barker et al. 1980).[10] This has been demonstrated clearly in the preparation of the porcine xenogeneic heart valve which when gluteraldehyde treated has functioned for at least ten years but when treated with formaldehyde started to break up after three years.

It was seen, while using C labelled formaldehyde, that after implantation, despite careful preoperative washing, formaldehyde escaped from the graft for a period of six weeks (Barker et al. 1980).[10] This may account for the greater initial cellular reaction found after implantation: later rejection has to be considered as a possibility in view of the work done by Van den Broek & Kuijpers (1974)[6] and Veldman et al. (1978).[4]

Both aldehydes are antimicrobial agents though gluteraldehyde is the more effective being used widely today as Cidex.

Cialit. Cialit, an organic mercurial compound, the sodium salt of 2-ethylmercurimercaptobenzoxazole 5-carboxylic acid, was originally used by orthopaedic surgeons to preserve bones (Guntz 1954).[11] Marquet in 1966[12] introduced it as a method of treating allogeneic tympanic membranes and according to Van den Broek and Kuijpers (1974),[6] grafts treated with it cause no reaction in the rats middle ear. It is also a very active antimicrobial agent.

The drawback to the use of Cialit alone is that the soft tissues are more difficult to dissect completely from the temporal bone. However, initial immersion of the temporal bone block in an aldehyde solution stiffens the tissues and permits a much easier dissection. The combined formaldehyde/cialit method has been used successfully by Marquet since 1971 (Marquet 1977)[13] and gluteraldehyde/Cialit by the author since 1974 (Ironside 1976).[14]

Tissues prepared in this way do not change their dimensions once the process has been completed and so it is possible to record the necessary measurements which will be important for the surgeon wishing to replace a tympanic membrane with an allogeneic graft of the same size. Sterility of grafts prepared in this way should not be in doubt as both substances are very active microbial agents.

Storage of grafts in Cialit is slightly less convenient than with freeze-drying as it is necessary to change the Cialit solution three-monthly. Providing these changes are made there is no deterioration of the graft for a year. Packaging and delivery are relatively simple.

Tissues used in reconstruction prepared in the Tissue Bank at Wakefield, Yorkshire.

Tympanic membrane ossicular blocks are prepared by initial immersion of the bone in a 0,5 % solution of gluteraldehyde buffered to 7,0 pH for 48 hours. After dissection of the block, the preparation is placed in a 0,02 % solution of Cialit until required.

Iliac cortical bone used in the reconstruction of the posterior meatal wall is freeze-dried. In this situation the slight initial tissue reaction is beneficial, while the packaging of these bones is simple and the shelf life excellent.

Cubes and granules of cancellous bone used in the mastoid cavity to support the new allogeneic posterior wall are also freeze-dried for the same reasons.

Dura in 16 cm^2 pieces. Two pieces are also freeze-dried. This can be placed on the posterior wall before returning the soft tissue wall, or be used to close the defect after opening the internal canal.

It is obviously necessary to keep a record of these allogeneic tissues in order to determine their usefulness and their long term results. Thus, every package issued by the Tissue Bank has a label in which there is a serial number of the item and details of the graft. Also with the specimen there is a form in three parts: one is placed in the patient's case notes, the second dispatched to the Bank at the time of surgery indicating which parts of the graft have been used and in what manner, and the third is returned from the Out-Patient Department at the two month follow-up with information about any reaction. Unfortunately, there is considerable difficulty in gaining the necessary co-operation of surgeons. They are only too keen to obtain these materials, but frequently it is necessary to send reminders and even cut off the supply unless the forms are completed.

For the surgeon to keep a record of how these grafts are used it is necessary to note those structures within the middle ear which have survived after the effects of disease and surgery and to indicate those which have had to be replaced by grafts. A computer takes the drudgery out of this scheme and a programme has been worked out with the Computer section of the Yorkshire Health Authority. Marquet has used now for many years a similar system which can be graphically represented and readily stored in a computer (Marquet and Graff 1982).[15]

As part of the computer programme, a record is made of other aspects of the utilisation of the grafts such as complications and long term results. Finally, when material becomes available, either through revision surgery or from the cadaver, it is still worth examining the graft materials histologically to determine their survival and growth and changes induced in surrounding tissues.

By these means it should be possible to build up a picture of the long term value of these materials in reconstructive surgery of the ear.

References:

1. KUIJPERS W., VELDMAN J.E. *Otolaryngology and Head and Neck Surgery 89*, 1. 142-152, 1981.
2. LINDENMANN J. Immunologie, ein Lernprogramm für Studierende und Ärzte (1972).
3. KINGMA M.J., HAMDE J.F. *Journal of Bone and Joint Surgery* 46B, 141, 1964.
4. VELDMAN J.E., KUIJPERS W., OVERBOSCH H.C. *Clinical Otolaryngology 3*, 93, 1978.
5. GLASSCOCK M.E. III, HOUSE W.F., *Laryngoscope* 78, 1219, 1968.
6. VAN DEN BROEK P., KUIJPERS W. *Acta Otolaryngologica* (Stockholm) 77, 335, 1974.
7. PERKINS R. *Laryngoscope* 80, 1100, 1970.
8. TAVIS J.J., HARVEY J.H., THORNTON J.H., WOODROOF E.A., BARLETT R.H. *Biomedical Materials Research 9*, 285, 1975.
9. COX R.W., GRANT R.A., KENT C.M. *Journal of Cell Science 12*, 933, 1973.
10. BARKER H., OLIVER R., GRANT R., STEPHENS L. *Biochimica et Biophysica Acta* 632, 589-597, 1980.
11. GUNTZ E. *Archiv für klinische Chirurgie* 279, 56, 1954.
12. MARQUET J. *Acta Otolaryngologica* (Stockholm) 62, 141, 1966.
13. MARQUET J. *Otolaryngologic Clinics of North America* 10, 479-485, 1977.
14. IRONSIDE W.M.S. *Journal of Laryngology and Otology* 9, 845, 1976.
15. MARQUET J., GRAFF A. *Audiology* 21, 20-32, 1982.

Xenogeneic material for tympanic membrane reconstruction

M. Sanna, C. Zini, R. Gamoletti

The modern reconstructive microsurgery of the middle ear greatly relies upon the use of grafting materials of biological origin. Autologous and homologous tissue transplants have found widespread application in otology; biological tissues of heterologous origin are being investigated and used in the clinical setting by some surgeons.

The terms autologous, homologous and heterologous are, however, improper ways of indicating the source of the transplant and the use of standardized terms should be encouraged. The suggested nomenclature should be:
— autografts: tissue transplants obtained and performed in the same individual,
— allografts: tissue transplants performed among individuals of the same species,
— xenografts: tissue transplants performed among individuals from different species.

As far as the tympanic membrane repair or reconstruction is concerned the use of tissue transplantation techniques is relatively recent: autografts of mesenchymal origin found their clinical application in 1960[1] and are still in use with very satisfactory results. Alternative methods of reconstruction were developed a few years later by Chalat,[2] Marquet,[3] Plester[4] and Perkins[5] with the use of allograft tympanic membranes. The search for a thin, vibratile, well-tolerated, packaged, commercially available biological material has led to the alternative possibilities offered by properly pre-treated xenografts.

The present paper deals with our experience with the clinical use of the moulded tympanic xenograft used at our Clinic since 1974.

Historical background

The history of xenograft transplants in otology is relatively recent. Flottes and co-workers[6] are generally given the credit of having been the first to have used such material: they repaired the tympanic membrane with dehydrated calf cornea in 20 cases but the postoperative course was discouraging because 11 grafts were eliminated within two months.

Salen and Simbach[7] in 1965 published a study of total membrane defect closure in cats with exogenous collagen obtained from the tail of the rat: they concluded that exogenous collagen was absorbed or transformed and participated in the tympanic membrane healing as a vector for the regenerative elements. Patterson[8] described in 1967 the results of experimental tympanic membrane closure in cats with the use of chrome-tanned and untanned collagen film obtained from cattle. Xenograft material had been chemically treated to remove non-collagenous proteins and fats but breakdown of collagen molecular structure had been avoided. Results showed that untanned collagen film was well tolerated and was gradually absorbed or replaced by host tissue.

In 1968 Jansen started the use of calf caecum serosa and published the first results in 1969.[9] In 1970 he reported the results in 150 cases:[10] no immunobiological or other reactions were observed. Cornish and Scott[11] reported the use of xenograft freeze-dried aortic valves as tympanic grafts in 5 patients in 1968. In the same period Kosoy et al.[12] reported experimental use of frozen human aortic valves xenografted into perforated guinea pig eardrums. Again in 1973 Jansen[13] described the possibility of calf's drum head use for repair of 25 human tympanic membranes: failure of the graft occurred in four cases.

Development of the Zini and Sanna moulded tympanic xenograft[14-18] started in 1974 following similar studies of vascular xenografts by Rosemberg et al.;[19] its clinical use was started in July 1974 and a ten-year experience of surgical practice has been accumulated by Zini and co-workers.

Characteristics of the moulded tympanic xenograft

Experimental use of connective tissue xenografts was started by Zini and co-workers at the beginning of 1974 and the calf jugular vein was selected because of its availability and easy removal. A method for preparation of the calf vein was developed according to similar methods used by North American surgeons in the preparation of vascular xenografts. The technique of preparation of the moulded tympanic xenograft has been described in detail elsewhere: in brief, the jugular veins are subjected to selective enzymatic digestion by treatment with a ficin solution (ficin is a proteolytic enzyme derived from the latex of the wild fig tree). Inactivation of ficin is carried out with a solution of sodium chlorite. The residual collagen structure of the jugular vein wall is subsequently tanned with dialdehyde starch. Tympanic xenografts are obtained by cutting pieces of the thinned vein wall and heat-moulding them over plastic moulds that reproduce the shape of the human tympanic membrane and of the adjacent walls of the external ear canal. The grafts are sterilized with ethylene oxide and packaged in glass vials. The tympanic xenograft consists mainly of denatured collagen fibers and it is absolutely non-viable (xenostatic graft). Its antigenicity has been reduced to minimum levels during preparation procedures.

Gamoletti et al.[20] have demonstrated that the moulded tympanic xenograft prepared according to this procedure consists mainly of collagen fibers arranged into a unique structure: the inner side of the graft is smooth in appearance, the outer (adventitial) side consists of coarse collagen bundles arranged in a wide mesh-like pattern. Such observations confirm that the moulded tympanic xenograft acts as a supportive structure for connective and vascular tissue regeneration.

Histological studies by Gamoletti et al.[20] of the implanted grafts have shown that the middle ear side of the graft becomes lined with normal middle ear mucosa and the canal side is covered with squamous epithelium. The grafted tissue becomes surrounded by young connective tissue and capillaries from the host in most cases; slow resorption is possible with time because fragmented graft teased by young connective tissue has been found in a few cases.

Clinical results

The moulded xenograft has been used in about 1800 cases of tympanic reconstruction over a period of nearly ten years from July 1974 to March 1984. We shall report herein the results of 1042 operations performed until December 1981. No selection of cases has been done with regard to the type of disease (table 1). The posterior auricular approach was used in all but 35 cases in which an endaural approach was used. A total tympanic membrane reconstruction was performed in 962 cases (partial in 80 cases only), the majority of tympanic membrane perforations being converted into total ones at the time of surgery. The three objectives of successful tympanoplasty have been defined as follows:

— eradication of pathological conditions,

— recovery of the anatomical conditions,

— preservation or recovery of auditive function.

The evaluation of postoperative records showed that postoperative suppuration was absent in 94% of cases. There was a 6% incidence of otorrhea that ranged from mild external temporary otitis to a severe middle ear infection with loss of the graft. The blunting of the anterior tympanic sulcus is a frequent problem with the lateral surface technique of tympanic grafting. We now prevent it by always removing the anterior canal wall bulge. Blunting still occurs in less than 5% of cases. The lateralization of the graft is practically absent in our hands. Minor anatomical prob-

Table 1. Moulded tympanic heterografts - Indications

Disease	Number	%
Cholesteatoma	370	35,52
Chronic otitis media	277	26,58
Sequels of otitis and tympanosclerosis	284	27,26
Reconstruction of old cavity	71	6,81
Glomus tumour	11	1,06
Trauma	16	1,53
Malformation	13	1,24
TOTAL	1042	100

lems may also affect the functional results and a second operation may be required. They include: canal stenosis (2,8%), excessive thickness of the tympanic membrane (0,5%) and retraction pockets (5%).

Anatomical results include graft failure rate with postoperative perforations. Table 2 shows six different groups of operated on ears with a follow-up ranging from three months to six years. Perforations have been divided into partial, total and temporary. The overall failure rate in the cases with a six months follow-up is 5,1% and only a very small number of cases failed later.

The graft take-rate was not influenced by the types of middle ear pathology: for example, cholesteatomatous ears had a 96,3% take while non-cholesteatomatous ears averaged 94,5% take-rate. The same was true when the presence of preoperative otorrhea was concerned. Whether the ear was draining at the time of surgery was of no consequence as the take-rate was 94% in draining ears and 95% in dry ears.

Discussion

The aim of tympanic membrane reconstruction is both the anatomical and functional recovery of the eardrum. The grafted membrane should be a barrier between the external ear and the middle ear spaces and also be a thin, vibrating, well-tolerated membrane for the transmission of the sounds. Clinical experience and histological investigations have confirmed the feasibility of tympanic membrane grafting with biological materials of xenogeneic origin. The moulded tympanic xenograft has shown good mechanical properties, resistance to proteolytic enzymes of bacterial origin and easy manipulation and insertion even in the presence of bleeding in the operative field. The high take-rate and the low incidence of postoperative complications which are unrelated to the middle ear pathology, have supported the use of this material for eardrum repair or reconstruction.

Table 2. Moulded tympanic heterografts - Anatomical results

	Postoperative perforations					
Type	**3 months (%)**	**6 months (%)**	**1 year (%)**	**2 years (%)**	**3 years (%)**	**6 years (%)**
Partial	16/781 (2,04)	25/643 (3,88)	20/520 (3,80)	13/292 (4,45)	6/138 (4,34)	—
Total	5/781 (0,64)	3/643 (0,46)	8/526 (1,52)	3/292 (1,02)	2/138 (1,44)	2/40 (5,0)
Temporary	7/781 (0,89)	5/643 (0,77)	4/526 (0,76)	2/292 (0,68)	—	—
TOTAL	28/781 (3,57)	33/643 (5,11)	32/526 (6,08)	18/292 (6,15)	8/138 (5,78)	2/40 (5,0)

References:

1. HEERMAN H. Trommefellplastik mit Fasciengewebe vom Musculus temporalis nach Begradigung der vorderen Gehörgangswand. *H.N.O.* 9, 136, 1960.
2. CHALAT N.I. Tympanic membrane transplant. *Harper Hosp. Bull.*, Detroit, 22, 27-34, 1964.
3. MARQUET J. Reconstructive microsurgery of the eardrum by means of a tympanic membrane homograft. *Acta Otolaryngol.* 62, 459-464, 1966.
4. PLESTER D. Skin and mucous membrane grafts in middle ear surgery. *Arch. Otolaryngol.* 72, 718-721, 1960.
5. PERKINS S. Human homografts otologic tissue transplantation: buffered formaldehyde preparation. *Trans. Amer. Acad. Ophtal. Otol.* 74, 278-282, 1970.
6. FLOTTES L., RIU R., LE DEN R. et al. L'utilisation des cornées de veau deshydratées dans les tympanoplasties. *J. Franç. ORL* 12, 955-958, 1963.
7. SALEN B, SIMBACH I. Exogenous collagen in the closure of tympanic membrane perforations. *J. Laryngol. Otol.* 79, 159-165, 1965.
8. PATTERSON M.E. Experimental tympanic membrane closure with collagen film. *Arch. Otolaryngol.* 86, 486-489, 1967.
9. JANSEN C. Heteroplastik des Trommelfells. *H.N.O.* 17, 238-240, 1969.
10. JANSEN C. Homo- and heterogeneous grafts in reconstruction of the sound conduction system. *Acta Oto. Rhino. Laryngol,* Belgica 24, 60-65, 1970.
11. CORNISH C.B., SCOTT P.J. Freeze-dried heart valves as tympanic grafts. *Arch. Otolaryngol.* 88, 350-356, 1968.
12. KOSOY J., SATALOFF J., LAUGHLIN L. Aortic valves in myringoplasty. *Arch. Otolaryngol.* 87, 364-367, 1968.
13. JANSEN C. Heterologous tympanoplasty. *Trans. Am. Acad. Ophthal. Otol.* 77, 111-116, 1973.
14. ZINI C., SANNA M., BACCIU S. Eterotrapianto conservato e modellato nella ricostruzione totale della membrana timpanica. Read at IX Congr. Nac. Otorrinolaring. j Cir. Cer. Fac., Malaga 1975 (unpubl. data).
15. ZINI C., SANNA M., BACCIU S. La ricostruzione della membrana timpanica mediante eterotrapianti. *Il Policlinico,* Sez. Chir. 83, 653-660, 1976.
16. ZINI C., SANNA M., BACCIU S. Hétérogreffes tympaniques en tympanoplastie fermée: technique et resultats. CR LXXIII Congr. Franç. ORL, Arnette Ed, Paris, 249-256, 1976.
17. ZINI C., SANNA M., BACCIU S. Une méthode alternative aux homogreffes: hétérogreffes tympaniques moulées. CR LXXV Congr. Franç. ORL, Arnette Ed, Paris, 451-457, 1978.
18. ZINI C., SANNA M., BACCIU S., Jemmi G. Cinq années d'expérience des héterogreffes tympaniques moulées. CR LXXVI Congr. Franç. ORL, Arnette Ed, Paris, 83-88, 1979.
19. ROSEMBERG G.N., HENDERSON J., LORD J.H. An arterial prosthesis of heterologous vascular origin. *JAMA* 187, 165-167, 1964.
20. GAMOLETTI R., LANZARINI P., ZINI C., SANNA M., BACCIU S. Moulded tympanic heterografts. Histological evaluation. *Ann. Otol. Rhinol. Laryngol.* 93, 132-135, 1984.

Reconstruction of the ossicular chain

J. Helms

The scientific and experimental basis for present day functional surgery of the ear was laid in the seventies of the last century. At that time European, mainly German, scientists and clinicians developed successful surgical procedures to treat inflammatory middle ear diseases. Authors such as Berthold[1], Kessel[2], Hoffmann[3], v.Tröltsch[4], Ely[5], and Tangemann[6] developed operations more than 100 years ago, which even then resembled todays concepts.

It is to their merit that Moritz[7], Wullstein[8], and Zöllner[9,10] developed modern standards for reconstruction of the ossicular chain, especially in inflammatory diseases.

General remarks for ossicular replacement procedures

In reconstructing the ossicular chain the following materials have proven highly valuable: patients' own ossicles or remains of them, human homo ossicles, steel wire, cartilage and bioactive ceramic prostheses.

Reconstruction in defects of the malleus

Isolated defects of the handle of the malleus are rarely observed. When this structure is fractured or eroded it has to be replaced in a way that an acoustically sufficient coupling between the tympanic membrane and the ossicular chain is achieved. The selected implant, be it the patient's own bone, human homo ossicle, cartilage or ceramic material, has to form a large contact area to the ear drum. This is also essential for a classical tympanoplasty type II.

Reconstruction in incus defects

Defects at the incus, mainly starting at the long process, have the highest incidence in ossicular chain defects.

When the long process of the incus is eroded so that its position is no longer superior to the head of the stapes, the whole incus should be removed. The defect between the head of the stapes and the handle of malleus or the ear drum has to be bridged directly.

In more than 50 % of our patients, the handle of the malleus is in a far anterior position to the head of the stapes. Bridging this distance directly results in a very oblique position of the implant. In this situation an angled construction of an implant is used. The posterior part of the implant contacts the posterior area of the tympanic membrane. The handle of the malleus is reached by the tip of the implant (malleus-incus-assembly after Austin[11]). In this situation, artificial prostheses have advantages, they have the necessary stability to transmit vibrations even in this angled form.

All implants used to replace the incus, remain situated only as long as the whole system exerts some pressure on the implant. This tension in the system is achieved by selecting an implant a little bit longer than the diameter of the defect itself.

The insertion of an implant slightly longer than the diameter of the defect causes a puffing out of the tympanic membrane. Postoperative scarring reduces this bulging of the tympanic membrane thus shrinking the ossicular system slightly together and giving stability. The billowing out of the tympanic membrane must remain minimal, otherwise an inserted implant might penetrate the membrane after weeks or months. Perforations occur earlier when less well tolerated materials are used.

The result of a tympanoplasty depends on optimal preoperative treatment, a qualified surgical technique and appropiate postoperative care. Under these conditions a well trained surgeon can obtain a postoperative conductive hearing loss of less than 20 dB in more than 3/4 of his patients. When larger numbers of patients are controlled, having been operated on by different surgeons, 2/3 of these patients show this small postoperative conductive hearing loss of less than 20 dB, as long as the stapes is preserved.

Reconstruction of incus and stapes defects

Combination of incus and stapes defects are frequently seen. The implant has to be inserted between the mobile footplate and the handle of the malleus or the tympanic membrane. Our results have been best using wire or ceramic implants. When using auto- or homo-ossicles for implantation, a fixation at the facial canal wall or promontory is a much higher risk.

In cases where the handle of the malleus is in an anterior position, so that a direct coupling of the footplate would result in a very oblique position of the implant, a columella should be inserted from the footplate to the posterior part of the tympanic membrane. A natural bony columella may incur the risk of being fixed to the facial nerve canal or the promontory. It is for this reason that the main part of the columella should be formed out of wire or, better, the whole prosthesis should be ceramic.

Ceramic implants, especially the biologically active preparations, are not fixed to the facial nerve canal or the promontory and gain solid contact to the tympanic membrane. When the surface of our ceramic material (Ceravital) is covered with small pieces of patients' own bone, this bone will spread over the surface so that the contact area finally is between patients' own bone and tympanic membrane. Long columellae made out of cartilage tend to weaken after months and years and are therefore recommended in this situation.

Reconstruction when all ossicles are defect

The technique to solve the problem when malleus, incus and the superstructure of the stapes are missing, is the same as in the case where the handle of the malleus is in a far anterior position. In these cases the transplantation of a complete homo-ossicular chain is additionally discussed. In these cases we recommend the insertion of cartilage after Heermann[12] to reconstruct the tympanic membrane. The cartilage is cut into strips of 2 mm diameter and these strips are implanted parallel, next to each other over the tympanic cavity. The cartilage should not be used in one piece because postoperative deforming processes are tremendously reduced by using the strip technique. The missing ossicular chain is replaced as already mentioned by ceramic or wire or a combination of wire and homo incus. This active ceramic material is called "Ceravital". It enables patients' own bone to spread over the surface in a layer up to 40 microns. This is done without intermission of connective tissue. The scientific research was done by Dr. Reck[13,14] in my clinic.

Results

When the stapes is missing and additional defects are present in the middle ear, tympanoplastic procedures remain insufficient. In only 30 to 40 % of these patients the air-bone gap is closed to 20 dB or less. Ceravital ceramic and wire implants have improved these results considerably. When the handle of the malleus is present, the insertion of the fork-like wire prosthesis between the handle of the malleus and footplate gives 2/3 of the patients a closure of the air-bone gap of 20 dB or less.

The most promising advance of the last years in microsurgery of the ear seems to be the introduction of ceramic materials for reconstruction of the ossicular chain. This material has been available to us for more than 5 years and the clinical results after more than 500 operations are most promising.[13,14]

References:

1. BERTHOLD E. Das künstliche Trommelfell und die Verwendbarkeit der Schleimhaut des Hühnereis zur Myringoplastik. *Mschr. Ohrenheilk.* 20:85, 1886.
2. KESSEL J. Über die Behandlung der chronischen eitrigen Mittelohrenentzündung. *Arch. Ohrenheilk.* 26:246, 1888.
3. HOFFMANN R. Über den chronischen Ohrenfluss. *Korrespbl. Allg.* Ärtzl. Verein, Tübingen 7:238, 1892.
4. V. TROLTSCH A. Lehrbuch der Ohrenheilkunde mit Einschluss der Anatomie des Ohres. Hirzel, Leipzig 1877.
5. ELY E.T. Hauttransplantation bei chronischer Eiterung des Mittelohres. *Ohrenheilk.* 10:146, 1881.
6. TANGEMANN C.W. Ersatz des Trommelfells durch Hauttransplantation. *Z. Ohrenheilk.* 13:174, 1884.
7. MORITZ W. Hörverbessernde Operationen bei chronisch-entzündlichen Prozessen der Mittelohren. *Z. Laryngol. Rhinol.* 29:579, 1950.
8. WULLSTEIN H.L. Operationen zur Verbesserung des Gehörs. Thieme Stuttgart, 1968.
9. ZÖLLNER F. The principles of plastics surgery of the sound conducting apparatus. *J. Laryng.* 69:637, 1955.
10. ZÖLLNER F. Hörverbessernde Operationen bei entzündlich bedingten Mittelohrveränderungen. *Arch. Ohr. Nas. Kehlkopf Heilk.* 171:1, 1957.
11. AUSTIN D.F. Ossicular reconstruction. *Arch. Otolaryngol.* 94:525-535, 1971.
12. HEERMANN jr. J., HEERMANN H., KOPSTEIN E. Fascia and cartilage palisade tympano-plasty: nine years experience. *Arch. Oto. Laryng.* 91:228-241, 1970.
13. RECK R. Bioactive glass ceramic: a new material in tympanoplasty. *Larnygoscope* 93: 196, 1983.
14. RECK R. Bioactive glass ceramics in ear surgery - animal studies and clinical results. *Laryngoscope* 94, 1984, supplement.

Literature:

1. EICHE T. TH. Ergebnisse einer modifizierten Malleoplatinopexie mit Draht. Dis. Tübingen, 1977.
2. HEERMANN H., HEERMANN J. Endaurale Chirurgie. Urban und Schwarzenberg, München-Berlin, 1964.
3. HELMS J. Vereinfachte Malleoplastinopexie. *HNO* 19:351-353, 1971.
4. HELMS J., HILDMANN H. Unpublished data. Univ. HNO-Klinik Tübingen, 1972.
5. HELMS J. Die Wiederherstellung der Schalleitungskette. *HNO* 31:37, 1983.

6. HOLMQUIST J. Size of mastoid air cell system in relation to healing after myringoplasty and to Eustachian tube function. *Acta Otolaryng.* (Stockh.) 69:89-93, 1970.

7. MARQUET J., v. CAMP K.J., CRETEN W.L., DECRAEMER W.F., WOLFF H.B., SCHEPERS P. Topics in physics and middle ear surgery. *Acta Otolaryngol.* (Belg.) 27:141, 1973.

8. PLESTER D. Myringoplasty methods. *Arch. Otolaryngol.* (Chicago) 78:310, 1963.

9. PLESTER D. Die Anwendung prothetischen Materials im Mittelohr. *Mschr. Ohrenheilk.* 102:105, 1968.

10. PLESTER D. Fortschritte in der Mikrochirurgie des Ohres in den letzten 10 Jahren. *HNO* 18:33, 1970.

11. PLESTER D. In: Hünermann Th., Plester D. (Hrsg.) Die Operationen am Ohr. Barth, Leizig, 1970.

12. PLESTER D. JAHNKE K. HEIMKE G. Aluminiumoxyd-Keramik, ein bioniertes Material für die Mittelohrchirurgie. *Arch. Ohr. Nas. Kehlk. Heilk.* 223:373-376, 1979.

13. RECK R. Bioaktive Glaskeramik in der Ohrenchirurgie. Tierexperimentalle Untersuchungen und klinische Ergebnisse. Habilitationsschrift, Mainz, 1981.

Restoration of the superior canal wall

M. Sakai, A. Shinkawa, H. Miyake

In the surgical management of a small attic cholesteatoma, surgeons always try to keep the entire superior bony canal wall intact as much as possible for preservation of the anatomically normal external auditory canal. However, one of the disadvantages of intact canal wall technique is the postoperative formation of retraction pocket, and recurrence of cholesteatoma from the bony defect at the scutum. When performing intact canal wall technique for cholesteatoma confined to the attic area, the bony defect must be repaired for prevention of the postoperative occurrence of retraction pocket.

There have been many reports concerning the restoration of the superior canal wall and a number of techniques and materials have been advocated in attempts to prevent the postoperative retraction pocket formation after the removal of attic cholesteatoma. Donald[1] presented the use of silastic sheet for reconstruction of the epitympanum. Kinney,[2] Brackman,[3] Sheehy,[4] and Pappas[5] reported the use of cartilage from the tragus or homograft cartilage to repair attic defect to prevent posterior retraction pocket. Pou[6] used a small curled bone plate to seal a defect of the scutum, and Sadé[7] described his combined approach tympanoplasty for attic cholesteatoma, and the scutum defect was reconstructed with a bone plate carved from the mastoid cortex.

We have been trying to repair a small defect of the scutum after intact canal wall technique was performed to eradicate diseased tissue and cholesteatoma from the attic. A silastic sheet was used to seal an attic defect from the external canal side in 10 cases of attic cholesteatoma. However, because of unsatisfactory results with silastic sheet, autogenous cartilage obtained from the tragus was used as sealing material. But the failure rate in a series of 25 cases was still higher than expected, and it was found that in many cases the cartilage was absorbed or retracted due to scarring behind the cartilage, producing a retraction pocket.

Then a piece of bone obtained from the mastoid cortex or the suprameatal spine of Henle was used. The bone plate was trimmed by rongeur to the size just large enough to wedge into the scutum defect, and the bone graft was covered with fascia. The short-term results were fairly satisfactory, but there were cases showing resorption of the bone wedge and reappearance of retraction pocket in one or two years postoperatively.

Finally the authors developed their own technique, named scutumplasty, using a rather large piece of bone plate, and this technique was applied in 79 cases of attic cholesteatoma. In this technique, intact canal wall technique was completed in the usual fashion to eradicate all abnormal tissue and cholesteatoma from the tympanum, attic and antrum, and the facial recess was opened from behind. The superior bony canal wall was entirely preserved. After the removal of the pathology, reconstruction of the ossicular chain was performed in the different methods. Then, an approximately 1 cm^2 area of cortical bone of the mastoid was lined and grooved by a small burr, and a bone plate was taken from the mastoid cortex with a flat chisel and mallet. At the anterior and superior edge of the scutum defect, parallel grooving was undertaken from the medial to the lateral portion of the superior bony canal wall by a burr to receive the bone plate. And the bone plate was trimmed and sculptured to the proper size and shape by a rongeur and burr to fit between two grooves. The bone plate should fit very snugly between the anterior and posterior grooves that have been made by the burr, but the medial edge of the bone plate should not be attached to the neck of the malleus so as not to disturb the ossicular mobility. A temporalis fascia graft was placed over the bone plate and the bare bone of the external canal wall.

The authors performed this technique in 79 cases, and the postoperative results were compared with those of the other techniques.

The results, according to the different methods used for the restoration of the superior canal wall, which was partially destroyed by cholesteatoma, are shown in table 1. Recurrent cholesteatoma was found in 80 % of the cases in which silastic sheet was used. It was assumed that the cause of retraction pocket and recurrent cholesteatoma was due to retraction of the silastic sheet

Table 1

FAILURE OF RESTORATION OF SUPERIOR CANAL WALL

	GRAFT MATERIALS			
	SILASTIC SHEET	CARTILAGE	BONE WEDGE	BONE PLATE
	N:10	N:25	N:37	N:79
RECURRENT CHOLESTEATOMA	8 (80.0%)	14 (56.0%)	8 (21.6%)	4 (5.1%)
RESORPTION OF GRAFT	0	5	8	1
RETRACTION OF GRAFT	8	9	0	3

into the attic space by the pulling force from behind caused by negative pressure in the attic or by scar tissue contraction behind the silastic sheet.

Choleasteatoma recurred in 56 % of 25 cases with reconstruction of the scutum with cartilage. In 9 of these cases cartilage graft had completely disappeared from the place where the graft was applied in the scutum defect. During revision surgery it was found that the cartilage had retracted and fallen into the attic space most likely due to scarring behind the graft. However, in 5 cases with recurrent cholesteatoma no cartilage graft was found in the attic in revision surgery, and it was thought that the cartilage was completely resorbed in the surrounding tissue.

In cases where a bone wedge was used to seal a small defect of the scutum, recurrence of cholesteatoma was found in 8 out of 37 cases, that is about 22 %. In revision surgery, we confirmed that the small bone wedge fixed in the scutum defect in the primary surgery had completely disappeared, most probably due to resorption of the bone graft.

Most of the 79 consecutive cases of scutumplasty were followed in outpatient clinics for more than two years. Recurrence of cholesteatoma in the attic area was found only in 4 cases, therefore, the recurrence rate of cholesteatoma was about 5 % of all scutumplasty cases in this series. All four recurrent cases received revision surgery and in 3 cases it was found that the bone graft was partially retracted into the attic space, and we considered that the reason for this retraction was probably due to the lack of support of the bony canal of the attic caused by bone necrosis, secondary to infectious osteitis which was accompanied by recurrent cholesteatoma. In one remaining case, there was complete resorption of the bone graft.

This scutumplasty technique represents a very useful addition to surgery for prevention of retraction pocket in intact canal wall tympanoplasty.

References:

1. DONALD P., McCABE B.F., LOEVY S.S. Atticotomy: a neglected otosurgical technique. *Ann. Otol. Rhinol. Laryngol.* 83, 652-661, 1974.
2. KINNEY S.E. Five years experience using the intact canal wall tympanoplasty for cholesteatoma: Preliminary report. *Laryngoscope* 92, 1396-1400, 1982.
3. BRACKMANN D.E., SHEEHY J.L. Tympanoplasty: TORPs and PORPs. *Laryngoscope* 89, 108-114, 1979.
4. SHEEHY J.L., BRACKMANN D.E., GRAHAM M.D. Cholesteatoma: Residual and recurrent disease. A review of 1024 cases. *Ann. Otol. Rhinol. Laryngol.* 86, 451-462, 1977.
5. PAPPAS J.J., BAILEY H.A.T., McGREW R.N. et al. Homograft septal cartilage for attic support in intact canal wall tympanomastoidectomy and tympanoplasty. *Laryngoscope* 91, 1457-1462, 1981.
6. POU J.W. Reconstruction of bony canal with autogenous bone graft. *Laryngoscope* 87m 1826-1832, 1977.
7. SADE J. Treatment of retraction pockets and cholesteatoma. Cholesteatoma and Mastoid Surgery. Sadé J. ed. Kugler Publications. 511-525, 1982.

Postoperative evaluation of restoration of the posterior-superior bony wall of the external auditory canal

E. Chiossone

Introduction

The inconvenience of a permanent exteriorized mastoid cavity has been recognized. This is the reason why many otologic surgeons prefer the intact canal wall technique[1, 2, 3,] and also the only reason to perform an obliteration of the mastoid cavity when a canal wall down technique has been used.[4,5]

Techniques for restoration of the posterior-superior bony canal wall have been advocated in cases of partial destruction of these walls, by disease or by surgery[6, 7] and even when total removal has been temporally performed by the surgeon[8] or when these walls do not exist as a consequence of a radical or modified radical mastoidectomy techniques.

The purpose of this study is to present a system for postoperative evaluation of permanent results with restoration techniques of the posterior and superior bony walls of the external auditory canal (EAC).

In order to evaluate the postoperative results of this surgical restoration, we should consider the posterior and the superior walls as a whole, since the surgical procedure cannot be applied to one of them individually ignoring the existence of the other. It is also very important to define first the etiology of the destruction, the degree of the lesion and the surgical procedure performed for restoration.

Although the restoration of the posterior-superior bony wall of the EAC can indirectly affect the functional results in tympanoplasty, we prefer to confine this evaluation only to the anatomical aspect. Hearing results are more in relation to the reconstruction of the ossicular chain, middle ear spaces and tympanic membrane.

Etiology of destruction

Destruction of the posterior-superior bony wall of EAC is in most instances the result of bone erosion produced by active disease as a cholesteatoma or any other bone- destructing disease of the temporal bone. But destruction of this wall in any degree can also be the result of a surgical procedure performed in an attempt to remove the pathology which has extended to the mastoid cavities.

Degree of lesion

It is important to define the degree of destruction produced by disease or by surgery. This destruction can be partial or total.

Partial destruction

We have divided it in four degrees:

GRADE I: It refers to lesions limited to the scutum in an extension not larger than 5 mm up in the superior wall (figure 1). This can be observed in attic cholesteatomas or as a result of drilling this area to explore the epitympanic region.

GRADE II: Destruction of the posterior-superior bony wall in a larger extension, remaining only an outer bridge of bone and usually a very high facial bony ridge (figure 2). Although a large cholesteatoma can produce this type of lesion, it is usually the result of surgery when a mastoid cholesteatoma is approached transmeatally or endaurally without a classical mastoidectomy.

GRADE III: There is absence of the outer part of the posterior-superior bony wall and there only remains a low bridge of bone usually with a high facial bony ridge (figure 3). This is almost always the result of demolition by surgery. Less frequent, it can be the result of recurrent cholesteatoma due to retraction of the posterior membranous wall of the EAC through a notch surgically made in the outer edge of the posterior bony canal wall when performing intact canal wall tympanoplasty.

GRADE IV: Isolated perforations of the posterior-superior bony wall varying in number, size and shape (figure 4) usually are the result of surgery when thinning down this wall in intact canal wall tympanoplasty. The number,

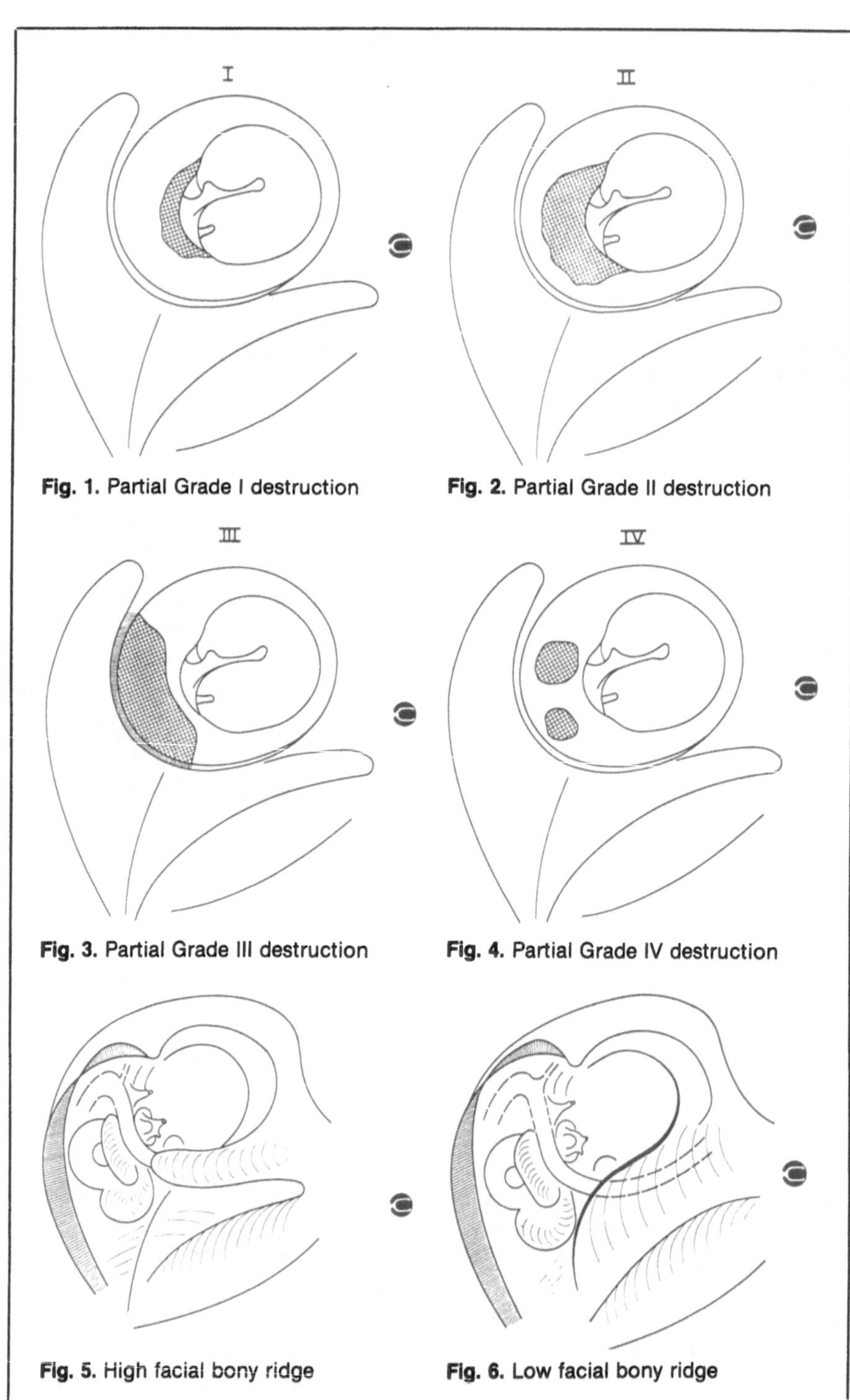

Fig. 1. Partial Grade I destruction

Fig. 2. Partial Grade II destruction

Fig. 3. Partial Grade III destruction

Fig. 4. Partial Grade IV destruction

Fig. 5. High facial bony ridge

Fig. 6. Low facial bony ridge

size and shape of perforations must be described in the protocol.

Total destruction
Total destruction is generally the result of a surgical procedure and is very seldom due to bone erosion by disease. In some cases, the opening of the mastoid cavity to the EAC is very narrow due to a *high facial bony ridge* which makes the cleaning of the cavity very difficult (figure 5). When a previous radical or modified radical mastoidectomy has been properly performed, there is usually a *low facial bony ridge* which makes the approach of the cavity through the EAC easier (figure 6).

Surgical technique
Different techniques and different material have been proposed for restoration of the posterior-superior bony wall of the EAC. We should consider here the most widely recognized.

Repositioning
In order to achieve a better exposure of attic region, facial recess and sinus tympani, careful removal of the posterior-superior wall has been advocated[8] and its repositioning after removal of disease. This is an elaborated procedure which has not been accepted by many otologists.

Reconstruction
Depending on the degree of lesion of the posterior-superior bony wall, the reconstruction can be partial or total. The material used for reconstruction will vary depending on the size of the defect to be reconstructed.

Material used
Autologous tissues (autograft) are the most common materials used for posterior-superior wall reconstruction. Homologous tissues (allograft) also have been used with success but to a lesser extent. Heterologous (xenograft) tissues have rarely been used but alloplastic materials continue to be reported as suitable material for posterior-superior canal wall reconstruction.

Autograft
Autologous tragal cartilage is suitable to repair minor defects. For major defects the autologous grafting of conchal cartilage is giving excellent results.[6,9] Autologous bone from the mastoid cortex,[10] iliac crest[11] and bone meal[4] have been used also.

Allograft. The following preserved allogenic materials have been used for repair of the posterior-superior auditory canal wall: septal cartilage,[7,12] conchal cartilage,[13] costal cartilage,[11] knee cartilage,[14] posterior walls of the external auditory meatus[13] and lyophilized dura.[15]

Xenograft. This type of graft has rarely been used for reconstruction of the posterior-superior canal wall[16] but it has to be considered as an alternative for reconstruction.

Alloplastic materials. Attempts to repair the posterior wall with plastic mesh have been reported unsuccessful and have been discontinued.[17] Other plastics such as Proplast and Plastipore have been used also but they extrude through the years.

Since 1979 bioactive glass-ceramic implants (Ceravital) have been reported to be used with great success.[18,19,20] They constitute a good alternative for posterior wall reconstruction but it is still necessary to wait for longer term results.

Postoperative evaluaton (anatomical)

We have already mentioned that the postoperative evaluation of the surgical restoration of the posterior-superior bony wall of the EAC must be in anatomical bases only. Hearing results should be considered only to know if the restoration wall procedure affects the functional results[6] but not as a postoperative evaluation of the surgical technique itself.

For the anatomical postoperative evaluation, two main parameters should be taken into consideration; the fate and the shape of the restored canal wall.

Fate of the restored wall: It should be considered if the restored wall is present or if it has been resorbed. If present, it is important to know if it has a healthy appearance or if it is involved by any disease as granulation tissue, dermal inclusions, etc.

Shape of the restored wall: With regard to the shape of the newly formed EAC, two main aspects should be considered: is the posterior wall restored or does the procedure fail to restore it?

If it is formed, it is important to know if it is regular and smooth or on the contrary, distorted due to displacement or healing problems. If it is not formed or partially formed, it is necessary to differentiate between retraction pocket formations or total retraction with an open mastoid cavity as it was before the surgical procedure.

It is of paramount importance that postoperative evaluation should not be done before six months after surgery and that definitive conclusions should not be established before five years of meticulous follow-up.

Conclusions

— The posterior and superior bony walls of the external auditory canal must be considered as a unit for postoperative evaluation of restoration results.
— It is important to clearly define the etiology of destruction, the degree of lesion and the surgical technique.
— Postoperative evaluation of restoration of the posterior-superior bony wall of the EAC should be done only in anatomi-

cal bases considering the fate and shape of the reconstructed wall.

— The postoperative anatomical evaluation should not be done before six months after surgery.

— Definite conclusions should not be established before five years of meticulous follow-up.

References:

1. SHEEHY J.L. Tympanoplasty with Mastoidectomy: Present Status. *Clin. Otolaryngol.* 8:391-403, 1983.

2. CHIOSSONE E. Importance of En Bloc Homograft in Intact Canal Wall Tympanoplasty. *Clin. Otolaryng.* 3:437-442, 1978.

3. JANSEN C. Evaluation of Surgery for Cholesteatoma. In: Cholesteatoma First International Conference, p. 352. Birmingham, Alabama: Aesculapius, 1977.

4. TABB H.C. et al. Reconstruction of the Mastoidectomized Ear (Panel Discussion) *Arch. Otolaryng.* 97:74-76, 1973.

5. PALVA T. Operative Technique in Mastoid Obliteration. *Acta Otolaryng.* 75:289-290, 1973.

6. CHIOSSONE E. "Three Cartilages" Technique in Intact Canal Wall Tympanoplasty to prevent recurrent Cholesteatoma. In publication. *Amer. J. Otol.*

7. JANSEN C. Cartilage Tympanoplasty. *Laryngoscope.* 73:1288-1302, 1983.

8. VASE P. et al. Posterior Meatal Wall Reconstruction in Tympanoplasty. *J. Laryngol. & Otol.* 95:893-898, 1981.

9. HEERMANN J.: Auricular Cartilage Pausade Tympano-Epytimpano-Antrum and Mastoid-Plasties. *Clin. Otolaryng.* 3:433-446, 1978.

10. MARQUET J. Personal communication.

11. WIGAND M.E. et al. Tympanomeatoplastik nach Radikaloperation: Mit Knochen oder Knorpel. *Arch. Otorhinolaryng.* 207:542-544, 1974.

12. PAPPAS J.J. Homograft Septal Cartilage for Attic support in Intact Canal Wall Tympanomastoidectomy and Tympanoplasty. *Laryngoscope* 91:1457-1462, 1982.

13. SHEEHY J.L. Otologic Homograft. *Trans. Am. Acad. Ophthalmol. Otolaryng.* 83:560-565, 1966.

14. WEHRS R.E. Reconstructive Mastoidectomy with homograft knee cartilage. *Laryngoscope* 82:1177-1188, 1972.

15. PALVA T., YLIKOSKI J., MAKINEN J. Use of Lyophilized dura in Aural surgery. 40:129-138, 1978.

16. GUILFORD F.R. Controlled Cavity Healing after Mastoid and Fenestration Operations. *Arch. Otolaryng.* 71:165-171, 1960.

17. GAMMERT C., EITSCHBERGER E.: Erfahrungen mit einem Kunststoffnetz bei der Rekonstruktion der hinteren Gehörgangswand. *HNO* 26: 100-103, 1978.

18. JAHNKE K., PLESTER D. Keramikimplantate in der Mittelohrchirurgie *HNO* 28:109-114, 1980.

19. WULLSTEIN S.R. Keramik und Humankleber beim Aufbau der Tympanoplastik. *Arch. Otorhinolaryngol.* 223-373, 1979.

20. RECK R. Bioactive Glass-Ceramics in Ear Surgery: Animal Studies and Clinical Results. *Laryngoscope* 94: Suppl. No. 33, No. 2, Part 2, Feb. 1984.

Post-traumatic restoration of the middle ear

A. Mazzoni

Traumatic injuries to the middle ear are produced by a variety of causes and mechanisms: sharp and blunt objects, head trauma with and without temporal bone fracture; surgery; obstetrical conditions (to mother or newborn); blast, barotrauma and burns.

Historical notes
Extensive temporal bone and middle ear injuries were known since the beginning of modern medicine. However, the limited middle ear involvement without clinical evidence of fracture or even without a known trauma in the patient's history started to be considered a possible occurrence by the late fifties.

Audiological studies on head trauma reported a high incidence of middle ear hearing loss, while surgical exploration described several types of middle ear injuries.

Increased awareness of the problem, audiometric and radiographic evaluation and microsurgery allowed a better diagnosis of the small tympanic injuries. Post-traumatic middle ear restoration techniques followed the progress of the surgery of chronic otitis media as well as of the more extensive pathology of the temporal bone.

Classification
Attempts at classification of middle ear traumatic injuries meet with two problems:
— multiplicity of middle ear changes,
— variance of the changes in relation to time between trauma and surgery.

These difficulties may be reduced by identifying a number of elementary changes, early and late, with the understanding that the different clinical pictures of the individual case are made up of one or more elementary changes.

Elementary surgical pathology in middle ear trauma
Early:
Canal: skin tears, bone steps;
Drum: tears, perforations, burns, deformities (by bone frame, dislocated ossicles), attic enlargement or dehiscence (gothic attic);
Tympanum: hemotympanum, dura tear, CSF leak, brain hernia; fracture, dislocations of attic, antri tegmen; foreign body, necrosis of mucoperiostium and ossicles;
Ossicles: incus-stapes disjunction; incus dislocation, fracture; fracture of stapes, footplate; stapes luxation; malleus luxation, fracture, dislocation;
Eustachian tube: fracture, foreign body;

Labyrinth: stapes luxation, footplate fracture, annular ligament rupture, round window membrane rupture, bony labyrinth fracture (promontorium, semicircular canals), perilymph fistula.

Late:
Canal deformity or stenosis; drum perforation, retraction; chronic purulent otitis; adhesive otitis or scarred tympanum; ossicles discontinuity or loss, cholesteatoma.

Surgical restoration requires different operations and lends different results according to the extension of the traumatic injuries. Thus, two categories or subgroups are advisable in reporting middle ear restorations:
— injuries limited to middle ear (ear drum and ossicles);
— extensive injuries of the temporal bone.

Surgery:
Conventional methods of closed tympanoplasty take care of the majority of the middle ear traumatic problems. The surgical guidelines are:
— first stage repair of eardrum, bony annulus and canal, revision of the middle ear cavity and walls, sheeting;
— second stage for transmission reconstruction;
— single stage repair is considered with minor injuries to drum, mucosa and ossicles. The type of exploration and repair includes: under-, over-lay myringoplasty, ossiculoplasty with auto- or homologous ossicles, with bio-synthetic prostheses.

Within this general frame there are important additions related to trauma-specific operative techniques.

Trauma – specific changes and repair
☐ Tympanotomy and cavity clearing: plain drum tear: repositioning of margins and splinting.
☐ Incus dislocation: malleus-stapes ossiculoplasty.
Incus-stapes disjunction: malleus-stapes ossiculoplasty (or incus repositioning and glueing?).
☐ Stapes crura fracture, incus intact: stapedectomy or malleus-footplate ossiculoplasty.
Fracture of footplate or annular ligament: stapedectomy or fistula repair.
☐ Malleus luxation (fracture) with deformity (tear) of drum: first stage restoration of drum.
Bony annulus disruption with deformed or torn drum: restoration of annulus, drum, attic.
☐ Fracture of ear canal with bony stenosis: canal calibration.
Cicatricial stenosis of canal: canalplasty.
☐ Stapes luxation with fistula: fistula repair.

Round window or bone labyrinth fistula: fistula repair.

In extensive injuries of the temporal bone, other surgical steps are considered, such as facial nerve decompression and repair, repair of tegmen of attic and antrum, repair of dura and brain hernia as well as of dura tear with CSF leak.

Timing of surgery
Several phenomena and processes related to time modify the anatomical and functional conditions, thus influencing the indication for surgery as well as its results. Spontaneous healing of a drum tear or spontaneous columella effect are positive events. On the other side are the scar tympanum, the cochlear losses by a fistula etc. Therefore, it appears to be important for the postoperative evaluation to indicate the time lapse between trauma, preoperative evaluation and surgery.

Postoperative evaluation
Anatomical evaluation
The anatomical condition of the ear drum, the attic wall and the external auditory canal are the data that can be collected. Radiological evaluation provides further data for anatomical follow-up.

Functional evaluation
Postoperative evaluation is based on the pure tone audiometry, as an internationally acknowledged standard for vocal tests and impedance is still lacking.

The data for evaluation are:
— air conduction (AC), preoperative and postoperative,
— bone conduction (BC), preoperative and postoperative.

The most representative figures of the functional condition are:
— hearing gain (AC postop. - AC preop.),
— AB gap (AC postop. - BC postop.),
— cochlear profile with difference in BC (BC preop. - BC postop.).

The common occurrence of cochlear losses due to trauma as well as to the operation recommends to include the 4K frequency in the audiometry evaluation.

Duration of follow-up
Stability of results has to be tested against time. A reasonable follow-up period should be longer than 5 years.

Literature:

1. BARTH H. Hörstörungen nach Kopfpellungen. *Ztschr. Hals-, Nasen-, Ohren-Heilk.* 50, 27, 1944.
2. GUERRIER Y., DEJEAN Y., GALY G. Les surdités de transmission dans les traumatismes fermés du crane. *Cahiers ORL* 1,11,1965.
3. HOUGH J.V.D. Malformations and anatomical variations seen in the middle ear during the operation for mobilisation of the stapes. *Laryngoscope* 68,1337,1958.
4. VOSS O. Die Chirurgie der Schädelbasisfrakturen. Barth, Leipzig, 1936.

Homograft tympanoplasty in perspective

ABSTRACT

S.G. Lesinski

Despite over 4 000 reported successful tympanoplasties using homograft (allogenous) preserved tympanic membranes and ossicles, general scepticism regarding this technique persists. Review of the literature indicates why:

— there are wide discrepancies for indications, preservatives, surgical techniques and results,
— several surgeons have not duplicated the 95 % success rate reported by Marquet and Wehrs,
— animal experiments have consistently failed,
— the host immunological response is still questioned,
— data on histological fate of the donor TM is limited,
— indications for instances when homograft tympanoplasty would prove superior to standard techniques have not been clearly established.

This study had limited the use of homograft TMs to those cases in which standard tympanoplasty techniques have already failed to produce a satisfactory anatomical or hearing result (recurrent perforations, lateralized TMs, draining radical mastoidectomy cavity) or to those cases where standard techniques have a high incidence of failure, (i.e. slag burns, total perforations with absent malleus, congenital atresia). Documentation of long-term anatomic and hearing results (4½ yrs mean follow-up) are presented for 125 consecutive patients in whom formalin-fixed homograft TMs were used to reconstruct the severely damaged middle ear.

At the completion of this study, 95 % (119/125) of the homograft tympanoplasties are currently intact. There were 13 immediate postoperative perforations, but 11 were repaired with a second-stage underlay fascia tympanoplasty. Long-term hearing results were analyzed according to the type of ossicular reconstruction employed (mean follow-up 4 yrs). In 87 patients with chronic otitis media, 94 % of the type I repairs maintained an air/bone gap of 25 dB or less, 85 % of type II, and 81 % of type III.

Forty-four patients presented with an absent malleus and TM and were reconstructed with a homograft TM with attached malleus and shaped incus columella. At 4 years postoperatively, 83 % of these patients maintained an average air/bone gap of 23 dB or better. A similar group of 38 patients presenting with absent malleus, incus and stapes were reconstructed with isograft temporalis fascia and a cartilage covered TORP. Only 18 % of the TORP patients maintained an air/bone gap of 25 dB 4 years postoperatively.

Thirty-three patients with draining radical mastoidectomy cavities were reconstructed; 97 % had a dry, self-cleansing ear with no activity restriction. Only 59 % maintained an air/bone gap closure of 25 dB or better in the long-term follow-up; 30 % developed persistent Eustachian tube dysfunction.

A one-stage surgical procedure utilizing homograft TM and ossicles combined with full-thickness host rotation flaps was developed for reconstruction of congenital aural atresia. Six ears were reconstructed. All have dry, self-cleansing external canals with intact TMs and no activity restrictions and have maintained a mean air/bone gap of 23.4 dB.

Formalin-fixed homograft TMs afford an opportunity for improving the anatomical and hearing results in reconstructing the severely damaged middle ear.

SYMPOSIUM III

Surgical procedures

SYMPOSIUM III
Surgical procedures

Chairman: G. Lacher

Surgical procedures

G. Lacher

Although many ideas have developed in the field of surgical techniques over the last few years, all the gaps are not yet filled. Our theme will give us the opportunity to base an appraisal of this evolution on the papers presented, and to derive from them several interesting surgical "improvements".

The presentation will be in three parts:
— The first part will be devoted to the eradication of lesions of the middle ear, and in particular of cholesteatoma, and to the delicate problem of the second look;
— the second will deal with the restoration of the apparatus of transmission in the middle ear, and of the Eustachian tube, using methods which, although not revolutionary, are nonetheless original;
— the third part, finally, will take stock of the latest developments in material: laser and fibrin seal.

The use of allograft stapes

T. Kumoi, T. Minatogawa, Y. Umetani

One of the most challenging problems to the otologic surgeon has been the reconstruction of the middle ear in which the only remaining tissue is the stapedial footplate or a membranous remnant of the oval window. Columellae such as polyethylene, shaped allograft incus, are generally accepted and commonly used but the results of this type IV modification are not as good as those of type II or type III modification because of poor contact between the columella and the footplate.

In cases where the stapedial arch or the stapes itself is absent, forming an ossicular chain from the tympanic membrane to the oval window does not offer satisfactory long-term results of improved hearing. For cases in which no remnant of the ossicular chain exists, other than the footplate of the stapes, a variety of methods using incus allografts, plastic or other synthetic materials, have been advocated to establish continuity of sound transmission.

Recently, allograft stapes have been used in otosurgery and Glaninger et al.[1], Tobeck[2], Hildyard et al.[3], Tos[4], Marquet[5], and Smith and Dobie[6] reported successful results, in which implanted allograft stapes was found to be vital. Since 1981, we have used the allograft stapes, singly or in combination with homograft incus in 20 cases and also in 7 cases of fixed stapes. All of the allograft stapes were procured, processed and stored by the Hyogo Ear Bank, a non-profit organization which was the first ear bank to be established in Japan in 1980.

Obtaining and preparing allografts

Temporal bone cores are removed from the cadaver within 24 hours of death. The cores are stored in 70 % alcohol or 4 % buffered formaldehyde for a week. Next, they are dissected and the de-epithelialized tympanic membrane and attached malleus, incus and stapes are removed together or separately under an operation microscope. Graft tissue is rinsed with an ample amount of saline, gas sterilized, prefrozen to –70°C and then freeze-dried for 5 days.

Materials and surgical techniques

The cases could be divided into two groups (table 1), of discharging or dry ears with missing stapedial structure and of fixed stapes. In the first group, the main objective was to obtain a dry ear and ossiculoplasty. In the primary surgery, as a rule the posterior bony meatal wall was

Table 1. Twenty-seven cases of allograft stapes surgery

footplate mobility	disease	No. of ears
without fixation	reoperation adhesive otitis cholesteatoma chronic suppurative otitis	12 4 2 2
	total	20
with fixation	postinflammatory otosclerosis congenital stapes anomaly	4 1 1 1
	total	7

preserved (closed method). With an open mastoid cavity (10 cases), the auditory meatus was restored using tragal cartilage and fascia and the cavity obliterated with a flap of temporalis muscle. After confirming the mobility of the footplate, the allograft stapes was placed on the middle of the footplate or on the oval window niche and then fixed with gel foam. Two modalities of positioning of the donor stapes were attempted:

— the allograft stapes was placed in the normal position and a shaped incus or cortical bone or tragal cartilage was placed on top of the stapedial head and connected and,

— the allograft stapes was placed upside down and the columella was placed on the stapes.

The size of the allograft stapes footplate could be easily adjusted by trimming the margin of the plate with a cutting burr.

In the second group of seven cases of fixed stapes (postinflammatory, congenital or otosclerotic), the allograft stapes was inserted as for primary otosclerosis. The oval window was exposed and a compressed vein graft was placed over the window. This technique was used in six of the cases, but in the seventh, after positioning of the vein graft, an allograft stapes was placed in the upside down position because of an overhung fallopian canal.

Results

All results were based on the mean hearing in the frequency range of 500 to 2 000 hertz. The

Table 2. Hearing results after ear surgery

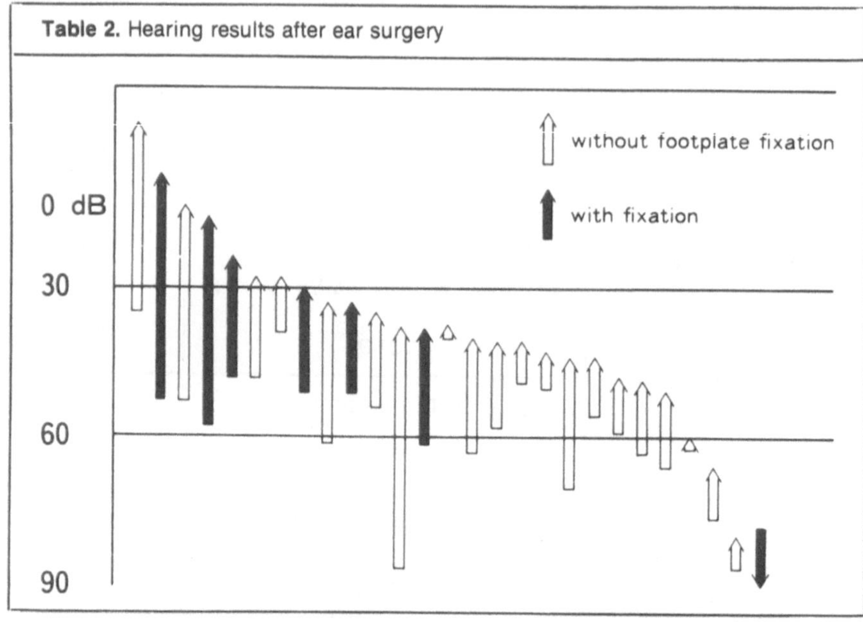

audiometric data represent a mean postoperative follow-up period of 12 months (minimum six months, maximum 26 months). Table 2, which gives the change in hearing level of all of 27 cases, shows a wide range of results ranging from a gain of 45 dB to a loss of 12 dB. As functional successes, we included patients who attained a mean hearing of 0 to 30 dB (social hearing), an air-bone gap of 0 to 15 dB, or a hearing gain of more than 20 dB (table 3). Satisfactory results were obtained in only 40 % of the cases with mobile footplate surgery, though 85,7 % was attained in the cases of stapes fixation. Our results are compared for the different ossiculoplasties in table 4. The group given the allograft in the normal position showed better results than the cases with upside down stapes.

Comment

The allograft stapes can be positioned in two ways on the patient's footplate or on the oval window niche: in the normal position[1,2,3,6] or in the upside down position.[4,5] Many modifications of ossiculoplasty can be considered with different graft positions, and in this series, seven ways of reconstruction of the sound transmission were used (table 4). Better functional results were obtained in the case of mobile footplate cases by placing the stapes graft in the normal position in combination with the columella or incus interposition compared with the upside down

Table 3. Hearing results in the present series			
	without footplate fixation	with fixation	total
1. air-bone gap <15 dB	4	3	7
2. air conduction <30 dB	4	4	8
3. hearing improvement >20 dB	6	5	11
functional success (1 or 2 or 3)	8 (40%)	6 (85.7%)	14 (51.9%)
average of hearing improvement	16.3 dB	22.8 dB	18.0 dB

position of the graft. The same results were observed in the fixed stapes cases for the stapes interposition.

One patient returned complaining of gradual loss of hearing, and revision surgery showed that the fascia had become separated from the planted cortical bone columella, while the grafted stapes columella assembly was in the normal position and the round window's light reflex was normal when the assembly was examined.

As already stated by Tos,[4] in the case of an allograft stapes placed with the head on the footplate, the contact surface is small and the transmission of energy to the footplate after a sound impulse cannot be as good as with an intact arch. Furthermore, an allograft stapes in the upside down position may more easily fall down after surgery. Generally, in Type III tympanoplasty, better functional hearing results are obtained with the stapes-columella assembly than with the stapes only. Our present results indicate that when the patient's stapes is missing, two-stage, rather than one-stage, middle ear surgery is a better way to achieve hearing improvement, i.e. the allograft stapes is first placed in the normal position with drumplasty and then ossiculoplasty is conducted.

A stapes graft could prove useful as a primary technique in surgery

Table 4. Ossiculoplasty and results

type of ossiculoplasty	without fixation	with fixation	functional success
normal position + columella	14		7
normal position	2		
upside down	1		
normal position + incus interposition	1		1
tympanoossicular graft (total replacement)	1		
upside down + columella	1	1	
interposition		6	6

for stapes fixation, as shown by our results and by Glaninger et al.[1], Tobeck[2] and Hildyard et al.[3] An allograft stapes interposition technique on the vein graft over the oval window niche could reduce the risk of fistula formation with concomitant disequilibrium. All of our seven cases have had no difficulties with either the cochlear or the vestibular function.

We conclude that use of the allograft stapes should contribute to surgical treatment for cases in which the stapedial structure is missing.

References:

1. GLANINGER J., NEUHOLD R. Eine Methode zur Konservierung menschlicher Gehörknöchelchen. *Mschr. Ohrenheilk. Laryngorhinol.* 102, 569-577, 1968. GLANINGER J. Freie Transplantation konservierter menschlicher Gehörknöchelchen. *Mschr. Ohrenheilk. Laryngorhinol.* 102, 609-623, 1968.
2. TOBECK A. Steigbügel Verstorbener als Steigbügelersatz bei der Otoskleroseoperation. *Z. Laryngol, Rhinol. Otol.* 41, 31-41, 1962.
3. HILDYARD V.H., ENGLISH G.M., DE BLANC G.B., HEMENWAY W.S. Stapes homograft - A report of four human cases. *Arch. Otolaryngol.* 88, 55-62, 1968.
4. TOS M. Allograft stapes-incus assembly. *Arch. Otolaryngol.* 104, 119-121, 1978.
5. MARQUET J. Human middle ear transplants. *J. Laryngol. Otol.* 85, 523-529, 1971.
6. SMITH M.F.W., DOBIE R. The use of homograft stapes. *Laryngoscope* 86, 1196-1202, 1976.

Eradication of cholesteatoma

P.H. Van De Heyning, J.F.E. Marquet

Introduction

Several approaches and techniques are advocated in order to remove cholesteatoma, some of them in view of reconstructing the middle ear. Comparison between the different techniques is made difficult by the absence of a universally accepted standardized descriptive terminology concerning these techniques and their real meaning, e.g. intrameatal removal, piece-meal removal, drill and suction removal.

Moreover there is an absence of a universally accepted way of reporting results. In our opinion,[1] this evaluation has to be done in terms of anatomical restoration, healing (and not only recurrence) and auditory function.

This paper gives a detailed description of our technique, called "en bloc resection", dealing with eradication of cholesteatoma.

The two main points of cholesteatoma surgery are:
— total eradication of all involved structures without compromise,
— full reconstruction of normal anatomy and the mesodermic barrier between external and middle ear, using tympano-ossicular homografts and posterior canal wall reconstruction.

Pathological basis of cholesteatoma surgery

A good knowledge of the pathogenesis of cholesteatoma is indispensible for understanding the method of eradication of the pathology. The basic pathological process of middle ear cholesteatoma consists of an ectopic presence of the basal proliferative layer of keratinizing

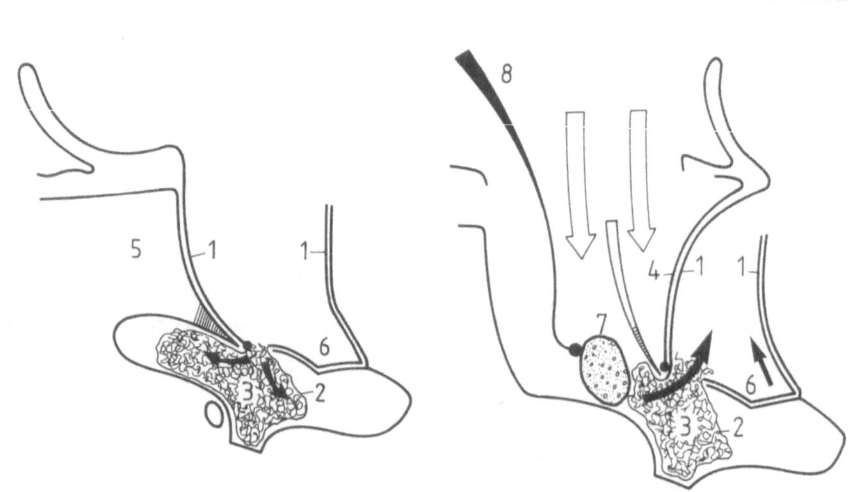

Fig. 1. The cholesteatoma (3) is invading (➤) the middle ear cleft, eroding the mastoid and epitympanic wall (5). Note the continuity of the epiderm of the external meatus (1) with the matrix (2) and the discontinuity of the mesodermic layer of the tympanic membrane (6).

Fig. 2. The whole cholesteatoma (3) and its matrix (2), including drum (6) and ossicular remnants are pressed out towards the meatus (➤). Dissection is aided by ball-point elevator (8) and plastic sponges (7). A combined approach (⇨) has been done, taking care to keep the periosteum of the meatus (4) and the epiderm of the meatus (1) and matrix (2) intact.

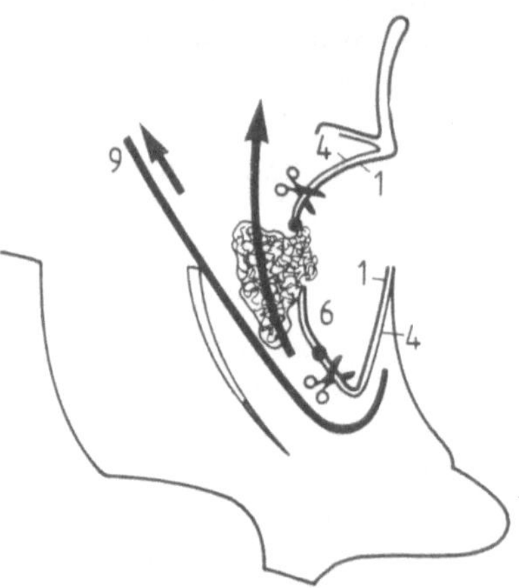

Fig. 3. The whole pathology is brought out of the meatus (➤) by a specially designed elevator (9) and is excised (✂) laterally to the fibrous annulus.

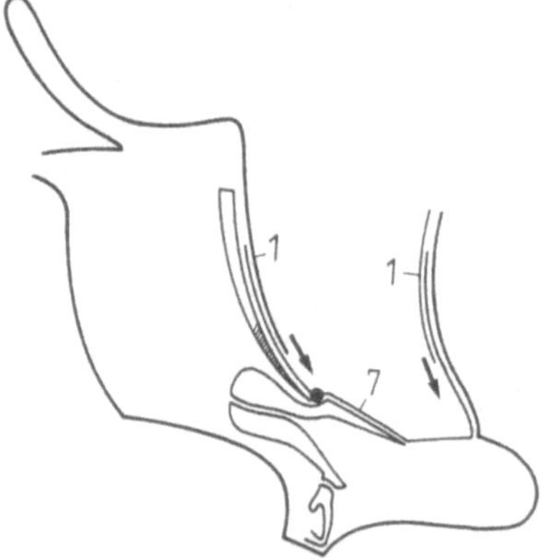

Fig. 4. Restoration of the bony annulus and lateral epitympanic wall (////). A total tympano-ossicular homograft (7) (in this drawing $HTMIS_p$) restores the mesodermic barrier, as well as the auditory function and middle ear anatomy. The epiderm of the external meatus (1) covers the meatal part of the graft.

squamous epithelium, called matrix,[2] lying in the middle ear cleft.[3,4] The most frequent modalities of development are the invagination, the immigration[5] and the papillary ingrowth.[6]
This implies (figure 1):
— a continuity of the matrix of cholesteatoma with the squamous epithelium of drum or drum remnants,[7,8]
— a discontinuity of the mesodermic barrier.[7]

Our technique[9] is based on the following main principles:
— all the pathology must be dissected and removed in one piece, including the drum remnants, the diseased ossicles and the surrounding pathology (permatrix), when necessary. Tearing the matrix by traction or drilling has to be avoided;
— the matrix and all the pathology must be dissected inside outwards towards the meatus, in fact, in the inverse way of the cholesteatoma ingrowth (figure 2).

We call this way of removal "monobloc" or "en bloc" removal.

Surgical technique: en bloc removal
The technique itself starts with a large combined approach with an attico-antro-mastoidectomy (figure 2). This approach allows the uncovering and visualization of the main poles of the cholesteatoma such as the anterior attical cells, the tegmen tympani, the posturo-superior angle of the mastoid, the tip of the mastoid and the sinus tympani and facial recess. Moreover, the combined approach makes an anatomical reconstruction possible, providing afterwards the advantages of the mastoid function.[10] The approach, including a large posterior tympanotomy[11] allows an exposition that is as good as a radical canal down technique. When the whole cholesteatoma is perfectly visualized, the pathway pattern by which the cyst itself has developed, is meticulously sought[12] and the planning of eradication is decided with respect to the anatomical and natural pathways.

After gentle elevation of the different poles of the cholesteatoma, rinsing with a 0,1 % aqueous solution of alfa-chymotrypsin is done. The enzymatic activity greatly facilitates later dissection, as it acts on the inflammatory granulation layers forming the perimatrix.

Dissection and elevation of the matrix is realized towards the meatus where the debris are collected and removed "en bloc" including the drum and ossicle remnants. This part of the surgery requires a meticulous technique in order to avoid tearing the matrix. The use of plastic sponges as well as the use of a specially designed ball-point elevator make dissection easier, pushing the sac towards the atrium. Particularly when the matrix is thin, or the underlying structures are fragile (facial nerve, labyrinth) is their use appreciated. In this way we are able to collect, through the meatus, an intact matrix of the sac with or without ossicle remnants. The meatal skin is then completely dissected from around the auditory meatus towards the bony sulcus (figure 3). With an elevator the whole cuff of skin is lifted "fingerlike" and rolled outwards through the meatus, so that the bony meatus is completely free of soft tissue. The whole pathology including the matrix, is then resected laterally to the fibrous annulus. This technique of total myringectomy is described in "Operative Surgery: Ear".[13]

Reconstruction

The eradication is followed by the reconstruction (figure 4). If the posterior canal wall or lateral epitympanic wall is partially destroyed, it is reconstructed with autogeneous mastoid cortical bone, in order to repair the anatomy and the function of the bony annulus,[14] and to provide support to the implanted tympano-ossicular homograft (TOH).

The ease of fixating the TOH in the bony meatus and in the middle ear, has been greatly facilitated by the use of human fibrin glue. A normal anatomy is built up in this way, restoring the important mesodermic barrier in order to prevent recurrence.

Second stage

Immediately after surgery, a prognosis is made and quoted:

1 — second stage excluded
2 — second stage improbable
3 — second stage possible
4 — second stage indispensible.

In stage 3 and 4, a second look is done 6 months after the first stage for early detection of recurrent or residual disease and for final functional adjustments.

References:

1. MARQUET J., GRAFF A. Postoperative evaluation of middle ear surgery. *Audiology,* 21, 20-32, 1982.

2. LIM D.J., SAUNDERS W.H. Acquired cholesteatoma: light and electron-microscopic observations. *Ann. Otol.* 81, 2-12, 1972.

3. GRAY J. The treatment of cholesteatoma in children. *Proc. Roy. Soc. Med.* 57, 769, 1964.

4. SCHUKNECHT H.F. Pathology of the ear, 225-228, Harvard Univ. Press, Cambridge, 1974.

5. FERNANDEZ C., LINDSAY J., MOSKOWITZ. Some observations on the pathogenesis of middle ear cholesteatoma. *Arch. Otolaryng.* 69, 537-546, 1959.

6. RÜEDI L. Cholesteatoma formation in the middle ear in animal experiments. *Acta Otolaryngol.* 50, 233-242, 1959.

7. MARQUET J., VAN DE HEYNING P.H. Cholesteatoma or keratoma "a pathological approach", *Belg. Tijdschr. Radiol.* 63, 251-258, 1980.

8. SCHAPER J., VAN DE HEYNING J. Cholesteatoma of the middle ear in human patients. *Arch. Otolaryngol.* 102, 663, 1976.

9. MARQUET J. Cholesteatoma: eradication of disease. Proc. II. Int. Conf. Tel Aviv 1981, 475-478, Kugler Pulb. Amsterdam, 1982.

10. AUSTIN D.F. On the function of the mastoid. *Otolaryngol. Clin. N.A.* 10, 541.547, 1977.

11. JANSEN C.W. Otitis media-closed techniques. *Acta ORL Belg.* 38, 1984 (special issue).

12. CLAES J., MARQUET J. Cholesteatomatous invasion of the middle ear. *Acta ORL Belg.* 38, 1984 (special issue).

13. MARQUET J. Human middle ear transplantation. In: Operative Surgery: Ear (ed J. Ballantyne) Butterworths.

14. ARS B. The rôle of the tympanic frame in sound transmission. Il. Valvassori, 1984 (in press).

LASER in otology

ABSTRACT

R. Perkins

The recent application of visible wave-length laser photo-surgical techniques has added a significant new dimension to otologic surgery. This paper describes the characteristics of a new 532 nanometer solid state laser recently introduced in the United States and its application in various surgical procedures.

Methods of achieving various surgical effects including cutting, vaporization and coagulation by beam parameter manipulation are described.

Various clinical applications are described with emphasis on applications in stapes and acoustic neuroma surgery.

Experience with freeze-dried dura mater and bone in tympanoplasties

ABSTRACT

W. Kup

In cases with very large perforations (subtotal defect) the reconstruction of the eardrum by free transplanted grafts of fascia can be difficult from the technical point of view. We try to master this problem by using a double graft consisting of an eardrum-like disk of freeze-dried dura mater (preserve), covered by normal endogenous temporal fascia. The dura disk, well adapted on the prepared limbus of the remaining eardrum, is not only a mechanical protection of the fascia but also a support of its nutrition, because it is quickly organized by granulation tissue well supplied with blood. The dura disappears after 3 weeks by absorption, leaving behind the meanwhile settled graft of fascia.

The implantation of freeze-dried bone into the tympanic cavity is always unsuccessful because the bone will not be tolerated and will be completely absorbed within a few days. Examinations on animals showed that there are no immunological and histological findings of an allergic response. The process of lyophilization seems to remove the premise of an immunological reaction.

Among a total of 240 myringoplasties we had 62 patients with large defects of the eardrum without suppuration. There were good results without any complication in 95 %. No relapsing perforations were observed for 2 years and the sound conduction became normal.

Second look after closed and obliterative techniques

ABSTRACT

M. Raivio

The indications for a second-look operation after closed and obliterative techniques are:

— postoperative cholesteatoma,
— planned second-stage reconstruction of the ossicular chain,
— inadequate closure of the air-bone gap, and
— postoperative infection of the obliteration material.

With the canal wall down technique used by the author, the frequency of the postoperative cholesteatoma is relatively low compared with experiences of the intact canal wall technique, but this harm cannot be completely avoided. In a long-term follow-up Ojala and Palva have shown how these few cholesteatomas grew in the meso- and epitympanum only, but none primarily in the obliterated mastoid. This can only be understood on the basis of complete radicalism of the surgery in the mastoid, with sufficient concern to every possible projection of the cholesteatoma within any little cell as well as into the Haversian canals in the bone. A golden rule to be kept in mind is therefore: "Never obliterate the mastoid without full reliability of your radicalism!" One ear with previous inadequate surgery in another hospital, reoperated on by the author, showed clearly the serious consequences forgetting this rule can have. A residual cholesteatoma on top of the labyrinthine massive advanced quickly resulting in a large fistula on the lateral semicircular canal. In the middle ear the radicalism of the primary surgery remains more or less questionable due to other demands. In order to improve the risk evaluation concerning the postoperative cholesteatoma, the author routinely takes specimens for histological examination from the hideaways of the middle ear, and from the mucosal borderlines when removing parts of the middle ear mucosa. However, keratinizing squamous cell epithelium is seen in these specimens far more frequently than the postoperative cholesteatoma which is to be expected, and the author does not consider such a finding as an indication for a second look. Due to the use of lyophilized dura on the bare bone surfaces in the middle ear the author waits nine to twelve months before the second look, due to persistent air-bone gap, or the second-stage reconstruction of the ossicular chain is performed. During this time the lyodura disappears as completely at it will do, and the regrowth of the middle ear mucosa can take place undisturbed.

Postoperative infection of the autogenous bone chips and the Palva flap is a seldom occurring complication. Two cases seen by the author were obviously infected by the bacterial strain grown even preoperatively. In both cases, an open cavity was made two months after the primary surgery. The reconstructed middle ears did not need to be touched, the ears became dry within a few weeks, and the hearing results were not worse than the average of the normal closed and obliterative technique.

Reconstruction of the Eustachian tube and the anterior tympanum

K. Murata, F. Ohta

Introduction

When the Eustachian tubal orifice shows ossification, proliferation of granulation, polyps and/or cholesteatoma, the ostium of the Eustachian tube needs curettage and enlargement for tubal patency. It is followed by adequate exposure of the bone surface. A one-stage reconstruction of the middle ear with bone exposure at the orifice will induce poor tubal

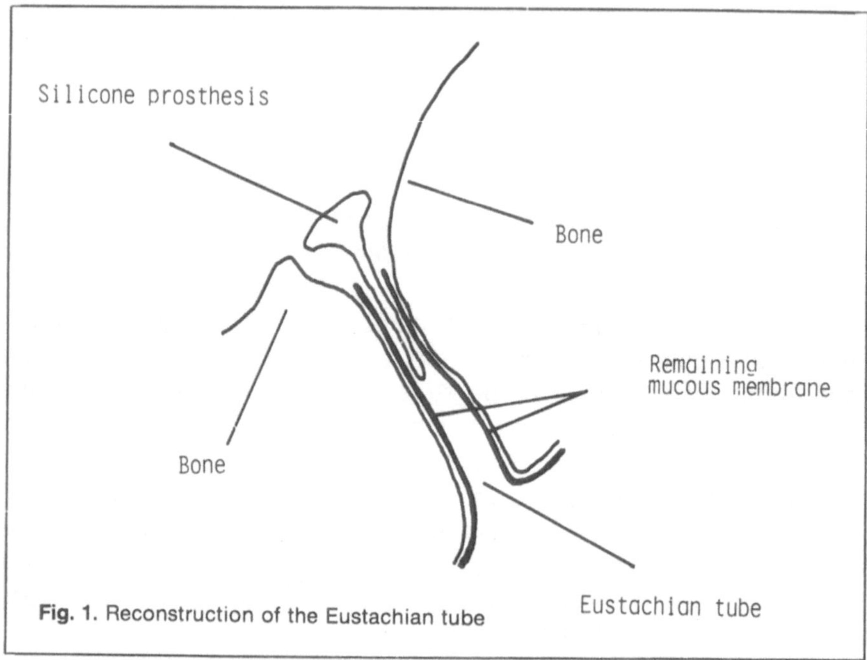

Fig. 1. Reconstruction of the Eustachian tube

function because of regrowth of granulation and loss of tubal patency.

The purpose of this study is to present our surgical techniques in management of the disease.

Materials and Methods

— Classical radical mastoidectomy is essental for this surgery. The posterior meatal wall is removed.

— A 0,2-0,5 mm thick Silastic sheeting is trimmed into a long T-shaped plate with a stem of ca. 20 mm in length. A bougie is sometimes passed from the middle ear to the nasopharynx to establish patency of the Eustachian tube. The silicone plate is placed in the Eustachian tube and pretympanum at the original surgery (figure 1). It runs a 2/3 length of the Eustachian tube so that it fully covers the denuded areas and extends over the area of remaining mucosa of the Eustachian tube. Nothing but gelfoam is placed over the proximal part of the silicone plate in the pretympanum.

— The exenterated antrum and tympanum are treated postoperatively as an open cavity. Caution must be paid to development of granulation (figure 2). Silicone plate is buried in the granulation tissue. The pretympanic epithelium must cover the granulation.

— The original surgery is followed by mucosal development from the normalized Eustachian tube. A small mucosal-lined air space is formed by the time of the second stage surgery, which is to

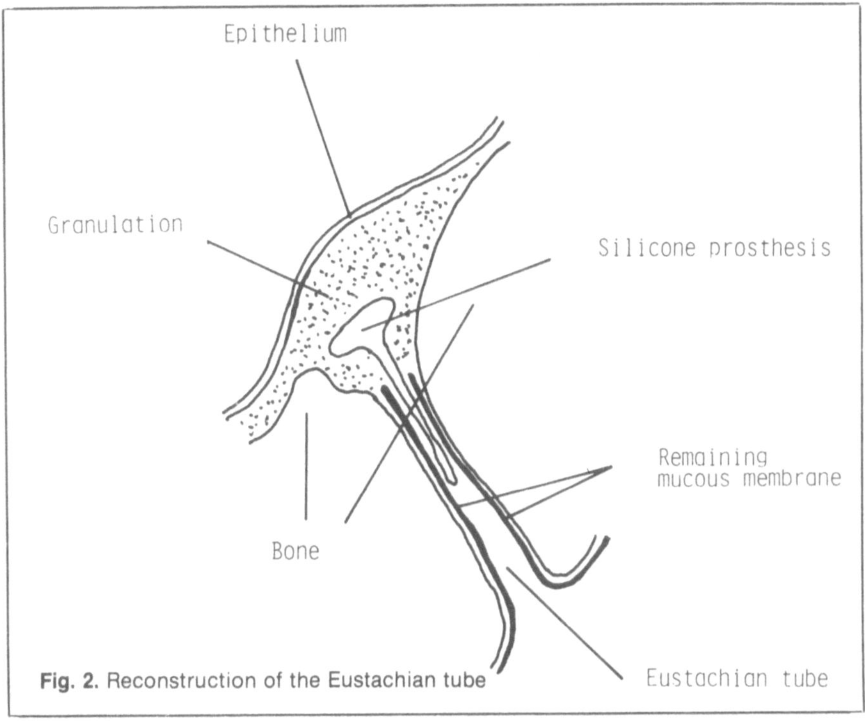

Fig. 2. Reconstruction of the Eustachian tube

be performed in half a year or later (AT in figure 3). It is communicated to the nasopharynx through the Eustachian tube (figure 3).

— The epithelium, which covers the open cavity, is ablated from the surface of the labyrinthine bone. At this postoperative stage, the mucosal cavity occupies the pretympanum, often reaching the mesotympanum and attico-antrum. The mucosa of the cavity is used as a pretympanic mucous membrane. The silicone plate is withdrawn from the Eustachian tube at the second stage surgery.

— The ablated epithelium is partially utilized as a tympanic membrane and the remainder may be used as a meatal skin of the reconstructed posterior wall.

— Continuity is restored between the new tympanic membrane and the stapes at the second stage surgery.

Results

Subjects

This new technique was performed during the last 5 years on 22 ears, ranging in age from 7 to 52, with a majority below 15. Twenty ears had cholesteatoma and 2 chronic purulent otitis media. Eighteen ears were of males and 4 of females. Right ears counted 10 and left 12.

Eustachian tubal patency

Eustachian tubal patency was evaluated by catheterization. Be-

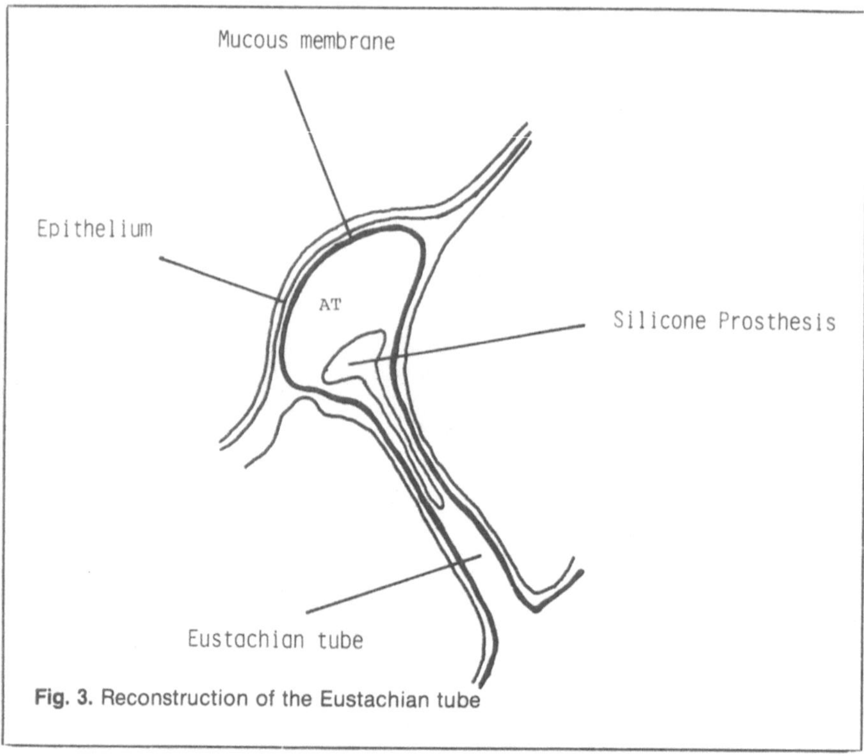

Fig. 3. Reconstruction of the Eustachian tube

fore the original surgery, adequate and dry patency of the Eustachian tube was found in 4 ears and poor patency in 12. Catheterization was not performed in 6. Ten of 12 ears with poor tubal patency before the initial surgery acquired the dry and patent Eustachian tube following the second stage surgery. All the patients were not old enough to endure catheterization. Nonperformance of catheterization amounted to 6 ears before the original surgery, of which one remained non-performed throughout the observation time. The dry and patent Eustachian tube was found in 19 ears following the second stage surgery.

Initial surgical findings in the tympanic orifice of the Eustachian tube

The Eustachian tubal orifice of 22 ears operated showed proliferation of granulation in 11 ears, polyps in 8, swollen mucosa in 5 and cholesteatoma in 5.

Development of a mucosal-lined cavity

The mucosal-lined cavity occupied only the pretympanic cavity in 9 ears, reached the mesotympanum in 4 and the attico-antrum in 8. Statistically significant correlation was not found between extension of the mucosal-lined cavity and the postoperative period following the original operation.

Audiometric results

At the second stage surgery, ossicle or cartilage was placed from the new tympanic membrane to the capitulum of the stapes on 13 ears, to the footplate on 8. A sound pressure transfer mechanism was not rebuilt in one ear because of impaired bone conduction following the original surgery. These ears were observed from one to 4 years following the second stage surgery. The mean air conduction hearing level and air-bone gaps for 0,5, 1,0 and 2,0 kHz were calculated for evaluation of postoperative hearing. The preoperative air-bone gaps were 10 dB or less in 2 ears, 20 dB or less in one, 30 dB or less in 4 and 30 dB or more in 14. The postoperative air-bone gaps were 20 dB or less in 8 ears, 30 dB or less in 8 and 30 dB or more in 5. Four ears showed the preoperative air conduction within 35 dB ISO level. Eleven ears gained postoperative air conduction within 35 dB ISO level.

Discussion

A small tube of various materials is placed in the Eustachian tube to discharge the exudate from the middle ear.[1] Its lumen, however, is easily occluded with mucous plug.[2] In addition, chronic stimulation of the Eustachian tubal mucosa and nasopharynx by the exudate may prolong normalization of them.

In our technique, the Eustachian tube is separated from the tympanum as a semiclosed duct with an orifice to the nasopharynx. Normalization of the Eustachian tubal mucosa and nasopharyngeal orifice can be expected because persistent inflammatory stimulus from the tympanum to this area diminishes.

In order to normalize the Eustachian tube, independently of the middle ear mastoidectomy cavity, the latter is necessary to be opened to the external acoustic meatus. Therefore, our new method is based on the concept of planned staged surgery.[3] Two staged surgery facilitates normalization of the Eustachian tube and exenterated open wound. Half a year or longer is estimated to be required for complete wound healing and for development of a mucosal-lined air space in the tubo-pretympanum. At the second stage surgery, rebuilding of the middle ear can be easily achieved including the pretympanic mucosal-lined cavity. Continuity between the new tympanic membrane and the stapes can also be easily restored with a good result of hearing.

References:

1. WRIGHT J.W. Jr., WRIGHT J.W. III. Preliminary results with use of an Eustachian tube prosthesis. *Laryngoscope* 87, 207-214, 1977.
2. LESINKSI S.G., FOX J.M., SEID A.B., BRATCHER G.O., COTTON R. Does the Silastic Eustachian tube prosthesis improve Eustachian tube function? *Laryngoscope* 90, 1413-1427, 1980.
3. RAMBO J.H.T. The use of paraffin to create the middle ear space in musculoplasty. *Laryngoscope* 71, 612-619, 1961.

Fibrinogen glue and packing techniques

F.E. Offeciers, J.F.E. Marquet

Introduction

Because of the specific anatomical construction of the ear, and even more because of the functional implications of complications in the early course of the postoperative healing process, the packing in reconstructive middle ear surgery is a delicate and important part of the surgical procedure.

Carelessness in the execution or removal of the packing can result in recurrent pathology (keratine pearls in the external auditory canal), or functional loss (blunting, lateralization of the graft, fibrin clots causing fibrous thickening of the tympanic graft or even a false second membrane, stenosis of the EAC).

Although it is clear that these complications are not solely due to packing problems, a number of them can be prevented by careful execution of the packing.

The recent availability of a two-component biological glue (Tissucol) has proven to be a major contribution in middle ear surgery, enhancing the postoperative stability of the tympano-ossicular reconstruction.

Packing technique

Rather than compare the various materials and techniques used for packing, we would like to establish a number of standard criteria:

— the packing should be easy to do, under good visual control;

— the packing should be perfectly adaptable to individual anatomical variations as in congenital ears, posterior wall reconstruction;

— the packing material should be sterile, antiseptic and biocompatible (non-toxic, inert);

— it should exert a constant and individually adaptable pressure on the entire graft surface as well as on the meatal wall. Thus, it should neutralize any effect of intratympanic pressure changes, caused by postoperative bleeding, coughing or sneezing, which could displace the graft;

— the packing should to some degree absorb, and be permeable to, serosanguineous liquid and instillated drops;

— it should be easy and painless to remove and, if necessary, as easy to replace as an office procedure.

All of these criteria are met by the packing technique we have been using for more than 20 years in our department.[1]

Description of the technique

After correct positioning and glueing of the tympano-ossicular graft, the meatal skin is replaced, partially covering the periosteal meatal cuff of the graft. Then a tubular concentric sheet of multi-punctured synthetic material (Melolin, Smyth & Nephew) is placed in the canal, touching the outer border of the tympanic graft near the annulus, and covering the periosteal cuff of the graft, as well as the meatal skin. In the center of this sheet, a number of synthetic sponges imbued with an antibiotic suspension, are carefully placed, one by one, starting in the anterior corner of the canal with small sponges, and progressively building up the size.

Because the used material is compressible and adapts itself perfectly to the available space, we obtain a firm, though mild and uniform pressure on the entire tympanomeatal graft and meatal skin. Thus, the packing prevents blunting or lateralization of the graft.

The multipunctured sheet prevents the adherence of the meatal skin's free border to the sponges when we take them out four to seven days after surgery. This allows an early suction cleaning of the canal, and a good look at how the graft behaves. The cleaning is repeated after three and ten days. The fact that this type of packing allows a very early post-operative control constitutes for us one of the major advantages.

Biological glue

The importance of the packing technique has been slightly diminished by what certainly is an old dream of many a surgeon and a major breakthrough in reconstructive middle ear surgery: the development of a non-toxic absorbable, thoroughly biological glue (Tissucol, Immuno Vienna).

The basic idea for this glue goes back to the first World War, when Harvey[2] and Grey[3] used fibrin tampons to staunch bleeding from parenchymatous organs.

Technological progress, and a better understanding of the biochemical processes involved in hemostasis and fibrinolysis, allowed the development and fabrication of a sufficiently concentrated and purified two-component glue out of human and bovine blood (Seelich 1982).[4]

Basic mechanisms, advantages and restrictions

The first component comprises highly concentrated human fibrinogen, factor XIII, plasma fibronectin, a small amount of plasminogen, and other human plasma proteins. This freeze-dried material is reconstituted by mixing it with an aprotinin solution. The second component consists of thrombin and $CaCl_2$.

When the two components are mixed, the material acquires a rubber-like quality, and adheres well to the tissue or bone surface where it is applied. Its rigidity increases quite fast as a result of the ongoing crosslinking reaction between the fibrin and fibronectin monomers. They form a solid polymer network, which crosslinks with the collagen of the surface to which it is applied.

This network, apart from glueing surfaces rapidly and rather tightly to each other, stimulates ingrowth of the fibroblasts. This accounts for a faster and better healing. The aprotinin of component I slows down the fibrinolytic process in such a way, that slow but complete resorption of the glue allows the physiological healing processes to take over. Listing the general advantages of this glue we find:

— biocompatibility and good tolerance,

— fast and firm glueing, and a definite hemostatic action,

— complete resorption during healing,

— a better and faster healing.

Compared to the previously used synthetic acrylates, the biological glue obviously has definite advantages. On the other hand, a few precautions should be taken:

— correct preparation of the glue is important, especially sufficient mixing while reconstituting the two components, under controlled temperature conditions;

— sufficient mixing of the two components after application on the surface to be glued is necessary;

— the glue should be used on a dry surface to prevent dilution, which would slow down the crosslinking process;

— the glue should be used sparingly, since it behaves as a blood coagulum with an abnormally long life. Especially in an infected or inflamed environment this could cause problems.

Method of application

Tympanic and tympano-ossicular allografts have been used routinely in our department for a long time.[5] For us, they are the material of choice in middle ear reconstruction, both anatomically and functionally. But until the introduction of the fibrin glue, some essential problems remained.[6]

• The contact between a vibrating membrane and any kind of organic or alloplastic material implanted in order to restore the columellar effect, remains the weakest point in reconstructive ear surgery. The unique structure of the drum as found in tympanic allografts, requested a very precise topographical positioning in order to function properly. The introduction of fibrin glue guarantees perfect positioning of the tympanic membrane, and its attachment all around the tympanic ring and along the manubrium.

• When a tympano-ossicular graft is used — e.g. a monobloc drum, malleus and incus — the lenticular process of the incus can be firmly glued to the head of the stapes.

• When only the stapes footplate remains, and we must use a full monobloc implant including the stapes, the functional result depends upon the acquired contact between the implanted stapes, and the remaining mobile footplate. The glue can be very helpful to secure this contact.

- In the reconstruction of the posterior canal wall by means of a remodelled autograft of cortical bone, the glue enhances the stability of the implant.

Illustrative of how well this glue works is the fact that impedance measurements carried out during surgery, just after positioning and glueing of the tympanic or tympano-ossicular graft, show a quite normal curve, without any sign of leaking at -300 to +200 mm H_2O. After surgery, the tympanogram often normalizes completely, and in quite a few cases of tympanic allograft we obtain clear stapedial reflexes.

References:

1. MARQUET J. Technique de pansement en cophochirurgie. *Acta Otorhinolaryng. Belg.* 19: 846-850. 1965.
2. HARVEY S.C. The use of fibrin paper and forms in surgery. *Boston Med. Surg. J.* 174: 658-659. 1916.
3. GREY E.G. Fibrin as hemostatic in cerebral surgery. *Surg. Gyn. Obstetr.* 21: 452-454. 1915.
4. SEELICH T. Tissucol (Immuno, Vienna): Biochemistry and methods of application. *J. Head & Neck Pathol.* 3: 65-69. 1982.
5. MARQUET J. Twelve years' experience with homograft tympanoplasty. *Otolaryngol. Clin. North Amer.* 10: 581-593. 1977.
6. MARQUET J. The fibrin seal in otorhinolaryngology. *J. Head & Neck Pathol.* 3: 71-72. 1982.

PLENARY SESSION

Medical ethics in postoperative evaluation reports

ABSTRACT
H. Diamant

So far there is no international agreement on the procedure for postoperative evaluation of results. The follow-up system is impaired by errors, where loss of cases is the gravest one. There are examples where more than 50 % of the cases were lost within 6 months. Another important fact is the lack of conformity in diagnosis in different materials. There are a few simple rules to be followed in order to reach comparable figures. These rules were published by Marquet and Graff, 1982, and include honesty, efficiency and standardization. Based on this proposition it is possible to construct a worldwide recognized follow-up chart, which will make a comparison between different reports meaningful.

The pathology of middle ear inflammation (otitis media)

M.M. Paparella

Before one can discuss the pathology of otitis media, it is necessary to begin with a classification of types of otitis media in order to have clarity of understanding. I had the privilege of chairing an international committee at the NIH Research Sponsored Conference held in Fort Lauderdale, Florida on May 21, 1983. This committee provided a report on definitions and classification of otitis media which, in brief, follows:

"Otitis media" is defined as inflammation of the middle ear
A. Myringitis

B. Acute suppurative otitis media (acute purulent otitis media, acute otitis media)

C. Secretory otitis media (otitis media with effusion, non-suppurative otitis media, catarrh), serous otitis media (serotympanum), mucoid otitis media (mucotympanum)

D. Chronic suppurative otitis media (chronic otitis media).

Based on my understanding of clinical, pathological, and basic scientific manifestations of otitis media, I find a modification of that classification to be helpful. The classification I currently use follows:

A. Suppurative (Purulent) Otitis Media
I. Acute Purulent (Suppurative) Otitis Media ("Acute Otitis Media") - POM
II. Chronic Suppurative (Purulent) Otitis Media - COM

B. Non-Suppurative Otitis Media ("Otitis Media with Effusion [OME], Secretory Otitis Media, Serous Otitis Media")
I. Serous Otitis Media ("Serotympanum") - SOM
II. Mucoid Otitis Media ("Secretory Otitis Media, Mucotympanum") - MOM

Complications of otitis media
Complications in temporal bone
a. Facial paralysis
b. Petrositis (Gradenigo)
c. Labyrinthitis, serous or suppurative (localized or generalized)
d. Acute mastoiditis and masked mastoiditis
e. Brain hernia (encephalocele)

Intracranial Complications
a. Extradural abscess
b. Subdural abscess
c. Brain abscess
d. Meningitis (localized or generalized)
e. Lateral sinus thrombophlebitis
f. Otitis hydrocephalus

Sequelae of otitis media
Clinical - pathological
A. Active sequelae
1. Frequent recurrent attacks of POM and OME
2. Chronic OME
3. Continuum: OME (POM-SOM-MOM) → COM (granulation tissue, cholesterol granuloma, cholesteatoma)
B. Inactive sequelae
1. Hearing loss (conductive, sensorineural)
2. Atelectasis
3. Tympanosclerosis
4. Otopathological findings

Developmental and behavioral sequelae
Otitis media, inflammation or infection of the middle ear, and its clinical subgroups are common problems throughout the world. In the United States it is esti-

mated that 95% of all children have had one or more middle ear infections before age five, and approximately 10% of all school children have otitis media with effusion (OME). In recent years, otitis media research has made important advances.

We have studied pathological, chemical, and bacteriological aspects of the pathogenesis of otitis media in human subjects and various animal models. Longitudinal studies of various forms of the disease, acute purulent otitis media (POM), serous otitis media (SOM), mucoid or secretory otitis media (MOM), and chronic suppurative otitis media (COM) were especially evaluated for evidence of interrelated changes of various groups. Purulent otitis media was produced in chinchillas by direct inoculation of less than one hundred Pneumococci into the middle ear space. Serous otitis media was produced in chinchillas and cats following the development of SOM in cats after two to four weeks of tubal occlusion. Material for evaluation of middle ear effusion (MEE) and serum was obtained from children with SOM and MOM after myringotomy for placement of ventilation tubes. Three components were studied: MEE (fluid), epithelium, and the subepithelial space (SES). Significant inflammatory changes in the SES, which characterized all forms of otitis media, were especially prominent in POM and SOM. Epithelial metaplasia of secretory cells was most prominent in MOM.

Pathology

The pathology of POM is characterized by the presence of pus in the middle ear (bacteria and polymorphonuclear leucocytes) along with acute inflammatory reaction throughout the organ, including the mucoperiosteum. Much inflammatory activity occurs in the subepithelial space. Serous otitis media, as seen in some children and adults with OME following barotrauma (aerotitis), or with nasopharyngeal tumors, is characterized by the presence of clear amber fluid. Here, the primary pathology occurs in the subepithelial space: transudation of fluid, demonstrated by direct visualization of vessels, rupture of the basilar membrane, and passage of fluid between cells, which was first demonstrated in our laboratory. MOM is characterized by the change of cuboidal epithelium into secretory epithelium, which is characterized by the presence of many goblet cells and secretory glands. The SES also participates in the changes of MOM. These types of otitis media overlap, and one can evolve into another. Either as a group or individually, they can lead to permanent sequelae, which include ossicular fixation or erosion, atelectasis, or tympanosclerosis resulting in conductive deafness. Inflammation of the round window can produce temporary or permanent sensorineural hearing loss. Another important sequela of OME in childhood is chronic otitis media and mastoiditis, characterized by cholesteatoma and/or persistent granulation tissue. Granulation tissue forms in the subepithelial space, while cholesteatoma results from migration of keratinizing squamous epithelium from the adjacent canal wall into the middle ear space. Metaplasia of mucoperiosteum of the middle ear cleft into squamous cells with keratin may also contribute to formation of cholesteatoma.

Sequential biochemical changes occurring with otitis media can also be studied in correlation with pathological changes. Levels of the enzyme lactate dehydrogenase (LDH) and of lysozyme were higher in effusions from POM than from SOM, indicating that the presence of micro-organisms enhances the release of cellular enzymes. The hexosamine content of middle ear effusions was higher in MOM than in SOM. In recent studies using combinations of models (SOM + POM), the levels of lysozyme in MEE were higher in animals whose middle ear infection was introduced after obstruction of the Eustachian tube than in those with primary purulent otitis media. The data strongly suggest that obstruction of ventilation through the Eustachian tube can enhance subsequent inflammatory changes of the middle ear cavity. Lysozyme, an enzyme found predominantly in neutrophils, is released in the process of phagocytosis.

In correlated human studies, levels of LDH, lysozyme, and hexosamine were higher in mucoid effusions than in serous effusions, corresponding to the finding in the animal models. In patients with recurrent disease (requiring repeated surgery within 18 months), lysozyme levels were higher than those found with first attacks. Thus, high levels of lysozyme in MEE indicate either severe inflammation or chronic disease. Reasoning from animal experiments in combination models cited above, we consider that the recurrent group with high lysozyme levels might have the combination of obstruction of the Eustachian tube and bacterial infection. The immunological characteristics of MEE in MOM are different than in SOM. The immunoglobulin content of MOM often is higher for IgA, IgG, and IgM than is similar fluid from SOM. Thus, bacteriological and biochemical study of fluids from the inner ear cleft assists in diagnosis and consequent treatment.

Prostaglandin studies conducted by Dr. Jung in our laboratory can also be studied relative to the otitis medias. The following summary and conclusions have recently been noted:

— A small amount of prostaglandin (PG) is produced in normal middle ear tissues. Prostaglandins may be involved in maintaining normal homeostasis, acting as a "fine tuning" agent of tissue metabolism, blood flow, and vascular permeability of the middle ear.

— In disease-states such as purulent otitis media and chronic otitis media, large quantities and abnormal combinations of PG may be produced, inducing acute inflammation, vasodilatation, increased vascular permeability, and bone resorption. Some of the non-PG arachidonic acid metabolites act as a chemotactic factor for polymorphonuclear (PMN) leucocytes, intensifying acute inflammation.

— Granulation tissue as well as cholesteatoma tissue can produce bone-resorbing PG.

— PG and arachidonic acid introduced into the middle ear induce mucoid otitis media in chinchillas.

— PG produced in the middle ear increases the permeability of round window membrane, allowing toxic substances to enter the inner ear.

Subepithelial space

Recently in our laboratory we have studied the rôle of the subepithelial space in the various forms of otitis media. This semiquantified study is most interesting in that it stressed the importance of the continuum of one form of otitis media leading to another type, and it also underscored the important rôle the subepithelial space plays in all forms of otitis media. The rôle of the subepithelial space (SES) has not received sufficient attention in assessing pathogenesis, pathology, and, therefore, clinical diagnosis and treatment of the various forms of otitis media (OM). Temporal bones from patients with OM were classified as cases of acute purulent (POM), serous (SOM), mucoid or secretory (MOM), or chronic otitis media (COM). Controlled morphometric studies were made of cellular components of the SES, along with studies of the epithelium and middle ear space. Corollary studies of biochemistry, cellular components, and prostaglandins (PGs) were done on fluid from the human middle ear. Middle ear effusions (MEE) from animal models of SOM, MOM, POM were analyzed biochemically. Findings are surprising in that the SES was more actively involved in all forms of OM than had been thought, especially in MOM and COM.

Based on that recent study, the rôle of the SES in the pathogenesis of otitis media can be categorized as follows:

— Production of effusion

o transudation (blood vessels)

o secretion (inflammatory cells and fibroblasts)

o absorption (blood vessels, lymphatic vessels)

— Production of granulation tissue (fibroblasts, blood vessels, and inflammatory cells)

— Production of tympanosclerosis (fibroblasts)

— Contribution to production of cholesterol granuloma (fibroblasts, macrophages, and red blood cells)

— Classification and continuum of otitis media

— Defense mechanisms

o phagocytosis (neutrophils and macrophages)

o humoral immune system (plasma cells)

o cell-mediated immune-mecha nisms (lymphocytes and macrophages)

o secretions from the inflammatory cells (lysozyme, hydrolases, prostaglandins, interferon, components of complement, lymphokines, etc.)

o secretions from fibroblasts (collagen and collagenase)

— Osteogenesis and destruction

— Influence on epithelial cells.

Otitis Media: a continuum

Although time here does not permit us to demonstrate in detail, all of our recent studies clearly point to otitis media as occurring along a continuum, that is, one form of otitis media can lead to another (figure 1). Thus, POM can eventually become SOM, and SOM can become MOM, although it is less likely that MOM will revert back to SOM. All of the forms of otitis media with fluid in the middle ear can eventually lead to chronic otitis media or chronic suppurative otitis media characterized by the presence of intractable tissue such as granulation tissue, cholesterin granuloma, or cholesteatoma. Moreover, the forms of otitis media having fluid in the middle ear frequently can have various sequelae, while suppurative otitis media, both of the acute and chronic varieties, can lead to the well established classic complications of otitis media. In addition to the concept of the continuum, our recent research has stressed the fact that the various otitis medias seem to have commonalities in terms of underlying considerations of etiology and pathogenesis. Foremost amongst these continues to be Eustachian tubal dysfunction, particularly as regards ventilatory dysfunction, host immunological response to bacteria, etc.

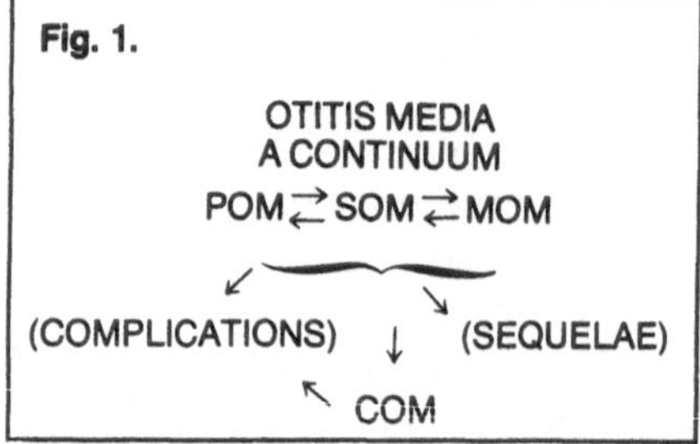

Fig. 1.

This paper is supported in part by Grant 1P50-NS-14538 and by the Bodman Foundation and the Guggenheim Foundation.

PANEL II
Middle ear pathology

Moderator: G.D.L. Smyth

Middle ear pathology

G.D.L. Smyth

C.D. Bluestone - Infection of the middle ear related to postoperative surgery

Streptococcus pneumoniae, Haemophilus influenzae, and Branhamella catarrhalis are the most frequently isolated pathogens in acute otitis media and chronic otitis media with effusion. Antimicrobial therapy is still indicated for children with acute otitis media and for selected patients with persistent effusion. Amoxicillen is the preferred antibiotic, except for Beta-lactamase-producing organisms. Cefaclor or erythromycin with sulfisoxazole and trimethoprim-sulfamethoxazole are useful alternatives. When chronic suppurative otitis media (without cholesteatoma) is caused by Pseudomonas aeruginosa, parenteral carbenicillin is recommended. When appropriate antimicrobial therapy fails, surgical treatment is usually indicated. The success of surgery may be enhanced by pre- and perioperative administration of antibiotics. Their efficacy in preventing complications requires long-term evaluation.

Y. Honda - Acquired and recurrent cholesteatoma

Experimentally, obstruction of the Eustachian tube leads to pars flaccida retractions and cholesteatoma. In humans a similar sequence occurs due to obstruction of the tympanic isthmus. This obstruction may be due either to persistent mucosal disease in the epitympanum or to retraction of the postero-superior pars tensa through the isthmus. A similar mechanism is responsible for recurrent cholesteatoma postoperatively.

M. Tos - Atrophy and dystrophy of the tympanic membrane

The most common cause of damage to the lamina propria is long-lasting negative middle ear pressure. Localised atrophy of the pars tensa, common in secretory otitis, may lead to partial or diffuse retraction, or as a consequence of subsequent acute otitis, perforation. Five types of change in the pars flaccida occur. The most extensive have important clinical significance due to irreversibility.

J. Sadé - Middle ear mucosa

Mucosal cells are derived from stem cells which mature into cell-producing glycoproteins and keratin, secondary to triggers and specific conditions. The histological character of middle ear mucosa reflects its past history of exposure to various diseases, especially inflammatory ones. The main questions of interest concern:

— the qualitative changes,
— the durability of these changes, and
— their reversibility.

A.G. Gibb - Tympanosclerosis

The clinical presentations of tympanosclerosis as "chalk patches" in the tympanic membrane and aggregates around the ossicles are described. The aetiology of tympanosclerosis is unkown. Recent work suggests that involvement of the tympanic membrane may be due to factors which reduce its mobility.

D. Plester - Congenital middle ear pathology (minor malformations)

Stapedial abnormality is the most common minor abnormality of the ossicular chain. Footplate fixation, the most frequent single finding, can be accompanied by defects of the incus and malleus. Persistent stapedial artery and anomalous course of the facial nerve are also encountered. The surgical technique used for stapedial malformations will be described in detail.

Infection of the middle ear related to postoperative surgery

ABSTRACT

C.D. Bluestone

The possibility of infection must always be considered in the post-operative evaluation of patients following middle ear surgery for otitis media-related conditions, since the etiology of otitis media is usually infection. Organisms gain access into the middle ear cavity from the nasopharynx by aspiration, insufflation, or reflux through the Eustachian tube. However, when the tympanic membrane is not intact, contamination of the middle ear cleft from organisms in the external ear canal is also possible. Acute otitis media is usually caused by *Streptococcus pneumoniae, Haemophilus influenzae, Branhamella catarrhalis,* and to a lesser extent, *Streptococcus pyogenes* and *Staphylococcus aureus.* The same organisms have been isolated from up to 50 % of middle ear aspirates from chronic otitis media with effusion ("secretory" otitis media). Beta-lactamase-producing strains of *H. influenzae* (20 %), *B. catarrhilis* (75 %), and *S. aureus* (50-75 %) have recently been identified from acute and chronic middle ear effusions. *Pseudomonas aeruginosa* or *S. aureus,* or both, are usually cultured from ears with chronic suppurative otitis media and from infected cholesteatoma. Anaerobic bacteria have been also isolated. Recently, *Candida albicans* has been the offending organism in chronic suppurative otitis media (without cholesteatoma). Antimicrobial treatment is still indicated for children with acute otitis media to eliminate infection/effusion and to prevent suppurative complications. Also, antimicrobial therapy is indicated in selected patients who have otitis media with effusion. Amoxicillin is preferred since it is effective against the common pathogens, but cefaclor is a reasonable alternative, especially when a Beta-lactamase-producing organism is identified or suspected, as are erythromycin with sulfisoxazole and trimethoprim-sulfamethoxazole. For children with frequently recurrent acute infection, antimicrobial prophylaxis is an attractive alternative to surgical intervention. When chronic suppurative otitis media (without cholesteatoma) is caused by *P. aeruginosa,* parenteral antimicrobial therapy (e.g. carbenicillin) may be successful in eliminating the infection. Myringotomy with or without tympanostomy tube, repair of tympanic membrane defects (myringoplasty/tympanoplasty), tympanomastoidectomy, and reconstructive middle ear surgery are performed to treat and prevent otitis media or its complications or sequelae, and to restore function. Appropriate and adequate antimicrobial therapy may prevent the need for such surgical procedures but, if medical treatment fails, surgery is indicated. Antimicrobial agents for preoperative treatment and perioperative prophylaxis may prevent postoperative complications following surgery for chronic suppurative otitis media and infected cholesteatoma. The success of surgical procedures for otitis media-related conditions should include, among other important outcomes, the rate of postoperative infection. This evaluation cannot be just for the immediate postoperative period but over many years, especially after surgery is performed in children.

Acquired and recurrent cholesteatoma

Y. Honda

I have been interested in the pathogenesis of cholesteatoma, since I experienced cases of postoperative recurrent cholesteatoma. It was better observed at the second revision surgery of staged tympanoplasty.

The common findings were as follows: although there was no perforation of the reconstructed tympanic membrane, the upper portion of the membrane adhered to the promontorium, and the attico-antral space was isolated from the tubotympanic space. Then the upper portion of the tympanic membrane was retracted into the isolated attico-antral space to form cholesteatoma. When the etiology of recurrent cholesteatoma is considered, the major cause might be the blockage of the middle ear cavity, which disturbs aeration to the peripheral cavities (figure 1).

Recurrent cholesteatoma is, in a sense, an artificial disease created in the ear of humans, so that it was thought possible to create similar cholesteatoma in animals,

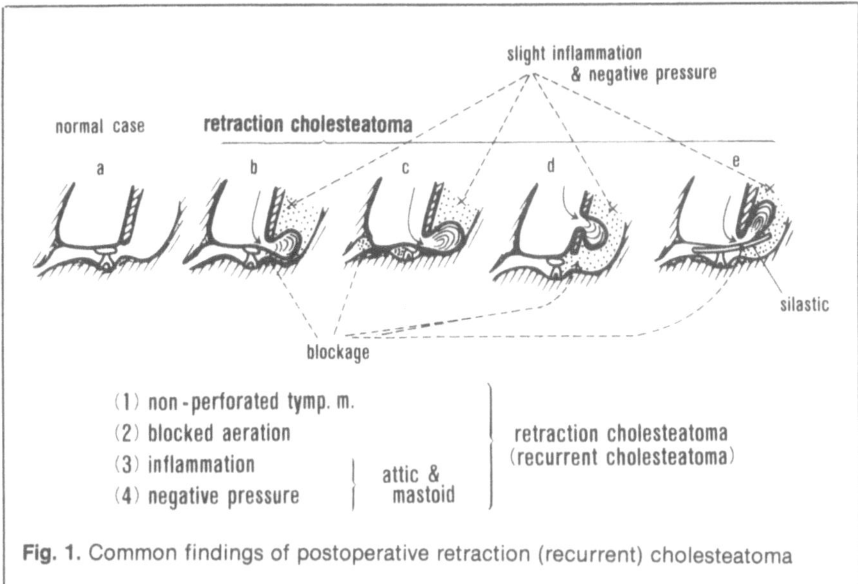

Fig. 1. Common findings of postoperative retraction (recurrent) cholesteatoma

and various experiments were conducted, (many of which are shown by our ENT department in the poster session).

The object of the experiments was to produce a continous but weak inflammation in the middle ear cavity of rabbits, not to damage the tympanic membrane, and to observe the morphological changes in the tympanic membrane.

• **Experiment 1:** obstruction of the tympanic orifice of the Eustachian tube. These cases were those in which the tympanic orifice of the Eustachian tube of rabbits was closed with a small piece of muscle in order to cause slight inflammation in the middle ear cavity. (The results are pointed out by Sano of my department in the poster session of these proceedings, p. 353.)

• **Experiment 2:** obstruction of the pharyngeal orifice of the Eustachian tube. (This experiment is pointed out by Mizorogi of my department in the poster session of these proceedings, p. 359.)

Summary of experiment 1 and 2: although there were tympanic perforations in many cases after obstruction of the Eustachian tube due to infection of the middle ear cavity, retention of effusion and inflammation cells was noted in the cavity in some cases of non-perforated tympanic membrane. And in these cases, in the pars tensa, no marked changes occurred, whereas in the pars flaccida, the thickening of the middle layers and the cell division of the epidermis became active, and marked retraction at the pars flaccida was indicated in nine ears. These findings are similar to retraction cholesteatoma in humans.

• **Experiment 3:** culture experiment of epidermal cells of tympanic membrane. The dermal epithelial cells at the pars flaccida and pars tensa of rabbits were cultured separately, and the difference of the growth of the two was compared. The research team was aware that hyaluronic acid was contained in great quantities around the cholesteatoma tissue. In this experiment, diluted hyaluronic acid was added to the culture solution to observe the proliferation of each cell. The activity of the cells was determined by the uptake of H^3-thymidine and H^3-leucine (figures 2 a and b).

Results: the volume of the uptake of H^3-thymidine and H^3-leucine by dermal epithelial cells at the pars flaccida was higher than that by the epithelial cells at the pars tensa. The addition of hyaluronic acid caused great changes in the uptake by epithelial cells at the pars flaccida. It was observed from the results of cell culture that the proliferation capacity of the dermal epithelial cells at the pars flaccida in rabbits was more active than that at the pars tensa. It was further

Fig. 2. Proliferation rate of epidermal cell of pars flaccida and pars tensa; **a)** indicates uptake of H^3-thymidine and **b)** indicates uptake of H^3-leucine. The vertical and horizontal lines indicate the uptake and the consistency of hyaluronic acid respectively.

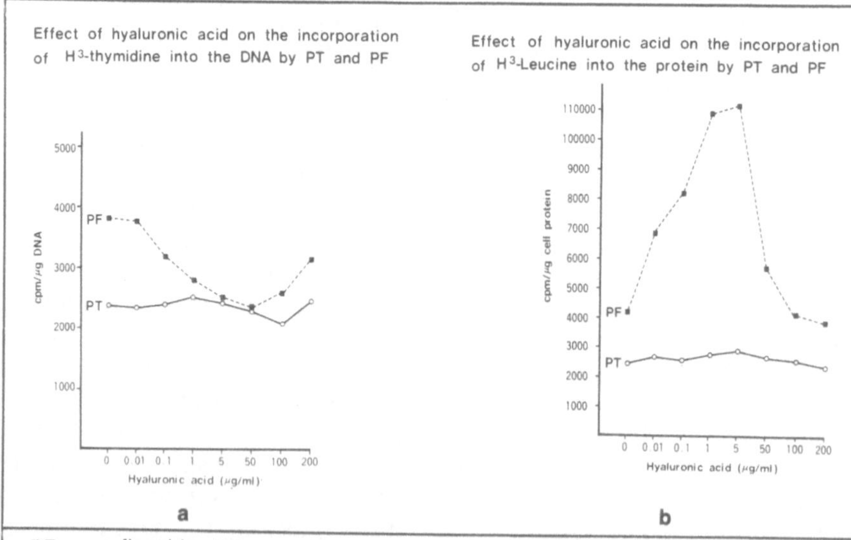

PF=pars flaccida PT=pars tensa

found that hyaluronic acid had a great influence on the proliferation and growth of the epithelium at the pars flaccida, while it had hardly any effect on the epithelium at the pars tensa.

• **Experiment 4:** stimulation of the tympanic membrane from the outside. (This experiment is pointed out by Mizorogi of my department in the poster session of these proceedings, p. 359.)

Results: the profileration of the epithelial cells at the pars flaccida in response to stimulation from the outside was rapid. It was believed that, when there was no difference of internal pressure between the middle ear cavity and external ear meatus, thickening at the normal site took place, whereas when the internal pressure of the external ear meatus was low, protrusion into the external ear canal in a balloon shape occurred, while, when the internal pressure of the middle ear cavity was low, retraction into the middle ear cavity seemed to occur. It was understood to be natural from these findings that, when the Eustachian tube was closed, the middle ear came under negative pressure, so that all proliferation at the pars flaccida took the form of retraction cholesteatoma.

• **Analysis of surgical findings** and observation of specimens of the human temporal bone: acquired cholesteatoma can be divided into two types, one originating from the pars flaccida and the other from the pars tensa. The point common to both types was the suppression of the growth of the mastoid cavity (experimental study of the mastoid pneumatization is introduced by Aoki of my department in the poster session of these proceedings, p. 363) and the inability of recognition of definite tympanic perforation. Even pus was drained. What looked like perforation, whether attic perforation or posterio-superior perforation, was nothing but the inlet for invagination of the tympanic membrane, and pus came out of it.

— *Pathogenesis of cholesteatoma originating from pars flaccida:* In cholesteatoma originating form the pars flaccida, the tympanic orifice of the Eustachian tube, the promontorium, and the pars tensa were almost normal. The tympanic isthmus at the boundary between the epitympanum and the mesotympanum was closed membranically, and the aeration from the Eustachian tube to the mastoid antrum was blocked at the isthmus. Cholesteatoma was formed by the retraction of the tympanic membrane at the pars flaccida, extending towards the direction of the mastoid antrum. The tip of the long process of the incus, and the stapes below the tympanic isthmus were intact in most cases. It should be postulated that the presence of chronic inflammation in the epitympanum before the formation of cholesteatoma and the resulting closure of the isthmus constituted an important mechanism of the formation of cholesteatoma.

With a view to examining the mechanism of the closure of the isthmus more accurately, 170 autopsy samples of wet temporal bones were studied. (This study is described by Miyajima of my department in the poster session of these proceedings, p. 347). Judging from the results of observation of these findings as well as the findings of a study of secretory otitis media in infancy, the etiology of cholesteatoma originating from the pars flaccida was considered as follows: if chronic secretory otitis media occurs in infancy, the growth of pneumatization of the temporal bone is inhibited, and retained fluids from the middle ear fill the mastoid antrum. With the growth of the child, however, the function of the Eustachian tube is being improved, and the retained fluids in the mesotympanum are excreted, restoring the tympanic orifice of the Eustachian tube and the mucosa of the mesotympanum to normal. In addition, the pars tensa in the tympanic membrane becomes normal. It takes a long time, however, for viscous substances retained in the narrow epitympanum to pass through the isthmus and to be excreted. In the meantime, the pars flaccida is exposed to mild inflammatory stimulation and negative pressure, retracting to the inside, as was observed in animal experiments, and proliferates there. As a result, dimples and retraction pockets are formed. If the retained fluid is excreted from the epitympanum, and aeration is given there, retraction at the pars flaccida does not progress. It has often been the case, however, that the old lesion in the epitympanum accelerated the proliferation of the connective tissue surrounding the isthmus and finally closed the isthmus. Under such circumstances, aeration to the mastoid antrum could not be undertaken in the cases of poor pneumatization, and the formation of retraction cholesteatoma was accelerated(figures 3 and 4). This is the etiology of cholesteatoma originating from the pars flaccida, starting from infancy and gradually appearing after puberty. In some cases, cholesteatoma was already apparent in childhood.

— *Pathogenesis of cholesteatoma originating frompars tensa:* in the following passages, the etiology of cholesteatoma originating from the pars tensa is explained. The cholesteatoma of this type comes from secretry otitis media in inflancy like the flaccida type cholesteatoma, as sequelae, in which the posterior-superior portion of the pars tensa becomes thinner and retracted, and simultaneously the proliferation of granulation tissue occurs in the middle ear cavity, and the long process of the incus and the superstructure of the stapes are melted with the retraction of the posterior-superior portion. Thus,

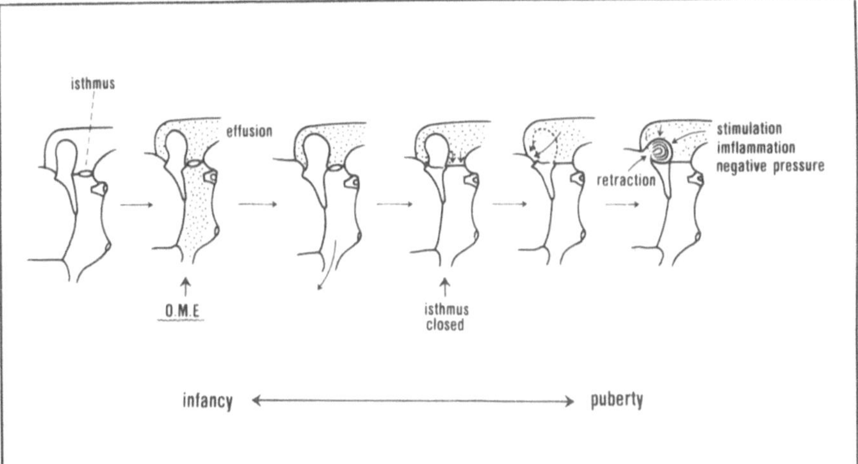

Fig. 3. The change from otitis media with effusion in infancy to pars flaccida type cholesteatoma

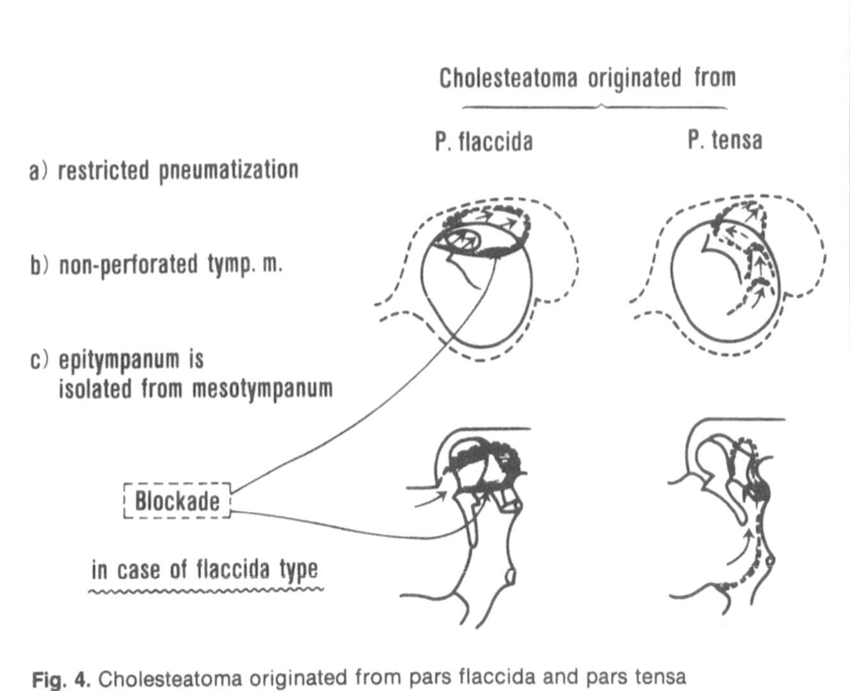

Fig. 4. Cholesteatoma originated from pars flaccida and pars tensa

the back surface of the retracted tympanic membrane comes in contact with the lower surface of the isthmus and closes it. As a result, the cavity of the epitympanum comes under negative pressure, and the tympanic membrane which closed the isthmus is retracted into the epitympanum to form cholesteatoma (figure 4).

In the chapter on cell culture, it was stated that epidermal cells at the pars tensa did not have too strong a proliferating power. This is attributed to the fact that the middle layer of the pars tensa has fewer blood vessels than that of the pars flaccida. It is considered that, since the epidermal cells in both portions are genetically of the same ectodermal origin, the potential of growth might vary in accordance with the changes in alimentary conditions.

Conclusion

Our concept of pathogenesis of cholesteatoma is considered to be as outlined above. This study had started with the discovery of the recurrent cholesteatoma after the posterior tympanotomy. It is most important for the prevention of the onset of recurrent cholesteatoma after posterior tympanotomy to secure aeration to the mastoid cavity. But the cholesteatoma ephithelium does exist in the epitympanum, irrespective of the origin — from the pars flaccida or from the pars tensa — and it must be removed. Consequently, defects of the mucosa occur in a wide area, and bone surfaces are exposed to the outside. Therefore, it is often the case that granulation tissue occurs on the promontorium after the operation, and the reconstructed tympanic membrane is adhered, and then aeration from the Eustachian tube to the mastoid antrum is inhibited. It also may result in the inhibition of aeration to construct the auditory ossicles, insert Gelfoam and perform underlay grafting.

Furthermore, although the facial recess is opened widely, the risk of reclosure by proliferated granulation tissue is not so small, especially in cases of cholesteatoma originating from the pars tensa.

So far, the author has reported on the pathogenesis of recurrent and acquired cholesteatoma, referring also to the prophylaxis of postoperative cholesteatoma.

Atrophy of the tympanic membrane

M. Tos

Definition

Atrophy of the tympanic membrane denotes a thin and pellucid eardrum. Histologically, the atrophic area is characterized by a thin lamina propria, containing abnormally few elastic and fibrous fibers which make it thin, unelastic, and slack. In severe cases, the lateral part of the pars tensa consists exclusively of keratinized squamous epithelium and the medial part of flat, cuboid mucosal epithelium with the basement membrane, whereas the laminia propria is completely lacking. The atrophy may be diffuse or localized, and it may occur as the only pathological change or in connection with tympanosclerosis.

Pathological manifestations of atrophy in the pars tensa

The combination of atrophy, retraction and tympanosclerosis as well as the different localizations of atrophy of the pars tensa result in more or less characteristic pathological manifestations, which will be described here.

— *Diffuse atrophy without retraction* indicates a membrane that is thinner than normal. It has almost normal mobility and elasticity. The atrophy comprises the whole of tensa.

— *Localized atrophy without retraction* often involves the inferior half of the tympanic membrane, i.e., below the umbo, or the posterio-superior quadrant of the pars tensa.

— *Diffuse atrophy with retraction.* The tympanic membrane is "too large", diffuse, and slack without elasticity. Owing to the constant retraction, the tympanic cavity is more or less atelectatic. At the same time there is myringo-incudopexy or myringo-stapediopexy. Adhesion of the tympanic membrane to the promontory is denoted *adhesive otitis.*

— *Posterior atrophy with retraction* is a frequent and well-known condition. The tympanic membrane is thin and slack in the posterio-superior quadrant. Soon, a *myringo-incudopexy* develops, bringing the tympanic membrane into contact with the long process of the incus and the lenticular process. We have observed a gradual resorption of the long process of the incus, resulting in *myringo-stapediopexy.*

The atrophic and slack tympanic membrane often adheres to the posterior and medial walls of the tympanic cavity, as is characteristic in *adhesive otitis.*

Prevalence and cause of atrophy

It has been demonstrated that 80 % of the population have secretory otitis during childhood and that sequelae changes of the tympanic membrane are caused by this disease.[1]

A randomized cohort of 222 healthy children were examined 7 times from age 4 to 7 years[2], atrophy occurred in 10 % of the ears (table 1). The prevalence of severe changes was quite high considering that this series was a cohort of randomized, healthy children.

In children with secretory otitis treated in our department with tubulation and adenotomy from 1970 through 1974 and, 5-8 years after treatment[3], re-examined with otomicroscopy, tympanometry, and audiometry, considerable changes of the pars tensa were found, including atrophy in 36 % of 527 ears (table 1).

The cause of atrophy of the pars tensa is, in my opinion, a long-lasting negative middle ear pressure. In our epidemiological studies, children with atrophy had a type B or C_2 tympanogram more frequently and for a longer period of time than had children with normal eardrums[2] or children with myringosclerosis. Owing to the long-lasting negative middle ear pressure, which often occurs in children without middle ear effusion, the fibrous and elastic fibers of the retracted eardrum are exposed to a constant pressure. The fibers lose their elasticity and become extended. When the eardrum is less elastic, even minor pressure changes may lead to further retraction and progression of the atrophy.

Risks of atrophy

The atrophic part of the pars tensa is a weak area that is constantly in danger of deteriorating either to a permanent perforation in connection with an episode of common acute otitis or to progression of a posterior atrophy to myringo-incudopexy, myringo-stapediopexy, adhesive otitis or sinus cholesteatoma, owing to impairment of the self-cleaning ability of the retraction. Usually, the desquamated epithelial cells are transported by migration from the retraction toward the meatus and even deep retraction pockets may be dry and peaceful for several years. If the migration for some reason is disturbed, e.g. by bathing, cerumen, external otitis, etc. infection and incrustation may develop in the retraction and the infection may further progress underneath the crust. A granulation formation — herodium[4] — posteriorly in the retraction is the direct result of a local-

Table 1. Prevalence of changes of pars tensa in a randomized cohort of 222 otherwise healthy 7-year old children (444 ears), compared with 527 ears treated with adenoidectomy and grommets for secretory otitis and reevaluated 5-8 years after treatment.

	Randomised cohort		Sequelae to secr. otitis	
	No. = 444	**%**	**No. = 527**	**%**
Diffuse atrophy	5	1,1	32	6,1
Localized atrophy	17	3,8	49	9,3
Atrophy with atelectasis	6	1,4	31	5,9
Posterior atrophy with pexi	9	2,0	17	3,2
Adhesive otitis			13	2,5
Atrophy with perforation	1	0,2	0	
Atrophy and myringosclerosis	6	1,4	48	9,1
Myringosclerosis only	32	7,2	99	18,8
Abnormal tensa	76	17,1	289	54,8
Normal tensa	368	82,9	238	45,2

ized infection and occurred in 2 of our 13 patients with adhesive otitis (table 1). It is evident that bone resorption is increased in an infected retraction pocket.

Perforation of the atrophic area in connection with an episode of common acute suppurative otitis is less likely to recover spontaneously than is a perforation of a normal eardrum, which explains the presence of perforations in many patients with no history of chronic otitis. Localized atrophy, e.g. anteriorly or inferiorly, which often accompanies tympanosclerosis, may explain the anterior and inferior perforations. In posterior perforations, the epithelial membrane often extends from the superior or posterior edge of the perforation toward an intact or defective induco-stapedial joint.

Diffuse atrophy may lead to total or partial perforation of the ear drum. The diffusely atrophic and retracted eardrum with atelectasis may, if infection intervenes, become adherent to the medial wall of the tympanic cavity. The most serious risk for an atelectatic ear is the development of tensa retraction cholesteatoma.

Definition of attic retractions

The Shrapnell's membrane is usually much thinner than the pars tensa, containing few fibrous fibers in a rather thin lamina propria. As it is usually quite transparent, there is hardly a

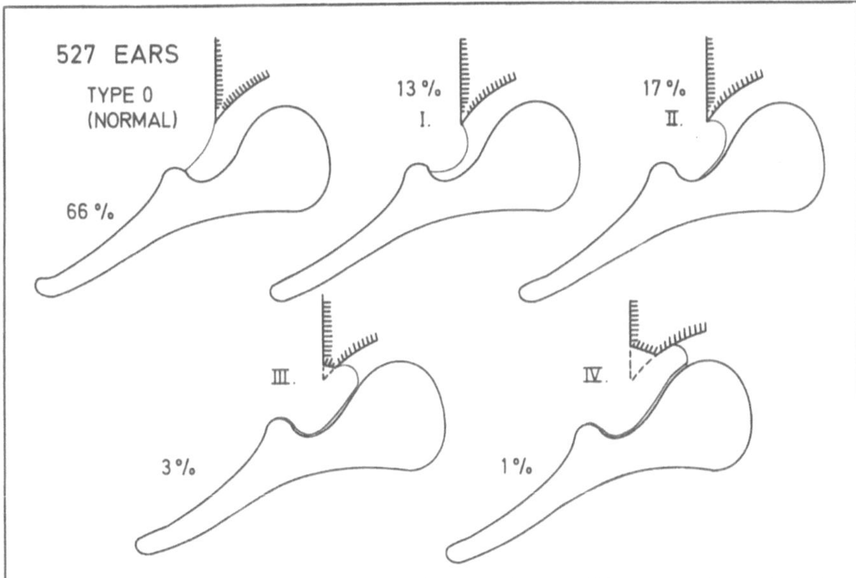

Fig. 1. The definition of four types of attic retractions and the percentage of each type seen 5-8 years after treatment of 527 ears with secretory otitis with adenoidectomy and grommets.

question of atrophy but rather of retraction. We have divided the attic retractions into 4 types[5] (figure 1): Type I indicates a slight retraction and air is visible between the Shrapnell's membrane and the neck of the malleus. In type II, the Shrapnell's membrane is retracted down to the neck of the malleus and no air is visible. The Shrapnell's membrane may adhere to the neck of the malleus, but this is not always the case. Type III indicates a retraction extending behind the osseous annulus, but, on tilting the patient's head, air is visible in the attic. There may be some resorption of the osseous annulus and the Shrapnell's membrane is thereby enlarged. Type IV indicates rather pronounced bone resorption, and the Shrapnell's membrane adheres to the head of the malleus and the incus, which are clearly visible. Because of bone resorption, the bottom of the retraction is still visible. When the bottom cannot be seen, even after cleaning of the pocket, the condition is denoted attic cholesteatoma.

Whereas a type I retraction is harmless and reversible, reflecting the actual negative pressure, a type II retraction may be irreversible if there are adhesions. Type III and IV retractions must be considered irreversible. We have previously discussed the stability of the attic retractions and their possible progression.[2] An attic retraction may constitute the basis for attic cholesteatoma.[1] Retention of desquamated epithelium in a retraction with disturbed migration may lead to infection, incrustation, and proliferation of the basal cells of the epithelium. By expansive growth this precholesteatoma condition may progress to the epitympanum.[6]

Prevalence of attic retractions

In a randomized cohort of otherwise healthy children observed with tympanometry and otomicroscopy from age 4 to 7 years, attic retractions occured in 15 % of the ears at age 5 years (table 2). The prevalence increased significantly from age 5 to 7 years (X^2 test, $p<0.05$). The most frequent

Table 2. Retractions of the Shrapnell's membrane in a cohort of 222 randomized otherwise healthy children, observed with tympanometry and otomicroscopy from 4 to 7 years of age.

Type of attic retraction	No. = 444 ears		
	5 years %	6 years %	7 years %
Type I (slight)	7,7	10,4	9,9
Type II	6,1	7,4	9,7
Types III and IV	1,1	2,0	2,0
Total	14,9	19,8	21,6
	├── p<0.05 ──┤		

retraction was type I, whereas types III and IV were rare, though occurring in 2 % of all 7-year-old children. In a consecutive series of children treated for secretory otitis with tubulation and adenoidectomy, attic retractions were found in 35 % of 527 ears 5-8 years after treatment (figure 1), but severe retractions occurred in only few ears.

Discussion

Owing to limitations of space, only the definitions of eardrum changes will be correlated to those presented by other workers.

Sadé et al.[7] proposed the term "metula", which is no better than the usually employed attic retraction. The graduation of attic retractions mentioned here appears to include the most frequently occurring conditions.[5]

The retractions of pars tensa are denoted atelectasis by Sadé and Berco[4], who proposed the following graduation: Stage I, slight retraction of pars tensa; stage II, retraction extending to the incus or the stapes; stage III, retraction extending to the promontory, and stage IV, adhesive otitis, when the eardrum is adherent. I agree on several points with this classification which does not deviate much from ours, though I would reserve the term "atelectasis" for a diffuse, slack, atrophic eardrum extending to the promontory, i.e. corresponding to Sadé[4] stage III. Our division aims at the permanent changes, such as atrophy and myringosclerosis, which is why we introduced the term "diffuse and localized atrophy without retraction", since these apparently are permanent changes. In contrast, we do not include the frequently occurring retraction of an otherwise normal eardrum (Sadé's atelectasis, stage I)[4], as this condition is extremely unstable and reflects the actual negative middle ear pressure. I do not think that a transient retraction of the eardrum should be denoted atelectasis. Our posterior retraction with pexis corresponds to Sadé's[4] atelectasis, stage II.

References:

1. TOS M. Relationship between secretory otitis in childhood and chronic otitis and its sequelae in adults. *J. Laryng. Otol.*95, 1011-1022, 1981.
2. TOS M., STANGERUP S-E., HOLM-JENSEN S., SØRENSEN C.H. Spontaneous course of secretory otitis and changes of the ear drum. *Arch. Otolaryng. 110, 281-289, 1984.*
3. TOS M., POULSEN G. Changes of pars tensa after secretory otitis. *ORL 41, 313-328, 1979.*
4. SADE J., BERCO E. Atelectasis and secretory otitis media. *Ann. Otol. (St. Louis),* Suppl. 25, 85, 66-72, 1976.
5. TOS M., POULSEN G. Attic retractions following secretory otitis. *Acta Otolaryng.* 89, 479-486, 1980.
6. TOS M. Can cholesteatoma be prevented? In: Sadé J. (Ed.): Cholesteatoma and Mastoid Surgery. *Kugler (Amsterdam),* 591-597, 1982.
7. SADE J., AVRAHAM S., BROWN M. Atelectasis, Retraction Pockets and Cholesteatoma. *Acta Otolaryngol.* 92, 501-512, 1981.

Middle ear mucosa

ABSTRACT

J. Sadé

For the last 20 years, the middle ear mucosa has been recognized to be essentially a respiratory or modified respiratory mucosa. As such it contains variable amounts of mature and specifically differentiated cells which can produce and synthesize various proteins and organelles. Glycoproteins, the backbone of mucus, is the most abundantly produced specifically proteinous substance - but lately keratin has been recognized to be a rather constant intracellular fellow traveller. The most prominent organelles are obviously the cilia. The mucosa cells have usually a relatively short life, and are reproduced again and again from stem cells which are active throughout the life of the organism. Thus, the stem cells divide and can mature into any specific mucosal cell - secondary to triggers and special conditions, and the mucosa can change the proportion of its various cell population accordingly.

Respiratory mucosa in general and therefore middle ear mucosa in particular, do not have a static cellular population. The mucosa is usually exposed during our life to various pathological influences, infections and differences in pressure and gas composition - and reacts accordingly. In fact, it may be correct to say that after birth, the mucosa in even the normal person is actually not quite "normal" - because most middle ear mucosa lining has been exposed to various influences and has reacted. Thus, what we usually find in man and animal is the reacting mucosa. This reaction, which is often mild, is however much more pronounced under inflammatory conditions. The main questions which confront us otologists are:

— the qualitative changes,

— the durability of these changes, and

— the reversibility of these changes in the middle ear mucosa.

The most frequent reaction in the middle ear is the appearance of more mucus-producing cells which produce more mucus than under non-irritative conditions. However, at times, cells appear which also produce more keratin than the mere traces found intracellularly, under normal conditions.

Often both types, mucus- and keratin-producing cells, are actually seen together, even side by side, as has been demonstrated by several investigators (Bendek, Palva, Friedman, Sadé, Lim, Paparella, Tos, Hentzer). This can be seen in secretory and in chronic otitis media. While the appearance of cells which synthesize more glycoprotein (mucus) or keratin is only a reaction to some influence, nevertheless, these reactions may prove to be the main manifestations of the pathological process. For us, clinicians, this chain of events is of great importance, but of even greater importance is the fact that at times the same or very similar reactions last for a short time - at others for a long time: months and years. Indeed, at times these alterations are irreversible, with major consequences to the integrity of the middle ear cleft and its future and treatment.

The pathology of tympanosclerosis

A. G. Gibb

Tympanosclerosis is an abnormal healing response characterised by the deposition of masses of collagen beneath the lining epithelium of the middle ear. It is generally agreed that the condition is the end result of previous inflammation of the middle ear cleft. Thus any of the tympanic structures may be involved in the process so that accurate classification is complicated and the assessment of results of treatment may be correspondingly difficult. I intend therefore first to discuss the pathology of the condition and thereafter attempt to devise a classification based on the pathological findings.

The pathological process can be considered from three different aspects:

— its extent and location,
— the histological appearances of the collagenous deposits,
— the interference with function.

Extent and location

Although an inflammatory process extending throughout the middle ear cleft could theoretically involve any of the tympanic structures, tympanosclerosis has a very distinctive and characteristic distribution. In certain areas it is distinctly common while in others it seldom occurs. It is frequently observed in the tympanic membrane as so-called "chalk patches". In the middle ear the most commonly involved area is the region of the oval window and the incudo-stapedial joint together with the adjacent areas of the promontory. Structures such as the stapedius tendon, horizontal part of the Fallopian canal and the shallow sulcus immediately inferior to the latter are also frequently affected. Plaques are also fairly common in the attic and around the malleus but are conspicuous by their absence over the lower promontory, the hypotympanum, the round window and the Eustachian tube areas. Involvement of the mastoid process is also thought to be rare, but the exact incidence is uncertain as this area is seldom explored in operations for tympanosclerosis. However, deposits are not uncommon in the mastoid aditus and undoubtedly occur from time to time in the air cell system.

The reasons for this somewhat odd distribution of tympanosclerosis remain obscure. In general, however, it will be observed that tympanosclerotic deposits tend to form mainly around the ossicles and especially in narrow or cul-de-sac areas, where glandular secretions and ciliary activity are virtually absent. This picture suggests possible failure in the clearance of inflammatory exudates following middle ear infection.

When considering the formation of plaques in the tympanic membrane, the recent work of Tos et al.[1] is worthy of mention. He believes that tympanosclerotic deposits develop in association with secretory otitis media and the incidence is increased when the tympanic membrane mobility is reduced, for example, by the splinting effect of the middle ear fluid or by the insertion of a grommet. Lack of tympanic membrane movement, e.g. on swallowing, combined with mild inflammatory oedema due to the otitis, causes stasis in the lamina propria of the membrane and increased fibroblastic activity resulting in tympanosclerosis. If this theory is correct it would explain why tympanosclerosis is so often encountered in the remnants of tympanic membranes where perforations are present.

Histological appearances

Tympanosclerosis is of mesodermal origin and affects the connective tissue of the middle ear. Secondary changes may occur also in the ossicles if they are surrounded completely by tympanosclerotic masses. Tympanosclerotic plaques occur either in the stratum fibrosum of the tympanic membrane or between the lining epithelium and periosteum elsewhere in the middle ear. On macroscopic examination the plaques appear as white patches in the tympanic membrane or as raised white masses in the tympanic cavity. It is possible, under the operating microscope, to recognise two distinct types of plaques:

— a softer creamy type, rubbery to the touch, which, on removal, tends to peel off in onion layers,

— a pure white, extremely hard,

dense plaque often firmly adherent to the surrounding bone. The latter, if thin, may crack if the plaque is removed.

On light microscopy the tissue is seen to consist of masses of collagen bundles, almost totally devoid of cells (even nuclei) and blood vessels, covered by an extremely thin flattened epthelium. The collagen is birefringent to polarised light, stains red with Van Gieson's stain and the bundles exhibit an irregular fibrillar appearance. The detailed structure of the collagen is seen clearly on electron microscopy. In some cases the structure of the bundles is lost and an amorphous hyaline mass results. The term "hyaline" indicating a glassy structureless mass on light microscopy is, however, appropriate only in a limited number of cases of tympanosclerosis. Deposition of calcium is common and areas of new bone may be distinguished. Usually plaques in which there is extensive calcium deposition are harder and whiter than the plaques of collagen.

Ossicles adjacent to tympanosclerotic tissue, especially the incus, frequently appear motheaten, porous and demineralised when viewed under the operating microscope. Histological sections confirm the presence of bone absorption with replacement by tympanosclerotic tissue. Absorption of considerable areas of bone is not uncommon so that ossicular discontinuity may result. While I do not believe that there is any active bone destruction in tympanosclerosis it appears nevertheless that this bone absorption is directly related to the tympanosclerotic process. The probable mechanism is as follows: while in the normal ear the overlying mucous membrane provides an adequate blood supply to the ossicles, the mucosa becomes displaced or destroyed in tympanosclerosis so that the ossicle loses contact with the mucous membrane and becomes encased in an avascular sheath of collagen. As a result, the blood supply is seriously impaired and a slow avascular necrosis results.

Interference with function

Tympanosclerosis is important as it is frequently associated with an impaired sound conduction mechanism due either to stiffness or discontinuity. The tympanic membrane and/or the ossicular chain may be affected. Plaques in the tympanic membrane may be unimportant if they are small but large plaques tend to impair the membrane's elasticity and its ability to vibrate. Large plaques also may gain attachment to the tympanic annulus or to the handle of malleus (or both) and when this happens, movement may be totally lost. Perforations of the tympanic membrane are frequently encountered in cases of tympanosclerosis. How exactly they relate to this condition is uncertain but their presence cannot be ignored and, indeed, the work of Tos suggests that perforations may actually play an important part in the development of tympanosclerosis in adjacent parts of the tympanic membrane. Thus, as far as the treatment is concerned, the repair of a perforation is just as important as removal of a large plaque.

In ossicular chain problems any or all of the ossicles may be affected either by stiffness or erosion. By far the most common area to be involved is the long process of incus, but the superstructure of the stapes and handle of malleus may also be affected. The latter, however, is less frequently eroded, probably due to the fact that the tympanosclerosis seldom surrounds the malleus and it continues to receive a blood supply from the vessel which runs along the manubrium in the substances of the tympanic membrane.

From the point of view of treatment it is important to decide whether tympanosclerosis, if excised, is likely to recur. The histological appearances suggest that the condition is essentially inactive and experience also suggests that recurrences, if they occur, are rare. The condition therefore is amenable to the standard tympanoplastic procedures, including stapedectomy. However, in very severe and extensive

Table 1. Recording of tympanosclerosis
According to: — Site — Structure (histology) — Effects on functional mechanism

Table 2. Site(s)

Tympanic membrane	Quadrant	Ant. sup. Ant. Inf. Post. Sup. Post. Inf.	**Diagram** ○	Code: Severity O=nil 1=mild 2=moderate 3=severe
Ossicles	malleus incus stapes	head handle L.P. S.P. body ant. crus post. crus footplate stapedius		Code: Severity 0-3
Cavity Walls	attic Fallopian canal promontory upper lower processus C. tensor tymp. round window Eustachian tube hypotympanum			Code: Severity 0-3

cases the old-fashioned fenestration of the horizontal semicircular canal may have to be considered as a possible method of treatment.

Classification related to evaluation of treatment

Based on the extent and sites of the tympanosclerosis, its histological nature and its effect on the sound conduction mechanism, I have devised a classification which might form a basis for the evaluation of results of surgical treatment. This is outlined in tables 1-5. A broad outline of the techniques employed in treatment is incorporated in table 6.

Table 3. Structure (histology)

	Code:
Collagen	Absent = 0
Calcification	Present = +
Ossification	Severe = +++

Table 4. Effects on functional mechanism

Tympanic membrane=	Code: S=stiffness E=erosion
M=	
I =	
S=	Severity 0=nil
Air space reduction	1=mild 3=severe (complete)

Table 5. Other relevant factors

1. Concomitant disease (active)
2. Ventilation tube(s)
   (a) present
   (b) previous
3. Other

Table 6. Treatment

Excision of plaques
  tympanic membrane
  middle ear
Reconstructive procedures
By-pass operations
Nil

Reference:

1. TOS M., BONDING P., POULSEN G. Tympanosclerosis of the drum in secretory otitis after insertion of grommets. A prospective, comparative study. *J. Laryngol. Otol.* 97:489-496.

Congenital middle ear pathology

ABSTRACT
D. Plester

During the last 15 years we have treated 184 patients with minor malformations of the middle ear. The stapes was most frequently affected. Forty-three per cent of the cases had an isolated stapes deformity, 32 % together with malformations of the long process of the incus, 13 % with the entire ossicular chain involved, and 2 % with the malleus. The stapedius tendon was missing in a third of the cases of stapes deformities. In 3/4 of the patients the stapes footplate was fixed due to defective development of the annular ligament. In the remainder of the cases the superstructure of the stapes was deformed or missing. In 12 cases of minor deformities we found the columella form of the stapes, frequently with a small footplate. Particulars concerning stapes surgery for malformations are covered in detail.

In only 4 patients we saw isolated deformities of the incus combined with osseus fixation to the posterior canal wall. Isolated fixations of the head of the malleus are considered in only a few exceptional cases in our statistics. In our opinion, the causes are only rarely congenital deformities, although a narrow epitympanum can be considered a constitutional predisposition. In 8 cases we found a persistent stapedial artery. Of these cases, one lacked an embryologically preformed oval window, two had a fixed stapes footplate, and one lacked a stapes head.

In 16 % of the cases there were anomalous courses of the facial nerve in the area of the oval window or over the promontory together with ossicular deformities, primarily of the stapes. In such cases the creation of a promontory window can lead to very good hearing results. Our own surgical techniques are described in detail.

SYMPOSIUM IV
Postoperative complications

Chairman: U. Fisch

Postoperative complications

U. Fisch

Postoperative complications are secondary conditions (or diseases) developing unexpectedly after a surgical intervention. As for the evaluation of postoperative results a subjective element casts its shadow over the "objective" evaluation of postoperative results. A surgical act remains a hybrid produced by the blending of scientific and artistic attitudes. To reduce surgery to pure science is as wrong as to elevate it to a pure act of artistic creation. In order to find a common language in the grey zone between art and science that characterizes surgical actions, one needs maximal transparency on the employed technique as well as on the criteria used to analyze the obtained results. The requirements for the "scientific" reporting of postoperative data - invariably joined to the unspoken accusation of "unscientific" behaviour for all those who do not comply with the established rule - fit well in the present day longing for unlimited, suffocating bureaucracy but may destroy individual creativity in the name of collective uniformity.

Keeping the above mentioned limitations in mind, any reasonable attempt to standardize the postoperative evaluation of complication in middle ear surgery has to be welcomed. In the excellent paper on "postoperative evaluation of middle ear surgery", J. Marquet and A. Graff[1] listed the requirements for adequate assessment of postoperative complications as follows:

— the precise **definition** of

anatomical or functional conditions that alter the expected postoperative course;
— the correct report of the **time interval** between surgery and the appearance of the complication;
— the distinction between **the total number of patients or of cases** having complications;
— the accurate **analysis of the cause of a complication** (surgical fault, residual or recurrent pathology, true postoperative problem).

In the following papers seven world-acknowledged experts brilliantly review the postoperative complications induced by infections and antibiotics, with respect to loss of hearing, vestibular and facial function, the fate of implanted materials and the study of recurrent and residual cholesteatoma after intact canal wall tympanoplasty. The papers will speak for themselves and have led to comments from the moderator.

The fact, that the infectious complications of middle ear surgery are more common when an operation is performed by a resident in training rather than by a member of the faculty staff, is not surprising. In view of the correct supervision of the residents, the observed complications have to be considered the price paid for learning. The question is whether this "necessary" price has to be paid for all residents undergoing training in our speciality when the decreasing number of patients requiring highly specialized interventions, such as stapedectomy, decreases at the point to hardly justify the performance of occasional operations.

Hearing loss due to postoperative adhesions in the middle ear mucosa will continue to defy all preventive measures as long as the basic problem of tubal dysfunction is not eliminated.

Vestibular complications of middle ear surgery are rare but very invalidating. Prof. Pfaltz is right in pointing out the dangers to the labyrinth, whenever surgery results in the unexpected opening of the labyrinthine spaces. Removal of cholesteatoma matrix over a labyrinthine fistula as well as excessive manipulations to free the stapes from pathology (granulations or cholesteatoma) should be avoided when they endanger the integrity of the perilymphatic space. There is always the possibility of coming back to the critical disease areas in a second-stage procedure later on.

The complications of stapedectomy have been extensively reviewed by Mr. Dowes. The only addition we would like to make relates to postoperative tinnitus and facial palsy. Severe postoperative tinnitus is rare but even in the presence of successful stapedectomy can disable the patient to a point that the sacrifice of the cochlear nerve must be considered. We do also believe that stapedotomy is a positive evolution in stapes surgery since it reduces the possible adverse effects of excessive surgical manipulations at the oval window in otosclerosis.

With regard to intraoperative facial nerve injuries we do not think that today "immediate exploration is indicated when in doubt about the extent of the lesion".

Repeated electrical testing, preferably by electroneurography, permits one to follow the course of denervation of the facial muscles (respectively degeneration of the facial nerve motor fibres). Experience[2] has shown that if denervation reaches less than 90 % within six days from the onset of the paralysis a perfect recovery can be expected without surgical revision. The few extra days required for the correct assessment of denervation of the facial muscles do not compromise the outcome of a successive surgical revision and may avoid unnecessary activism.

The search for the best biocompatible material for ossicular substitution continues. It may be questioned whether the appearance of a single giant cell around or in an implanted material is sufficient to disqualify its clinical use. Consideration should be given to the fact that a limited amount of tissue reaction is necessary to provide fixation of the implant. That the "best may be enemy of the good" may prove true also when using implanted materials.

Finally, the appearance of recurrent or residual cholesteatoma one year after intact canal wall tympanoplasty cannot be blamed on the operation only but also on its indication and on the surgical technique used. (For instance, the reinforcement of the postero-superior quadrant of the drum with cartilage considerably reduces the number of new retraction pockets.)

In conclusion, the general analysis of the presented papers shows that there is a great need for a more transparent documentation of conditions altering the expected postoperative course. Adequate guidelines standardizing reports on postoperative complications will improve multicentric evaluation of surgical procedures.

References:

1. MARQUET J., GRAFF A. Postoperative evaluation of middle ear surgery. *Audiology* 21: 20-32, 1982.
2. FISCH U. Prognostic value of electrical tests in acute facial paralysis. *Amer. J. Otol.* (in press).

Postoperative infections secondary to ear surgery - Antimicrobial therapy

A. J. Maniglia

Introduction

Surgical procedures involving the temporal bone are performed mainly for the following reasons:
— eradication of infectious processes,
— improvement of hearing,
— control or cure of vertigo or tinnitus,
— removal of neoplasms, cysts or arterio-venous anomalies involving the temporal bone, skull base or cerebello pontine angle.

Fortunately acute infections manifesting as postoperative complications are not common. The cause of such postoperative infections are:
— virulence of micro-organisms following residual infections which did not respond to postoperative antibiotic therapy,
— low resistance as in cases of diabetes mellitus, immunocompromized hosts etc.,
— contaminations in the operating room or during the immediate postoperative period,
— iatrogenesis due to poor surgical technique or excessive duration of the procedure.

These contribute to trauma and contamination of inner ear, temporal bone adjacent structures such as dura, subarachnoid space, major vessels or even brain tissue. The postoperative infections following ear surgery may be: otitis externa, otitis media, mastoiditis, labyrinthitis, meningitis, cerebritis, brain abscess and lateral sinus thrombosis with infection. In spite of adequate surgical technique and even if all precautions are properly taken, postoperative infections following temporal bone surgery may happen in the hands of the most experienced surgeons.

The review of the literature reveals a paucity of reports dealing with specific postoperative infections following otologic surgery. Several papers allude to complications secondary to previously done surgery involving the temporal bone![1,9]

Our clinical experience

From 1968-1984 we have had a rather extensive surgical experience with procedures perfomed in the temporal bone and adjacent structures. Our complications of serious postoperative infections are described on table 1 and 2. Regarding stapedectomy we have reviewed the experience at our institution, University of Miami, Jackson Memorial Medical Center[8]. From 1978-1980, 95 stapedectomies were performed. Sixty-six cases were residents' cases and 29 were private cases performed by the faculty. The series

TABLE 1. Serious postoperative infections following temporal bone surgery (1968-1984)

Procedure	No. cases	Labyrinthitis	Meningitis	Perichondritis
Stapedectomy	> 500	6	0	0
Tympanoplasty	> 1000	3	2	2
Glomus tumors	15	0	1	0
Temporal bone cancer	11	0	1	0

TABLE 2. Postoperative meningitis (1968-1984)

Procedure	No. Cases	Meningitis	%
Endolymphatic sacmastoid shunt	100	0	0
Removal of CPA tumors	89	8	9

of cases performed by the resident physicians in training with supervision, indeed, show a far greater rate of complications compared with the series done by the faculty members. Table 3, summarizes these complications. Seven out of 19 complications which occur in the residents' group were infectious processes. It is fair to conclude that inadequate surgical technique and the duration of the surgical procedure are the main factors responsible for the difference in the complication rate between the two groups. We have the temerity to go so far in recommending that a resident physician should do at least eight stapedectomies during his training with a reasonable success rate in order to incorporate such procedure in his surgical armamentarium. Stapedectomy in the hands of the very occasional operator may very well lead to disastrous results.

Surgery for chronic ear disease may also result in serious complications. Meningitis has occurred in two of our cases (0,2 %). Those cases were of extensive cholesteatoma with infection and dural exposure. Both patients recovered without any neurological deficit. We strongly feel, advocate and teach that the posterior canal

TABLE 3. Complications of stapedectomy, n = 95 operations (1978-1980)

Complications	Resident	Faculty
Suppurative otitis media	5	0
External otitis	1	0
Perforations	8	0
Facial paralysis	1	0
Anacusis	2	0
Serous otitis media	0	1
Labyrinthitis	1	0
Total	19	1

TABLE 4. Intracranial abscesses secondary to ear and sinus infections

Case No.	Age	Sex	Etiology	Surgical treatment	Organism isolated	Comments
01	30	M	Cholesteatoma	Radical mastoidectomy Drainage cerebellar abscess	Bacteroides fragilis	Alive and well
02	41	M	Cholesteatoma	Radical mastoidectomy Drainage cerebellar abscess	Proteus morgani	Alive and well
03	15	M	Cholesteatoma	Prior mastoidectomy canal wall up	Proteus mirabilis	Fulminating cerebellar abscess brain stem compression and hemorrhage Expired before neurosurgical procedure could be done
04	19	M	Cholesteatoma	Mastoidectomy Posterior fossa craniectomy for drainage of subdural empyema	Proteus mirabilis Peptostreptococcus	Alive and well
05	54	M	Mastoiditis Granulation tissue	Prior mastoidectomy	Klebsiella	Temporal lobe abscess. Died of bacterial endocarditis before neurosurgical procedure
06	19	F	Cholesteatoma	Prior mastoidectomy canal wall up Radical mastoidectomy drainage middle fossa Epidural abscess	Escherichia coli	Alive and well

wall should be removed in cases of cholesteatoma involving the mastoid. Those who advocate preservation of the posterior canal wall stress the fact that the follow-up must be very close and second or third "looks" may be necessary. Table 4 describes our experience in treating intracranial abscesses secondary to ear infections.[9] Cases no. 3 and no. 6 (which came from elsewhere) had tympanomastoidectomy with preservation of the posterior canal wall for removal of cholesteatoma. Case no. 3 died, due to a fulminating cerebellar abscess with brain stem compression and hemorrhage before any neurosurgical procedure could be contemplated. Case no. 6 developed an intracranial abscess (epidural) and was successfully treated by undergoing radical mastoidectomy and adequate intravenous antibiotic therapy. Even in the hands of experienced surgeons there is a 10 to 20 % recurrence rate of cholesteatoma, even much greater in the pediatric age group. The patient population of teaching hospitals is far from being reliable regarding compliance with follow-up visits. Dreadful complications and even death may occur due to unchecked recurrent or residual cholesteatomas. Intracranial abscess secondary to ear infection occurring in the cerebellum, temporal lobe or epidural space may be successfully surgically

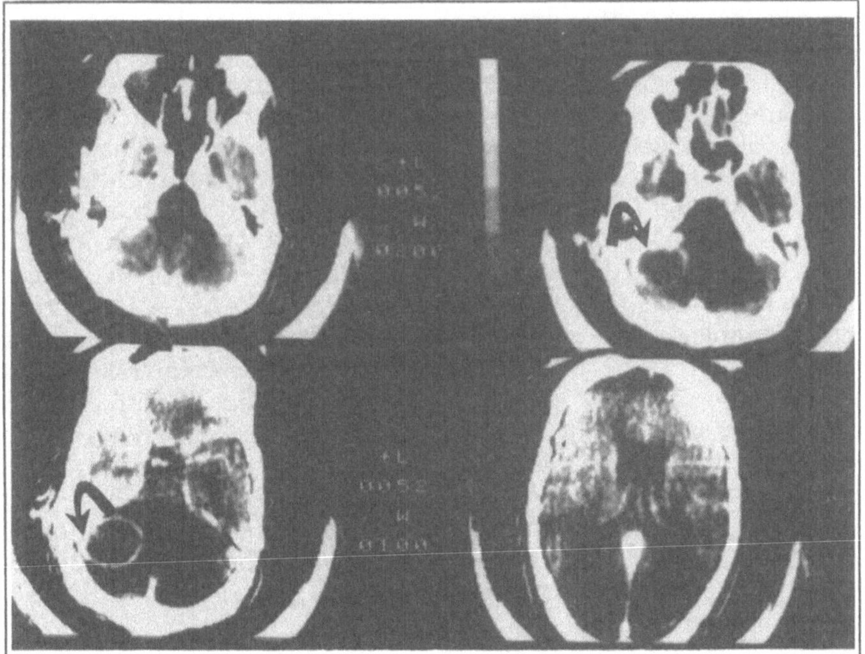

Fig. 1. This horizontal cut CT scan illustrates the cerebellar abscess with capsule and ring formation (arrow).

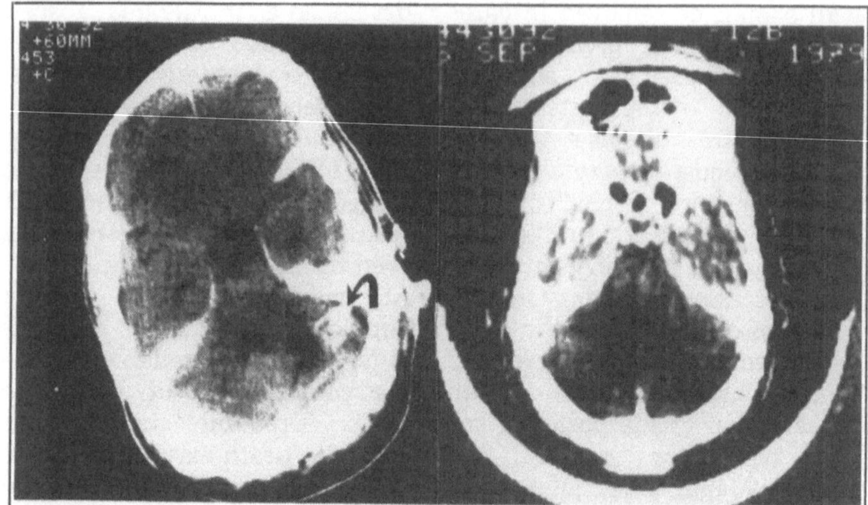

Fig. 2. Left side: cerebellar abscess drained through the mastoid approach. Procedure performed by the otologic surgeon with neurosurgical cooperation (arrow).
Right side: control CT scan (postoperatively). This patient has been doing well four years after drainage of the cerebellar abscess.

treated through the temporal bone by the otologic surgeon with close neurosurgical cooperation. Computerized axial tomography has revolutionized the treatment of intracranial abscesses optimizing the timing for medial and surgical management. Figures 1 and 2 illustrate the approach, successfully used, to treat patient no. 2 of table 4.

Discussion

Tympanomastoidectomy using the intact wall technique for removal of cholesteatoma, in our opinion, should not be taught in residency training programs. Endolymphatic sac drainage procedures are quite popular in the treatment of intractible vertigo in cases of Ménière's disease.[10,11,12] Endolymphatic sac subarachnoid shunt may also carry the complication of cerebro-spinal fluid leak and meningitis.[4] It is known that one case of death secondary to such complication had occurred.[13] It is well documented in the literature that addition of the subarachnoid shunt does not statistically improve the success rate of control of vertigo in cases of Ménière's disease.[14] Most authors favor decompression of the endolymphatic sac with drainage into the mastoid cavity.[14,15] The results are just as good as subarachnoid shunt procedure but it carries a much lesser risk of infections, affecting the central nervous system.[16,17]

House and Hitzelberg have reported a 15,5 % incidence of meningitis following acoustic neuroma surgery.[5] Some cases have resulted in death! Our experience in a much smaller series is similar (table 2). In order to reduce the incidence of meningitis we feel that intraoperative irrigation of the wound with bacitracyn powder is indicated. Small tumors occurring especially in the older age group of patients should be followed by periodic CT scan with contrast.[6] Yearly CT scans appear to be adequate because vestibular schwannomas are known to be very slow growing neoplasms. We feel that surgery should be reserved mainly if there is convincing evidence of rapid growth of the tumor. Computerized axial tomography provides a non-invasive technique for evaluation of these posterior fossa tumors and indeed has changed the indications of the surgical management of these tumors.

Perichondritis as a postoperative complication is rare.[18] The incidence is about one to every five hundred cases (table 1). It is more prone to occur in cases of diabetic patients or with a history of a previous surgical procedure.[19] Small vessel disease and scar tissue secondary to previous surgery results in poor blood supply of the perichondrium with possible perichondritis. The treatment of choice is appropriate intravenous antibiotic therapy, usually carbenicillin and tobramycin, cephalosporin or oxacillin. Pseudomonas aeruginosa, Proteus and Staphylococcus are the most commonly cultured organisms. Surgical debridment or tubal drainage may often be necessary.[18]

Postoperative ear infections should be recognized early and treated adequately. Collection of materials for culture and sensitivity should be done before antibiotics are started. Knowledge of the incidence of bacterial infection in different clinical pictures is very helpful to speculate what kind of micro-organism will probably be cultured and what kind of antibiotic should be started even before the culture and sensitivity result is available. Anaerobes are known to be slow growers and difficult to culture. Gram stain are very important to identify anaerobic organism causing infection. The principles and the uses of antibiotic therapy in postoperative infections of the ear are very similar to those applied to other infections affecting the temporal bone and other adjacent structures.[20,21,22] Knowledge of the bacteriology of chronic otitis media, acute purulent otitis media, serous otitis media are of utmost importance in the planning of treatment. Figure 3 describes the most common bacteria cultured in purulent otitis media and its complications with attention directed to the appropriate use of antibiotics. Second and third generation cepholosporin are effective against Pseudomonas. Needless to say, one ounce of prevention of infection is indeed worth one

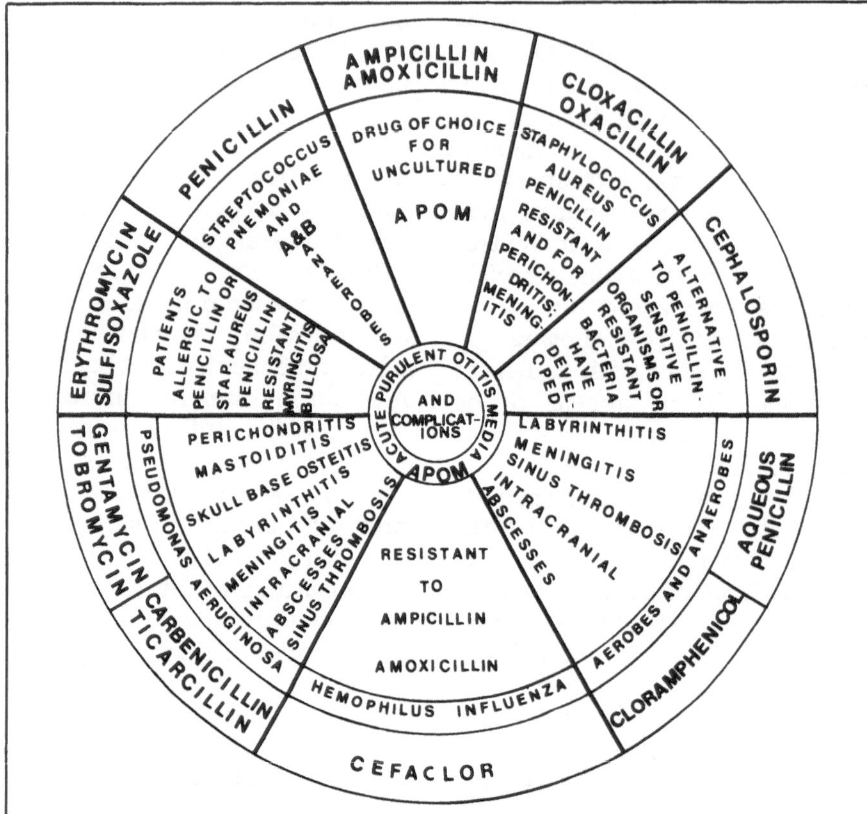

Fig. 3. Description of the antibiotics of choice used in the treatment of acute purulent otitis media, its complications and other infections involving the temporal bone. Second and third generation cephalosporin are very effective in the treatment of Pseudomonas infections.

pound of antibiotic therapy and hours of secondary surgery.

Properly chosen surgical techniques which statistically carry the lowest complication rates but yet afford comparable successful results should minimize the incidence of postoperative infections. Adequate removal of pathology and appropriate choice of antibiotics to be used in the postoperative period should prevent infectious processes which may cause dreadful complications or even death.

References:

1. PALVA T., PALVA A., KARJA J. Fatal meningitis in a case of otosclerosis operated bilaterally. *Arch. Otolaryng.* 96:130, 1972.
2. JABLOKOW V.R., KATURIA S. Fatal meningitis duct to serratia marcescens after stapedectomy. *Arch. Otolaryngol.* 108:34-35, 1982.
3. GRAHAM M.D. Meningitis following stapedectomy. *J. Otolaryngol. 5:42-43, 1976.*
4. PAPARELLA M.M., HANSON D.G. Endolymphatic sac drainage for intractible vertigo (method and experience). *Laryngoscope,* 85:697, 1975.

5. HITSELBERGER W.E., HOUSE W.F. Diagnosis and Management of Acoustic Tumors. *Otolaryngology* (Editor G. English) Vol. 1, Chapter 55, 1983 Harper & Row, Philadelphia.
6. MANIGLIA A.J. Diagnosis and Surgical Treatment of Cerebello pontine angle tumors. *Ear Clin. Intern.* Vol 2, Chapter 31, 193:201, 1982 (Williams & Wilkins, Baltimore/London).
7. MANIGLIA A.J. Intra- and Extracranial Meningiomas Involving the Temporal Bone. *Laryngoscope* Vol. 88, No 9, part 2, Supplement 12, 1978.
8. CHANDLER J.R., RODRIGUES O.T. Changing Patterns of Otosclerosis surgery in teaching institutions. *Otolaryngol. Head Neck Surg.* 91:239-245, 1983.
9. MANIGLIA A.J. et al. Intracranial Abscesses secondary to ear and paranasal sinuses infections. *Otolaryngol. Head Neck Surg.* 88:670-680, 1980.
10. ARENBERG I.K., BALKANY T.J. Prevention of complications and failures in endolymphatic system surgery. *Otolaryng. Clin. North Am.* 15:869-82, 1982.
11. CODY D.T., McDONALD T.J. Endolymphatic subarachnoid shunt operation for idiopathic endolymphatic hydrops. *Laryngoscope* 93:1018-21, 1983.
12. BRACKMAN D.E., ANDERSON R.G. Ménière's disease: Treatment strategies and Results of endolphatic subarachnoid shunt in 125 cases. *Otolaryng. Clin. North Am.* 13:737-44, 1980.
13. BRACKMAN D.E. Personal communication.
14. SNOW J.B., KIMMELMAN C.P. Assessment of surgical procedures for Ménière's disease. *Laryngoscope* 89:737-747, 1979.
15. MEYERHOFF W.L., PAPARELLA M.M. Ménière's Disease and Its various surgical therapies. *Otolaryngol. Clin. North Am.* 13:767-773, 1980.
16. GLASSCOCK M. et al. Surgical Management of Ménière's disease with endolymphatic subarachnoid shunt. *Laryngoscope* 87:1668, 1977.
17. GARDNER G. Endolymphatic sac shunt operation in Ménière's disease. *Trans. Am. Acad. Ophthalmol. Otolaryngol.* 80:306, 1975.
18. BASSIOUNY A. Perichondritis of the Auricle. *Laryngoscope.* 91:422-431, 1981.
19. BELLUCCI R.J. Personal communication.
20. PARKIN J.L. Antimicrobial Treatment of otitis media: Penicillins, cephalosporins, sulfonamides. *Otolaryngol. Head Neck Surg.* 89:376-380, 1981.
21. FAIRBANKS D.N.F. Topical Therapeutics for Otitis media. *Otolaryngol. Head Neck Surg.* 89:381-385, 1981.
22. BROOK I., FEINGOLD S.M. Bacteriology of Chronic Otitis Media. *JAMA* 241:487-488, 1979.

Strategies of overcoming unsuccessful reconstruction of the middle ear air space — Nasal mucosa transplantation

J-I. Suzuki, Y. Kano, H. Hashimoto, A. Kodama

Facilitation of postoperative drainage of the reconstructed middle ear.

Postoperative drainage of the reconstructed middle ear has to be mostly through the Eustachian tube. In the normal middle ear, the Eustachian tube and its orifice area in the tympanum have the densest populations of ciliated cells, which are the major factor promoting the drainage of the whole middle ear cavity. Succesful experiences with tympanoplasty with very fast recovery were usually in those cases with near normal tympanic mucosa, while unsuccessful experiences were mostly in those with defective or wholly pathological tympanic mucosa. Even in the latter cases, the Eustachian tube and its tympanic orifice frequently have near-normal populations of cilia cells, indicating that even this level of such cells in these areas was not sufficient for postoperative drainage of the whole middle ear cavity. Probably, then, the tympanic cavity itself should have a lining of cilia cells for effective drainage of the middle ear cavity. *Drainage should precede ventilation.*

Two methods of facilitating the growth of cilia cells in the reconstructed tympanum can be considered:
— preservation of the mucous membrane in the tympanum as much as possible even if it would appear pathological, and
— transplantation of the ciliated mucous membrane to the area where the mucous membrane is defective. Easy access to the ciliated mucosa to be transplanted is through the use of the nasal mucosa.

In our tympanoplasty, the former, the preservation of even pathological mucosa, has been one of the routine manœvres and we believe that this has been proved to be a useful and important strategy for air cavity recovery.

The latter, the transplantation of the nasal mucosa to the tympanum, is a new idea. The inferior turbinate and the nasal septum are most easily accessible. The mucous membrane should be thinned by shaving the submucosa as thinly as possible just to leave the germinal layer of the epithelium intact and to eliminate nasal glands. The access to the inferior turbinate is easier than to the septum. Although the mucosa over the tip of the inferior turbinate frequently does not have cilia, the renovated epithelium from the germinal cells is expected to be ciliated. For transplantation, accordingly, the inferior turbinate mucosa is recently of routine use in our department.

Since August 1982, nasal mucosa transplantation has been conducted in 25 cases (26 ears) presenting almost complete adhesion of the eardrum and/or wide defective mucosa in the tympanum. Among these cases, those which were operated on between August 1982 and December 1983, 18 (19 ears) in total, were carefully evaluated by microscopic observation, audiometry, CT scan, revision operation, etc.

Table 1 indicates the results of nasal mucosa transplantation. Of the 19 ears, 4 involved adhesive otitis media, 6 cholesteatoma with tympanum adhesion, 5 were referred reoperation cases with tympanum adhesion and 4 presented postoperative adhesion. Evaluation studies revealed that there was no adhesion in 13 cases, partial adhesion at the promontory in 2 cases, and partial adhesion at the posterior wall of the

TABLE 1. Cases of nasal mucosa transplantation

	Cases	Evaluated cases
Adhesive otitis media	4	4
Cholesteatoma with adhesion	8	6
Referred reoperation cases with tympanum adhesion	9	5
Cases with postoperative adhesion	5	4
Total	26	19

TABLE 2. Results after nasal mucosa transplantation

Case / Outcome	Adhesive otitis media	Cholesteatoma with adhesion	Referred reoperation cases with tympanum adhesion	Cases with postoperative adhesion	Total
No adhesion	2	4	3	4	13
Adhesion at the posterior portion of the eardrum	1	2	1	0	4
Adhesion at the promontorium	1	0	1	0	2
Total	4	6	5	4	19

eardrum in 4 (table 2). For proper evaluation, we need still more accumulation of cases and also a comparative study of those without transplantation as well. The present data, however, are quite promising as shown in table 2.

Scanning and transmission electron microscopic as well as light microscopic pictures of the promontorium mucosa where the inferior turbinate mucosa was transplanted six months earlier showed near-normal recovery of the middle ear mucosa. Some specimens showed an impression of denser population of ciliated cells and less population of goblet cells compared to normal tympanic mucosa. No nasal glands were demonstrated.

Removal of attic blockades and assurance of attic routes

In more than 75 % of chronic otitis media and in almost all attic cholesteatomatous otitis media, there are attic blockades. The blockades in the attic have to be removed to drain and to ventilate the mastoid cavity and then to normalize the pathology in the cavity. The pathology in the antrum in chronic otitis media is usually a thickening of the mucosa and a retention of exudates. Thick mucosa in the antrum may not have to be eliminated. In other words, the elimination of blockades in the attic is necessary to facilitate and to secure attic patency and is a sufficient manœuvre for normalization of these cavities, as for the antrum, only massive granulation tissues or extremely thickened mucosa may need to be removed.

The removal of attic blockades without removing or disconnecting the ossicular chain may not always be easily accomplished when blockades are extensive or when there is a cholesteatoma. To remove attic blockades without disconnecting the ossicular chain, some special convenient instruments, such as small flexible curettes of different sizes and the smallest cup forceps, may have to be used.

Type I tympanoplasty as the surgical method of choice

The evaluation of postoperative hearing conducted on 1 051 tympanoplasty cases in our university hospital definitely indicated that the type I tympanoplasty was the best. Consequently, our efforts have been applied to the removal of the blockades in the attic to conduct type I tympanoplasty, if possible, instead of other operations, such as type III with columella.

Postoperative patency of the attic may be better maintained in type I than in type III, probably because of the near-normal supporting framework of the eardum. Attic patency in type I, however, may not be easily maintained postoperatively because of the narrow passages among the framework, especially when attic blockades are partially removed and when postoperative inflammation causes tissue or cellular reactions to reobliterate the attic routes. Although there are successful cases in both type I and III, the percentage of success was higher in the former. We compared the success rate by measuring the air-bone gap decrease within 30 dB and found that it was 89 % in type I, but 75 % in type III with columella.

A spacious antrum cavity should be reconstructed

The whole air space in the middle ear cavity should be reconstructed as spaciously as possible, exactly as in the normal temporal bones. When the air space is limited, for example, only in the tympanic cavity, even minimum changes of the middle ear air pressure, which can be easily caused by Eustachian tubal dysfunction, would affect the mucous membrane physiology and would induce pathological reactions in the cavity. This may be seen in those cases of tympanoplasty with remaining attic blockades, in those of open-method tympanoplasty or in those of modified radical operation.

In the light of these considerations, postoperatively the whole middle ear cavity should be reconstructed to be as large as possible by reconstructing or pre-

serving the antrum and by removing the attic blockades. Postoperative inflammations or infections in the tympanum, which may occur even to the minimum extent, could be better attenuated when a greater amount of air exists in the spacious middle ear cavity.
In view of this speculation, neither oblitaretion nor elimination of the antrum cavity should be undertaken, even with rare exceptions.

Conclusion
As a conclusion to the above considerations and their applications, reconstruction of a spacious middle ear cavity, which should include the antrum, is the first and most important step of tympanoplasty. Ossicular chain reconstruction, as the next step, will then be most successfully accomplished and will result in a stabilized level of expected improvement of hearing.

References:

1. SUZUKI J. The Approaches to Conductive Hearing Loss, Examinations-Diagnosis-Tympanoplasty-Hearing Aids, Shinohara Publishers, Tokyo, 1983.
2. SUZUKI J. et al. Clinical Observations on the Physiology of Mastoid Antrum and Cells (in preparation).

Vestibular complications following middle ear surgery

C.R. Pfaltz

The vestibular part of the inner ear may suffer accidental injury either from mechanical energy (direct traumatization by surgical instruments, indirect traumatization by transmission of high energy sound) or it may be injured by thermal energy, due to unskilful drilling close to the osseous labyrinth.

Acoustic trauma
The contact between the rotating burr and an intact ossicular chain (particularly incus and stapes) will cause a transmission of high energy sound and produce inner ear lesions very similar to gun shot trauma (brief exposure to a very loud sound). Paparella placed 4 mm sharp cutting burrs (6 grooves) rotating at 15 000-18 000 rpm, as commonly used in ear surgery, on the body of the incus for periods of time varying from 5-20 seconds for the different animals. On behavioural audiograms these animals exhibited severe high frequency hearing losses. Histological studies showed cochlear injuries characteristic of acoustic trauma. However, as a rule, this type of surgical lesion does not induce vestibular symptoms.

Dislocaton of the stapes and incus

Accidental luxation or fracture of the stapes associated with fistulization of the oval window may occur during mastoid and middle ear surgery and was more common prior to the development of surgical microscopes.[2] With modern surgical techniques this type of injury occurs less frequently, but should it occur it ought to be recognized by the following symptoms:

Table 1. Symptomatology of stapes dislocation
• Combined conductive and sensorineural hearing loss (the former involving the lower and middle frequencies, the latter frequencies above 2 000 cps). • Tinnitus. • Constant, permanent dizziness, increased by head movements and changes of position. • Horizontal-rotatory spontaneous nystagmus towards the normal ear, increased by quick head movements and in a position with the operated ear uppermost.

The symptoms are due to a progressive serous, i.e. non-infectious labyrinthitis, caused by chronic perilymph leakage and bleeding into the perilymphatic space. Immediate revision of the tympanic cavity, particularly the oval and round window niche, is indicated. According to the severity of the lesion, the following microsurgical procedures must be carried out (table 2).

Table 2. Surgical management of stapes dislocation
• Reposition of the dislocated stapes - or • stapedectomy and closure of the oval window by a perichondrial or fascia graft, followed by a replacement of the extracted, fractured stapes (cartilage or plastic strut) - or • in case of a dislocated incus with dislocation and fracture of the stapes: stapedectomy (eventually only the suprastructure) closure of the oval window with perichondrium or fascia, transposition of the incus (columellization).

Surgical fistulization of the labyrinth

Probably the most common injury to the inner ear during mastoid surgery is inadvertent opening of the lateral semicircular canal. The canal is vulnerable because of its prominent position in the floor of the mastoid antrum. The creation of a small fistula without tearing of the membraneous semicircular canal may be tolerated without incident.[2] If, however, the membraneous canal is injured by tearing the membrane with the tip of the suction, or with a needle while removing granulations from the antrum, the usual result is a profound hearing loss and a moderate to severe loss of vestibular function.[3] The cochleo-vestibular disorder shows the following subjective and objective symptoms in cases of a subtotal or total inner ear damage (table 3).

Immediate surgical revision of the labyrinth, particularly of the horizontal semicircular canal, is absolutely indicated in order to save the remaining function and to prevent the development of a progressive labyrinthitis (closure of the fistula by cartilage, temporalis fascia and fibrin glue).

Table 3. Symptomatology of surgical fistulization of the labyrinth
• Severe permanent vertigo with turning sensations. • Severe nausea. • Tinnitus and complete deafness in the operated ear. • Spontaneous nystagmus, horizontal-rotatory, directed towards the normal ear. • Ataxia. • Severe partial or total loss of cochlear function.
In cases of a partial damage of the inner ear: • Positional vertigo. • Tinnitus. • High tone hearing loss (sensorineural type). • Positional nystagmus with the operated ear uppermost, mainly horizontal-rotatory, directed towards the normal ear, persistent.

Surgical fistulization of the labyrinth may occur more rarely at the level of the *posterior* or *superior semicircular canal* in case of the removal of a large cholesteatoma. Postoperative symptoms are less characteristic because initially the patient will only complain about a slight constant dizziness, increased by rapid head movements or by change of the position, which are sometimes accompanied by tinnitus and a mild hearing impairment. After some time the patient will develop progressive instability which is due to a *non-infectious, serous labyrinthitis* and as soon as the operation cavity is filled up by granulation tissue the patient will suffer from a *positive labyrinth fistula symptom,* whenever he touches or pulls his external ear, because the shearing forces are transmitted via the fibrous tissue to the open fistula and induce a mechanical (pneumatic) irritation of the membraneous labyrinth. Surgical revision of the mastoid cavity is absolutely indicated. The granulation tissue has to be removed, the fistula must be cleaned and sealed with a lid of tragal cartilage, perichondrium or fascia, fixed by fibrin glue.

Inflammatory labyrinthine fistula

A labyrinthine fistula is most commonly the sequel of a cholesteatoma. The most frequent location is again the dome of the horizontal semicircular canal. The fistula may be total, with complete exposure of the perilymphatic space or subtotal, with bone erosion but only marginal exposure of the endosteum, covering the perilymphatic space.[4]

The most common symptom is vertigo, accompanied by a discrete spontaneous vestibular nystagmus, and a *positive fistula phenomenon:*

Subjective symptoms: Attacks of severe vertigo, induced by sneezing, blowing the nose, straining, sudden head movements, Valsalva manœuvre or by manipulation of the auricle.

Objective symptoms: Fast beating nystagmus, induced by applying positive or negative pressure to the external auditory canal or Siegle's otoscope. Characteristically, the nystagmus elicited by positive pressure is directed to the side of the fistula, as soon as positive pressure is changed into negative pressure nystagmus reversed to the normal ear and disappears as soon as the pressure is relieved. Vertigo is produced when movement of the soft tissue, bridging the fistula, displaces endolymphatic fluid, with resultant cupular deflection.

The *surgical management of the fistula* requires delicate techniques to remove the cholesteatoma matrix. If the squamos epithelium is adherent to the connective tissue covering the perilymphatic space, it is recommended to leave the fistula open and remove the matrix at a second stage operation. In the course of time the inflammatory process around and within the fistulous area will regress and gradually heal more or less completely. At this stage it will be much easier to peel off the matrix from the fistula without damaging the membraneous labyrinth. The fistula must then be closed with a bone chip or a cartilage graft, covered by temporalis fascia or perichondrium, fixed with fibrin glue.

If a lesion of the membraneous labyrinth (in most cases of the horizontal semicircular canal) occurs inadvertently, this incident is either due to the careless application of the suction or to the unskilled use of the sharp hook, employed for peeling off the matrix. The surgeon will sometimes not even notice the damage but postoperatively the patient will either develop the symptoms of a *progressive serous labyrinthitis,* if the lesion is only partial, or in the case of a total destruction of the membraneous canal he will show signs of a *sudden loss of cochleo-vestibular function.*

Table 4. Symptomatology of sudden loss of cochleo-vestibular function

- Ipsilateral total deafness
- Vertigo and nausea
- Spontaneous nystagmus towards the normal ear
- Ataxia

The leading symptoms of a postoperative serous labyrinthitis are:

Table 5. Symptomatology of serous labyrinthitis

- Ipsilateral progressive deafness
- Tinnitus
- Vertigo (permanent) and disequilibrium
- Spontaneous nystagmus towards the normal ear, increased by head movements and in a position with the operated ear uppermost

Management: i.v. application of low molecular dextrane, cortisone and antibiotics.

Thermal injuries may be caused by careless intensive drilling in close vicinty to the labyrinthine capsule without water cooling of the burr. Both cochlear and vestibular symptoms may result from this type of traumatization. Generally, they are mild and transitory. Irreversible damage has not yet been reported.

Postoperative traumatic disorders of the neck may be caused in elderly individuals by an extreme hyperextension and torsion of the cervical spine during a long-lasting ear operation.

Table 6. Symptomatology of post-operative disorders of the neck.
• Headache • Pain in the neck • Dizziness and light-headedness • Stiffness of the neck • Postural vertigo and nystagmus • Vertigo and nystagmus induced by neck torsion

Pathogenetic considerations: The long-lasting, extreme passive torsion of the patient's neck results in a traumatic irritation of the cervical sympathetic nerves, inducing hypertonicity of the erector muscles of this region, which for its part can be an aetiological factor too in causing vertigo. Hypertonicity of the deep nuchal muscles and dysfunction of the brainstem reticular formation may have a trigger-target relationship in bringing about vertigo of cervical origin.[5] This happens particularly in elderly patients, whose cervical spine shows already degenerative alterations (cervical spondylosis) and who suffer at the same time from a more or less compensated vertebro-basilar insufficiency.[5]

Therapy: Improvement of brain circulation, myotonolytic drugs to reduce the hypertonicity of the deep cervical muscles and physiotherapy of the neck, carried out very cautiously in order to prevent further mechanical trauma.

References:

1. PAPARELLA M. Acoustic trauma from the bone cutting burr. *Laryngoscope* 72, 116-21, 1962.
2. SCHUKNECHT H.F. Pathology of the ear. *Harvard University Press* Cambridge Massachusetts, 291 ff, 1974.
3. ALTMANN F. Healing of fistulas of the human labyrinth; histopathologic studies. *Archives Otolaryng.* 43, 409-15, 1946.
4. GOODHILL V. Ear diseases, deafness and dizziness. Harper and Row, New York, San Francisco and London 381-82, 1979.
5. PFALTZ C.R. Vertigo, edited in disorders of the neck. In: Vertigo, edited by M.R. Dix and J.D. Hood, J. Wiley, Chichester, 179-197, 1984.

Complications of stapedectomy

J.D.K. Dawes, A.R. Welch

The effectiveness of stapedectomy is well proven, producing an immediate success rate of 97,5-98 % but complications do occur even with the most expert surgery. Total loss of hearing in the operated ear has a reported incidence of 0,6-4 %.[1,2,3] Less severe degrees of sensorineural hearing loss as a consequence of cochlear damage during or after surgery occur in 1,4 %.[1] Conductive hearing loss follows 5 % of stapedectomies perhaps long after a succesful operation.[4] Other complications such as perforation of the tympanic membrane, alteration of taste and facial palsies are briefly considered.

Sensorineural hearing loss may be an immediate or delayed complication. The usual cause of immediate senorineural loss is faulty operative technique.[2] Direct trauma to the membranous labyrinth follows clumsy instrumentation, the use of too long a piston, failure to correctly trim the wire of a wire-fat or wire-gelfoam prosthesis, excessive suction, or attempts to remove fragments of bone from the vestibule itself.

Excessive movement of the stapes, pulling it out of the oval window like a cork from a bottle, or overmanipulation of a floating footplate may indirectly severely injure the cochlea. These problems can usually be avoided by perforating the footplate prior to fracturing the crura or manipulating the stapes. If this cannot be done, very careful handling of the stapes may be needed to prevent a "floater". For the inexperienced stapedectomist and perhaps even the experienced, it is wisest not to attempt removal of the floating footplate, particularly if thick but to leave it in situ, allow it to refix and reoperate six months later. Oval window granulomas cause inner ear changes probably by producing a serofibrinous labyrinthitis.[5] Symptoms of progressive hearing loss usually begin six weeks after stapedectomy and may be accompanied by an increasing severity of tinnitus and vertigo. Left untreated, the sensorineural loss progresses to a "dead" ear. These granulomas are not thought to be infective in nature and have most commonly followed the use of wire-fat or wire-gelfoam prostheses.[6,7] Glove powder was implicated in one of two cases described by Dawes, Cameron and Curry (1973).[8] The incidence of oval window granulomas has significantly decreased since using the small fenestra technique.[9]

Immediate or late severe sensorineural hearing loss may follow otitis media, or perilymph fistulae. A "dead" ear may follow otitis media or labyrinthitis and in the few individuals with a patent cochlear aquaduct[10] meningitis may develop. A perilymph fistula may occur immediately because the oval window fails to seal and some surgeons prefer to cover the window with vein, fascia or perichondrium prior to inserting the prosthesis to prevent this. Unfortunately, if the sealing tissue becomes displaced during insertion of the prosthesis and a leak develops it is very likely to be persistent. A perilymph "gusher" is said to occur in the ratio of 1 in 300[5,11] and it is essential to seal off the oval window to prevent cochlear damage.[12]

Late sensorineural losses follow the development of perilymph fistula and when seen should be treated urgently. Hemenway et al. (1968)[13] found it occurred in

2,4 % of the cases they reviewed. Sudden fistulas may follow rupture of the oval window seal by barotrauma, a direct blow to the ear or by frequent displacement of the tympanic membrane in self-treatment of external otitis. Others seem to result from a shearing movement of the piston which is possible if the whole footplate had originally been removed. The small fenestra technique may prevent this shearing action but does not prevent rupture of the sealing membrane by a direct injury or barotrauma. Experience had shown that early closure of major ruptures stand the best chance of preserving hearing.[14] Occasionally, the patient only complains of repeated minor giddiness with a fluctuating hearing loss for some weeks or months prior to closure of the fistula with hearing preservation, but the risk of delay to the hearing is greater than if once diagnosed repair is undertaken within 24 hours.

Late sensorineural loss may be due to cochlear involvement by cochlear otosclerosis or senile presbyacusis. Slowly progressive hair cell degeneration of the basal turn of the cochlea is a common post-stapedectomy feature.[2]

Conductive hearing loss following stapedectomy may also be immediate or late in occurrence. Early failures tend to result from poor surgical techniques and the later failures from biological phenomena.

Faulty surgical technique may produce tears and perforations in the tympanic membrane, the long process of the incus may be fractured during the act of crimping and the incus can be dislocated if its body is exposed at surgery. An incorrect or inadequate exposure of the oval window region may not allow adequate assessment of piston length, and too short a piston may be used. Covering the window with too thick a tissue may prevent correct placement of the piston within the window and so it catches on the window edge. If the crura are not fully visualized, a crus remnant may interfere with movement of the prosthesis. A shortish long process of incus or a deformed incus can test the ingenuity of the best surgeons. Manipulation of the handle of the malleus after division of the incudostapedial joint tests mobility of the incudo-malleal block and prevents overlooking a fixed malleus head or incudal body by tympanosclerosis or bone. Occasionally, a facial canal overhang or a bulging facial nerve or a stapedial artery may prevent access to the footplate or satisfactory placement of a prosthesis.

Late conductive losses usually follow biological phenomena. The long process of the incus normally receives its blood supply through mucosal and Haversian vessels of the long process and from the anastomotic vascular ring around the incudo-stapedial joint which is supplied by vessels descending along the long process of the incus, ascending the crura and travelling in the stapedius tendon.[15, 16] Division of the stapedius tendon and removal of the crura jeopardise the blood supply to the lenticular process and the end of the long process in those cases where the Haversian vessels finish short and the mucosal vessels over the long process of the incus are damaged. Therefore there is a great need to care for the mucosal vessels on the long process of the incus and whenever possible to preserve the stapedius tendon. In some cases, due to poor vascular supply, the lenticular process and even the tip of the long process necrose and the piston falls off. Constant irritation of the wire or teflon loop may erode the shaft of the long process if the blood supply is poor particularly when a minor infection is associated with it; often the patient's sudden development of a conductive hearing loss follows an upper respiratory tract infection. These pathological abnormalities of the long process and lenticular process are not the only cause of late piston displacement. Particularly when a large opening is made through the footplate or the whole footplate is removed the mucous membrane grows beneath the piston and as it regains its tension over a prolonged period of time the biophysical force exerted upward against the piston may open the wire loop and free the piston from the long process. Similarly, the regrowth of otosclerotic bone, admittedly an uncommon occurrence, may displace the piston.

The development of adhesions in the sinus tympani following infection, or more frequently the use of gelfoam, may pull the piston backwards as the adhesion scleroses. Reoperation does not hold the terrors attributed to it and a successful result is frequently obtained.[4]

In my experience (JDKD) approximately 7-10 pistons of all types have been seen to be rejected. Checking the original operation notes shows that a tear occurred in the tympanic membrane. The tympanic membrane at the site of the tear adheres to the piston's wire or teflon loop and then rejects the piston to the exterior as is common with all foreign bodies.

Even more rare has been disintegration of the posterior segment of the drum without infection some months or years after the original successful stapedectomy — a simple careful myringoplasty solves the problem.

Many patients complain of disturbance of taste following surgery; 32 % have abnormal taste sensation after section of the chorda tympani compared with 7 % if it has only been stretched.[17] Far less disturbances of taste occur if the nerve is carefully dissected from its canal before displacement so that even stretching is avoided. The facial nerve should never be permanently damaged in capable hands[3] but undoubtedly to say "never" means "very rarely".

Stapedectomy is a highly skilful operation and to do it with low morbidity requires experience, a delicate touch and a proper training. It is not the field for the occasional surgeon - he can cause irreparable damage.

References:

1. DAWES J.D.K., CURRY A.R. Types of stapedectomy failure and prognosis of revision operations. *J. Laryngology & Otology* 88(3) 213-226, 1974.
2. SMYTH G.D., HASSARD T.H. Eighteen years experience in stapedectomy. The case for the small fenestra operation. *Ann. Otol.* 87, Suppl. 49. Pt. 3, 1978.
3. MORRISON A.W. Scott Brown's Diseases of the Ear, Nose and Throat. 4th Edition. Ed. J. Ballantyne and J. Groves, London, Butterworths, 1979.
4. PEARMAN K., DAWES J.D.K. Post-stapedectomy conductive deafness and results of revision surgery. *J. Laryngology & Otology* 96 (5) 405-410, 1982.
5. SCHUKNECHT H.F. Stapedectomy. Boston. Little, Brown & Co. 1971.
6. HARRIS I., WEISS L. Granulomatous complications of oval window fat grafts. *Laryngoscope* 72, 872-885, 1962.
7. KAUFMAN R.S., SCHUKNECHT H.F. Reparative Granuloma following stapedectomy. Ann. Otol. 76, 1008-1017, 1967.
8. DAWES J.D.K., CAMERON D.S., CURRY A.R. Post-stapedectomy granuloma of the oval window. *J. Laryngology & Otology 87* (4) 365-378, 1973.
9. MARQUET J., CRETON W.L., VAN CAMP K.J. Considerations about the Surgical Approach in Stapedectomy. *Acta Otol.* 74, 406-410, 1983.
10. MATZ G.J., LOCKHARD H.B., LINDSAY J.R. Meningitis following stapedectomy. *Laryngoscope* 78, 56-63, 1968.
11. CAUSSE J., CAUSSE J.B. Eighteen years report on stapedectomy. Problems of stapedial fixation. *Clin. Otol.* 5, 49, 1980.
12. GLASSCOCK M.E. The Stapes Gusher. *Arch. Otol.* 98, 82-91, 1973.
13. HEMENWAY W.G., HILDYARD V.H., BLACK F.O. Post-stapedectomy perilymph fistulas in the Rocky Mountain area. *Laryngoscope* 78, 1687-1714, 1968.
14. DAWES J.D.K., WATSON R.T. Perilymph fistula. *Clin. Otol.* 4, 291, 1979.
15. ALBERTI P.W.R.M. The blood supply of the long process of the incus and the head and neck of the stapes. *J. Laryngology & Otology,* 79, 964-970, 1965.
16. ALBERTI P.W.R.M., DAWES J.D.K. Necrosis of the lenticular process of the incus after stapes surgery and its treatment. *J. Laryngology & Otology* 75, 821-825, 1961.
17. BULL T.R. Taste and the Chorda Tympani. *J. Laryngology & Otology* 79, 479-493, 1965.

Facial nerve injuries in middle ear surgery

J.-M. Sterkers

The rate of facial nerve (7N.) injuries in middle ear surgery is astonishingly low when one realises how numerous the operations on the ear are and how the 7N. is exposed to injury.

All textbooks expose how to avoid, diagnose, and treat this disagreable complication, yet every otologist has some personal experience on this subject, which might be interesting to discuss.

Some hidden factors may predispose to a facial injury:
— the anatomical factors depend on the mastoid, cellular or condense, and also on congenital anomalies of the trajectory of the 7N., or of the bony canal of the nerve; a lack of the Fallopian inferior wall in the tympanic segment is a predisposing cause of injury, in the surgery of the ovalis fossa;
— the pathological factors are the existence of a hidden granuloma under the second genu of the nerve in a chronic otitis, and osteitis or sequestra of the Fallopian canal wall.

Predisposing diseases to facial injuries are:
— cholesteatoma, particularly when there exists a fistula of the lateral semicircular canal, or a deep extension in the petrous bone;
— tympanosclerosis with lesion in the fossa ovalis, and on the Fallopian canal;
— glomus tumors when extended under the mastoid segment of the nerve; the tuberculosis of the ear;
— tumors (neuro-fibroma, carcinoma, rhabdomyosarcoma in children);
— foreign body in the ear;
— malignant otitis.

Injury to the nerve recognizes many causes:
— traumatic, by direct injury with instruments (chisel, curette, burr, hook);
— compression, by hematoma, chip of bone, ossiculoplasty, prosthesis, packing;
— thermic, by coagulation, drilling, electrical stimulation (> 1/2 volt);
— inflammatory, by granulomas, allergy to antibiotics;
— ischemic, by the vaso-constrictor effect of adrenaline;
— chemical, by too strong an antiseptic, which gives an inflammatory reaction or
— by cauterisation near the 7N.

Prevention of injuries to the 7N needs:
— an identification of the landmarks of the nerve in the middle ear: the lateral semicircular canal, the digastric groove, the cochlear process;
— if the nerve is hidden by the disease, its trajectory must be identified distally and proximally to the disease. This means that sometimes, to identify the proximal segment of the nerve, a middle fossa approach must be created in addition to the middle ear approach;
— to avoid any traumatism to the nerve, all the work of the instruments must be parallel to the direction of the nerve and away from it.

Diagnosis and the prognosis of the facial injury is done during the operation or after:
— during the operation, if an injury is recognized, the nerve is uncovered proximally and distally to the lesion. A decompression, a partial or a total graft, an end-to-end anastomosis are done according to the lesion;

— after the operation, the facial palsy is recognizable as soon as the patient awakes. The closure of the superior eyelid is never a sign of a good prognosis. The symmetry of the motility of the zygomatic muscles is the only reliable test.

If possible, the wound is immediately reopened to identify the site of injury of the nerve. If the asymmetry is very slight, and if an injury has not been observed during the operation, the decision of reoperation can be delayed to the next day.

The first postoperative day: if the palsy is total or severe, the nerve is exposed and treated. If the palsy is slight or partial, the state of the facial motility is followed by clinical testing and minimal electrical stimulation (Hilger apparatus).

If there is no response to the electrical stimulation, the nerve is exposed.

When the difference between the two sides is less than 2,5 mA, and is identical on the following days, it can be assumed that the nerve will recover spontaneously and there may be no sequelae at all. But, in some selective cases it can be preferable to reoperate, when one wants to make sure that there will be no sequelae. In these cases the objective of the revision is to expose the nerve by unroofing the Fallopian canal and making an incision of the fibrous sheath of the nerve.

Treatment

— *Medical:* anti-inflammatory alone. It is not indicated as there is always a possibility of infection in middle ear surgery. Antibiotics alone or with anti-inflammatory drugs: in some very septic cases, it can be preferable to give a 24 hour antibiotic cure before reoperating. In all cases, antibiotics are administered during and after the reintervention.

— *Surgical:* It depends on the severity of the lesions. A decompression is made if the nerve is swollen and not interrupted. A nerve graft is done if the nerve is interrupted, and if it is not possible to make an end-to-end anastomosis by rerouting the nerve. A difficult case is partial interruption of the nerve. If the facial palsy is not complete, a partial graft is applied between the interrupted fibers. Finally, it must be kept in mind that only the cases of complete palsy, where a restitution ad integrum without sequelae is observed, are the ones where a decompression of the nerve is done rapidly, after the onset of the palsy.

Extrusion of implanted materials

ABSTRACT
K. Jahnke

Generally, extrusion is interpreted as a reaction of the body to non-tolerated implants. This applies to many uses of various materials in different surgical fields. Middle ear implants are used for very different purposes (e.g. ossicular replacement prostheses, grommets, sheatings, posterior canal wall implants, materials for obliteration). We consider the following factors important for the phenomenon "extrusion":

— biocompatibility of the implant material including surface properties,
— implant biomechanics (design, intraoperative modelling, applied tension after insertion, etc.),
— quality of tympanic membrane (atrophic, reinforced by cartilage; with or without handle of malleus),
— tubal function (a dysfunction may lead to retraction pockets, may change the biomechanics and the quality of tympanic membrane),
— quality of middle ear mucosa (infection, residual or recurrent disease),
— fixation of the implant (e.g. osseous binding of a bio-active ceramic material).

Many of these factors may influence the selection of cases, depending on the experience of the surgeon, some may be apparent only after a longer period of time. Our experiences are based on the use of different materials such as ossicles, cartilage, different metals, plastics, bio-inert as well as bioactive solid and porous ceramics and carbons. Results, including histology, are discussed in detail.

SYMPOSIUM V

Patho-anatomy

Chairman: L. Manolidis

Chairman's comments

L. Manolidis

In this symposium we have the pleasure of discussing current aspects of very serious and laborious subjects of otology such as
— chronic inflammations of the middle ear, including granulomatous lesions,
— tumoral processes of the middle ear
— otosclerosis which always remains a problem, demanding further research and clinical investigation and
— immunology of the middle ear diseases, and particulary immunology in tympanoplasty.

Experts in each one field will contribute greatly with their personal experience and their extensive knowledge.

The discussion which will follow each presentation, will clarify even more every detail of the techniques and the current conception of the above mentioned subjects. We hope that the symposium will contribute greatly to the clinical and laboratorial knowledge of the middle ear pathological processes and to schedule new orientations for further enlightment in the future.

Frootko M.J.

Allograft tympanoplasty is extensively used currently with considerable success due to graft preservation techniques and to advanced knowledge of tissue interaction and human histocompatibility.

The proper analysis of HLA antigens on the one hand and the proper preservation techniques of the tympanomeatal dura mater and ossicular bone allografts on the other hand, are of crucial importance for an uncomplicated tympanoplasty.

Some techniques like formaldehyde fixation, immersion in cialit, or dehydration in alcohol as well as freeze-drying preservation, counteract the immunogenicity of the grafts preventing their rejection by the recipient. It must be said that sites such as the external auditory meatus and the middle ear are more receptive to allografts, than many other sites of the body, ensuring therefore a prolonged survival of the allograft.

In general, a tympanoplasty should be successful, unless an Eustachian tube malfunction, a chronic otitis media or a cochlear damage as well as a technical failure, abbreviate the life of the allograft and reinduce the same clinical problems as previously.

The responsibility of the surgeons who perform a tympanoplasty is based on
— a careful and detailed histocompatibility study of the recipient
— the right preservation and the proper selection of the allografts
— on the proper clinical assessment of the recipient particularly as far as the middle ear is concerned and
— the correct application of the appropriate surgical technique.

Münzel M.A.

Inflammatory granulomatous lesions of the middle ear are not an uncommon phenomenon. Tuberculosis, Wegener's disease, sarcoidosis, syphilis and amyloidosis are the most frequent types of granulomatous transformation of the anatomical structures of the middle ear. In addition to the appropriate pharmaceutical treatment in cases of tuberculosis and syphilis, an operation could improve the condition of the patient aiding a hearing recovery.

It is of paramount importance to make a differential diagnosis between tuberculosis, sarcoidosis, Wegener's disease, generalized or localized amyloidosis and syphilis. The laboratory investigation, including tissue biopsy contributes greatly to the right diagnosis of the underlying disease.

The diagnosis might predict whether a surgical intervention is essential in the hearing restoration of the patient or whether a conservative pharmaceutical treatment is enough for an amelioration of the acoustic perception of the patient. The general condition of the patient and the stage of the disease play a very important rôle in the possibility of eventual hearing recovery. From the otological point of view, the extent of granulomatous alterations of the middle ear structures determine the type and mode of the surgical operation and predispose the efficacy of the operation or the consequent complications.

Niho M.

Cholesterol crystals are frequently found in the middle ear, particularly in cases of cholesteatomas, chronic suppurative otitis media, chronic non-suppurative otitis media such as blue eardrum and hemotympanum.

The fatty degeneration of the mucosa is the main pathogenetic factor for the presence of cholesterol crystals in the middle ear. The connective tissue proliferation frequently leads to a cystic transformation of the mucosa with a subsequent increase of the fatty degeneration and a considerable accumulation of cholesterol crystals.

Crystals are commonly found in the obstructed parts of the middle ear. The obstruction could be the result of the connective tissue proliferation, of fluid accumulation, or of the development of a cholesteatoma. In the case of blue eardrum, numerous foam cells containing crystals of cholesterol are accumulated in large numbers in the tympanic cavity. The diagnosis of the accumulation of cholesterol crystals in the middle ear is feasible by a microscopic examination of the fluid or by histological examination of the mucosa of the middle ear. The presence of the foam cells is a pathognomonic criterion of the accumulation of cholesterol. For an effective treatment, reduction of the pathogenetic mechanisms and recovery of the non-suppurative pathological process is always essential. Mastoidectomy should always be carried out at an earlier stage since crystals appear very early in the mastoid due to obstruction. The lesion in the middle ear is properly treated by aspiration of fluid and Eustachian catheterizations.

Ribári O.

The pathogenesis of otosclerosis is a very disturbing problem. Long discussions and long debates after prolonged research and experimental work have tried to bring light to the whole subject.

The histopathology offers some valuable information concerning the various stages of the process, the morphological alterations of the tissues and the functional structures. Light microscopy contributed a great deal to the understanding of the rough pathology of otosclerosis. Electron microscopy and scanning electron microscopy enable us to throw some light on the fine structure of the disease and to understand clearly the series of the pathogenetic process. Histochemistry, on the other hand, revealed the rôle that several enzymes play in the various phases of the disease. It is well known that otosclerotic focus assumes a mosaic-like appearance with reabsorption and remodellization of the tissues at the same time. Electron microscopy revealed that otosclerotic microfoci always develop close to larger foci of otosclerotic alterations. The otosclerotic process involves mainly the non-collagen proteins of bone tissue.

In the active phase of the disease the bone matrix is extensively vascularized and contains a large number of osteoclasts resulting in an otospongiosis due to increased reabsorption of the bone. The blood vessels and the pericytes play a very important rôle in the process. It is well known that otosclerosis often develops in areas where embryonic material such as cartilage still remains. The production of new bone is initiated by an intensive enzymatic activity around small capillaries. Further histochemical and morphological research will enlighten even more the pathogenesis and the etiological background of the diseases.

Hildmann H.

The histological examination of the middle ear epithelium after a tympanoplasty offers valuable information on the condition of the middle ear tissues in cases of mechanical trauma, chronic inflammations and vascular lesions. In a large number of biopsies, partial or multilayer epithelial proliferation is commonly seen. This represents a common type of reaction of the epithelium towards chronic irritation or prolonged inflammatory process. Very often in addition, connective tissue proliferation is also seen, consisting of collagen fibers and reticular fiber accumulation in a matrix of a vascular tissue.

Although light microscopy has been extensively used in middle ear histology, it does not give sufficient information on the fine processes which occur in middle ear structures whenever a pathogenetic factor acts upon them.

Electron microscopy and scanning electron microscopy contribute greatly in the further approach of the middle ear tissue reaction to chronic irritation.

The application of current histochemical techniques enable us to understand clearly the enzymatic and biochemical aspects of the tissue proliferation.

Patho-anatomy

L. Manolidis

The pathological alterations in the middle ear which occur during the various diseases, determine the extent of the underlining lesion and subsequently indicate whether a histological recovery to the normal status and/or the functional rehabilitation of the tissue following the application of the appropriate treatment is feasible. In addition, they enable us to determine preoperatively, whether the surgical reconstruction of the acoustic organ will be effective or not.

The knowledge of the histological alterations in the various diseases of the middle ear could determine the effectiveness of the microsurgical reconstruction immediately after the lesion or at a second time. It is clear, therefore, that the estimation of the type of the surgical procedure must be based on the histological data of the existent lesion.

The pathological study of the acoustic organ is divided into two main fields:
— the study of the histological structures of the peripheral part of the acoustic organ and
— the neuro-otological study of the central part, extending centrally to the spinal ganglion.

The recent use of the electron and the scanning electron microscopy brings to light new information explaining the clinical phenomena, resulting in a marked reassessment of the treatment procedures and surgical methods in favor of the patient.

The patho-histological estimation of the alterations of every individual structure of the middle ear, the histological assessment of the pathological findings pre- and postoperatively, the estimation of those findings in relation to the applied surgical procedure, the estimation of the histological findings in relation to the material which was used according to the applied technique (alloplastic, autoplastic or homoplastic) could lead us to useful information on the treatment of otological diseases and on the validity of surgical rehabilitation of the affected hearing ability of the patient.

To know the side effects and the consequences of the application of alloplastic material in operations of reconstruction of the conductive system, following the immunological reactions, is very important for the selection of the appropriate material and the assessment of the appropriate case and appropriate time for its application.

The postoperative histological study of the middle ear mucosa would bring useful information on the efficacy of our method in a large number of operations and would demonstrate whether the mucosa has recovered and whether its function is restored.

The otosclerotic alterations under the light of electron microscopy are discussed in relation to the latest data.

Our discussion extends to several other diseases of the middle ear, such as tympanosclerosis, connective otitis etc. In all these diseases, the pathological findings play a very important rôle for further and deeper understanding of the etiological background of the clinical phenomena.

Tympanic allografts - Immunopathology

ABSTRACT

N.J. Frootko

Most complications of allograft tympanoplasty have been attributed to technical failure, recurrent and/or residual disease, cochlear damage and Eustachian tube malfunction, while those complications which may be due to immunological rejection have received little attention.

In our investigations of immune responses in allograft tympanoplasty in the rat and in man, we have found that
— the deep external auditory meatus and middle ear are sites where tissue allografts in tympanoplasty enjoy prolonged or even indefinite survival and
— the preoperative graft preservation techniques currently used, appear to alter or destroy the immunogenicity of the grafts, thus preventing their early destruction.

Formaldehyde, Cialit, alcohol and freeze-drying preservation techniques impart different physical, chemical and immunological characteristics on tympanomeatal, dura mater and ossicular bone allografts. This influences not only the magnitude of specific immunological and non-specific inflammatory responses to these grafts, but also the rate and degree of revitalisation and/or resorption by host tissues.

Inflammatory granulomatous lesions of the middle ear

M.A. Münzel, W. Frank

Inflammatory granulomatous lesions in various mucosal areas are found in several diseases. In the case of the mucosa of the middle ear, this applies in particular to:
— lues
— leprosy
— tuberculosis
— Wegener's granulomatosis.

As it is a very special clinical entity, leprosy shall be excluded from the following considerations. Even luetic infection of the middle ear mucosa is doubtless exceedingly uncommon. It has also only been reported in the literature many years ago. These publications always point out that an acute otitis media is observed remarkably frequently in syphilis. However, this inflammation is mostly non-specific, and is caused by common pathogen germs.[1,2] It is a concomitant manifestation. Attention is repeatedly drawn to the fact that specific and non-specific inflammations in the middle ear can be distinguished from each other either insubstantially or not at all in lues. Thus, middle ear conditions have been reported which quite resemble a mucosus otitis or a tuberculous inflammation. Besides the histology of an inflammatory granulomatous lesion, it is also necessary to detect spirochetes in the mucosa to demonstrate a syphilitic otitis media. For the vast majority of cases of luetic infection, involvement of the inner ear is very much more characteristic than involvement of the middle ear mucosa.[1,2]

Compared to luetic infection of the middle ear mucosa, the clinical picture of middle ear tuberculosis has been very much better documented and described. Nevertheless, clinical diagnosis of the disease gives rise to repeated difficulties, especially when a primary pulmonary tuberculosis is not present. In terms of pathological anatomy, a distinction is made between primary and secondary middle ear tuberculosis.[3,4] Primary middle ear tuberculosis occurs exclusively in neonates and infants. The penetration of tubercle bacteria via the Eustachian tube into the middle ear is considered as the route of infection.

Secondary or post-primary middle ear tuberculosis of the older child and the adult is very much more frequent. Here, the canalicular and hematogenous dissemination of tubercle bacteria into the middle ear cavities are considered as routes of infection. In an open pulmonary tuberculosis, the route of infection via the Eustachian tube is also possible in principle in that the disease organisms are passed into the upper airways in coughing, and are conveyed into the middle ear by the route specified. Just as the clinical picture of tuberculous infections has undergone a general change in recent years, this applies in particular to mucosal tuberculosis of the middle ear. The exudative ulcerating necrotizing specific inflammation of the entire middle ear cavity with caseous degradation of bone and mucosa, which was frequently described in former times, has become exceedingly rare. Nowadays, the productive reaction form is much more frequent. In terms of pathological anatomy, it is characterized by subepithelially situated specific granulation tissue with extensive superficial spreading.[4,2]

Typical clinical signs in the presence of middle ear tuberculosis are:

— multiple perforations of the tympanic membrane (which are observed very rarely, however) or

a rapid alteration of form and size of the perforation of the tympanic membrane,
— an often remarkably good pneumatization in the X-ray,
— therapy-resistant otorrhoea,
— pain in the region of the mastoid,
— a whitish staining of the tympanal mucosa or the development of thick coagulated white granulations in the mastoid,
— strikingly frequent spontaneous occurrence of facial nerve paresis.

However, when there is suspicion of tuberculosis due to the additional presence of tuberculous infection of an other organ or due to the clinical picture of the ear, appropriate detection is possible as a rule by smear investigations. In such cases, middle ear tuberculosis is actually hardly a major therapeutic problem today. It can be healed with relative certainty with a specific tuberculostatic chemotherapy. If, for any reason, it is necessary to carry out a surgical revision of the diseased middle ear in known tuberculosis, the operation can also be completed in accordance with the principles of tympanoplasty with appropriate postoperative treatment, when the local finding is not too extensive. Specific tuberculostatic chemotherapy allows the mucosa in the newly formed tympanic cavity to heal in most cases.

The situation becomes problematic when suspicion of presence of middle ear tuberculosis only arises during a planned tympanoplasty. In these cases, an attempt will be made to verify the diagnosis during the operation by smear investigations and frozen-section histology. Tuberculostatic treatment can then follow immediately after the operation. Only in very extensive processes will the decision be made to attempt to improve auditory function in a second session after healing of the infection.

Middle ear tuberculosis should be considered especially when a spontaneous necrosis of the fascia transplant occurs after a tympanoplasty for reasons which are otherwise obscure.

Finally, Wegener's granulomatosis is an inflammatory condition which as a rule starts in the upper respiratory tract. A disease of the organs in the lower respiratory tract, generalized vasculitis and finally involvement of the kidney, occur. A simultaneous involvement of the middle ear was already mentioned in the first descriptions.[5,6] Recent publications have frequently pointed out that a corresponding disease of the middle ear mucosa is also possible as a first symptom besides the simultaneous involvement of the middle ear structures.[7,8] Whereas the concomitant manifestations are as a rule an acute otitis media or a serous otitis media which can be explained by the tubal dysfunction caused by the inflammation of the nasopharyngeal space, there are doubtless cases with a primary involvement of the middle ear mucosa. The typical granulomatosis of the middle ear mucosa is then observed histologically before pathological changes in other parts of the upper respiratory tract can be found. Both the macroscopic and the histological appearance resemble that of a mucosal tuberculosis. A facial nerve paresis also occurs here very early, and as a rule a well pneumatized mastoid system is also found.[6,8]

Naturally, it is not possible to demonstrate tuberculosis in these cases. The course is characterized by relatively early appearance of corresponding granulomatous alterations of the mucosa in the upper respiratory tract and in the lungs. Because of the generalized vasculitis, an inner ear reaction also occurs relatively early here. Of course, a surgical treatment is not possible in the generalized underlying condition. In these cases, the treatment must consist of appropriate chemotherapy with corticosteroids and cyclophosphamides after establishment of the diagnosis.

References:

1. SCHÄTZLE W., HAUBRICH J. Pathologie des Ohres in: DOERRSEIFERT-UEHLINGER. Spezielle pathologische Anatomie, Springer, Berlin-Heidelberg-New York 1975.
2. SCHUKNECHT H.F. Pathology of the ear. Harvard University press, Cambridge 1974.
3. KAMIO T., KAMIO T., IWASA H. Clinical observations of infection route of otitis media tuberculosa. *HNO (Berlin)* 30, 350-353, 1982.
4. MÜNZEL M., PATUTSCHNICK H. Mittelohrtuberkulose und Tympanoplastik *Laryng. Rhinol.* 54, 198-201, 1975.
5. FAUCI A.S., WOLFF S.M. Wegener's granulomatosis: Studies in eighteen patients and review of the literature. *Medicine* 52, 535-561, 1973.
6. KARMODY C.S. Wegener's granulomatosis: Presentation as an otologic problem. *Otolaryng.* 86, 573-584, 1978.
7. RISTOW W., MARTIN H. Zur Wegenerschen Granulomatose. *Arch. Otorhinolaryng.* 213, 431-432, 1976.
8. KORNBLUT A.D., WOLFF S.M., FAUCI A.S. Ear disease in patients with Wegener's granulomatosis. *Laryngoscope* 92, 713-717, 1982.

Cholesterol crystal in the middle ear

M. Niho

During the last 33 years, 107 patients (139 ears) with cholesterol crystals (CC) deposits were operated on and 1 036 pathological specimens were obtained during surgery (table 1) at the Niho Clinic. Examinations of these patients and their specimens were performed, in order to describe:

— manifestations of CC deposits in the temporal bone,
— diagnosis and
— treatment of patients with CC deposits.

Manifestations

The occurrence is 11 % of 152 patients with chronic suppura-

Table 1. Case material										
	Non-suppurative OM		Suppurative OM		Reoperation		Cholesteatoma		Total	
Age	Case	Ear	Case	Ear	Case	Ear	Case	Ear	Case	Ear
1-10 yrs	55	81	1	1	0	0	1	1	57	83
11-20 yrs	6	8	7	8	8	8	4	4	25	28
21-52 yrs	2	3	9	11	7	7	7	7	25	28
Total	63	92	17	20	15	15	12	12	107*	139

*Seven cases with two diagnoses

Table 2. Occurrence of granuloma in each part of temporal bone

	Non-suppurative OM	Suppurative OM	Reoperation	Cholesteatoma	Total
Mastoid part	50/51	15/15	7/10	9/12	81/88
Squamous part	3/19	0/1	0/3	0/1	3/24
Petrous cells of the perilabyrinth	8/23	1/1	0/4	0/2	9/30
Tympanic part	2/8	2/10	6/9	6/11	16/38
Petrous apex	0/3	0/5	1/7	0/8	1/23

Table 3. Length of follow-up in all cases

Years	% of cases with non-suppurative OM	% of cases with suppurative OM	% of cases with reoperation	% of cases with cholesteatoma
< 1	16	12	7	17
5	41	41	13	33
10	24	29	33	17
< 27	19	18	47	33

tive otitis media (OM), 50 % of 24 with cholesteatoma and 28 % of 54 with reoperation. Although the occurrence is 38 % of 162 with chronic non-suppurative OM (middle ear effusion, blue ear drum and hemotympanum), 87 % of them, including all patients with blue eardrum (9 patients, 12 ears) and hemotympanum (one ear) were between 1 and 10 years old (table 1). Large amounts of CC deposits were found in non-suppuration and small deposits were in others. Blue eardrum and hemotympanum were far-advanced stage findings of non-suppuration with CC deposits. Presence of CC was found in the obstructed part. The part might be obstructed due to fluid, connective tissue, cholesteatoma and graft materials.

Diagnosis

Diagnosis is established by

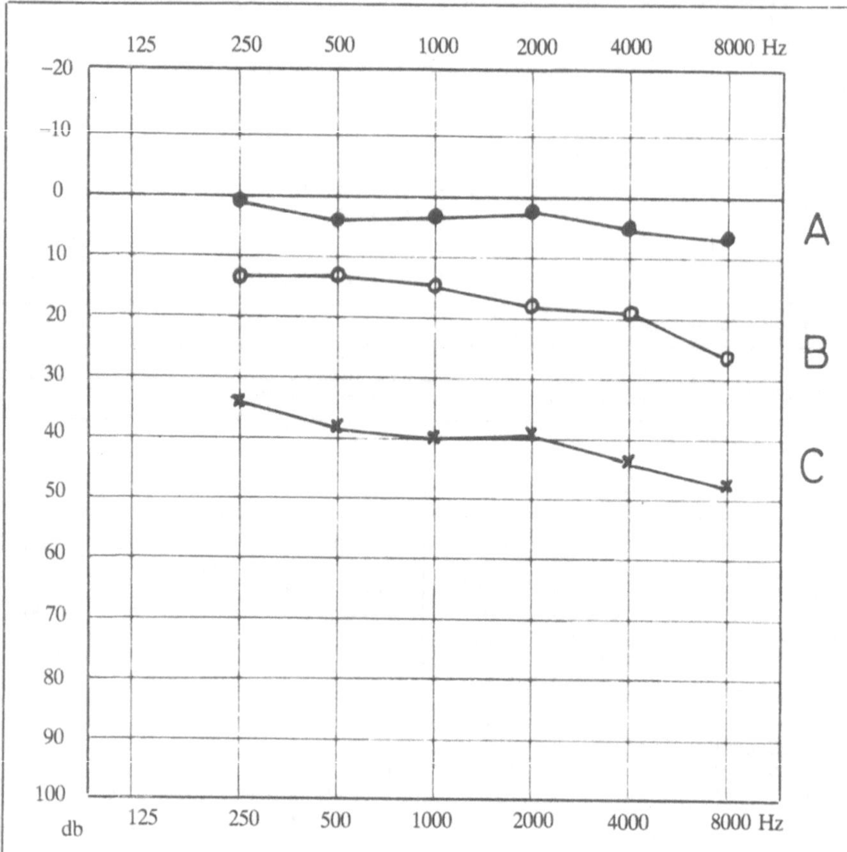

Fig. 1. Hearing results (N=99)
A: 60 ears with non-suppurative OM performed mastoidectomy
B: 12 ears with suppurative OM performed mastoidectomy
C: 27 ears performed radial operation

discovery of CC in the temporal bone due to microscopic examination of smears of fluid or granulation, and from pathological specimens. CC are almost always found in glistened or brown fluid and occasionally in yellowish or gluey fluid.

Treatment

Not only removal of cyst or cystic structure including CC but also recovery from chronic ear diseases are the desired treatment. Occurrence of granuloma in these diseases, which indicates sites of obstruction, is presented in table 2. Length of follow-up of the patients is presented in table 3. Hearing results are summarized in figure 1. When we performed a radical operation, we usually proceeded directly to petrosinectomy in the case where the air cells of the petrous apex developed. Tympanoplasty was not performed on these patients, since we considered it much better to have an open cavity than to close it because of delayed healing and follow-up examinations.

In infants and children, inflammation of the paranasal sinuses, adenoid and Eustachian tube is usually involved. Frequent irrigations of the maxillary sinus are effective for sinusitis. Amelioration of sinusitis leads to that of adenoiditis and salpingitis caused by sinusitis.

Chronic non-suppurative otitis media and mastoiditis

Serous OM is thought to be similar in kind to secretory OM, blue eardrum and hemotympanum. Conditions of their occurrence may be similar to those of suppuration, except that an advance in chemotherapy must be included. Accordingly, my concept of treatment of non-suppurative OM is that for inflammation.

Occurrence of cholesterol granuloma in the middle ear was usually found in patients of a far-advanced stage. No relapse of inflammation or these deposits have been seen in 2 of these patients (2 ears) with blue eardrum and one (one ear) with hemotympanum during the follow-up years between one and 19, who had a radical operation. Among 7 patients (10 ears) with blue eardrum having a complete mastoidectomy, no relapse has been seen in 2 of these patients (2 ears) during the follow-up years between 9 and 19, but there was a relapse in 3 of these patients (5 ears) who have been seen during the 4 years postoperatively.

Intraoperative findings in the middle ear of relapse patients were retention of a large amount of brown mucinous fluid and presence of scattered granulomatous structures in the strongly swollen mucous membrane with similar color. Middle ear orifice of the Eustachian tube may have been obstructed. Since the operative results of such patients are not so successful in general, surgery should be performed during an earlier stage in which CC deposits probably occur in the mastoid. Among 55 patients (79 ears) with chronic non-suppurative OM and mastoiditis, excluding patients with blue eardrum and hemotympanum, a complete mastoidectomy was done 54 (78) and radical operation on one. Operative results were all successful. However, frequent observations of infant and child patients were required until about 8 years of age because of acute repeated infection in the nose, pharynx and ear. With proper treatment given as early as possible, they healed successfully.

Chronic suppurative Otitis media and mastoiditis

A complete mastoidectomy was performed on 11 patients (13

ears) and radical operation on 6 (7). Occurrence of granuloma in the middle ear was found in patients in the far-advanced stage (table 2). A relapse of otorrhoea appeared in 2 of these patients.

Reoperation. Prior to visiting the Niho Clinic, radical operations had been performed on 8 patients (8 ears), a simple mastoidectomy on one, simple mastoidectomies with tympanoplasty on 5 (5) and an atticotomy with tympanoplasty on one. Radical operations were performed on 14 (14) and a complete mastoidectomy on one in the Niho Clinic. Occurrences of granuloma in the mastoid and in the middle ear were almost with the same frequency (table 2). Both the mastoid air cells, which had not been removed previously, and the middle ear were obstructed by the connective tissue and/or graft materials. A relapse of otorrhoea appeared in 3 patients.

Cholesteatoma. Radical operation was performed on all of 12 patients (12 ears). All cholesteatomas were extended to the mastoid. Occurrence of granuloma in the mastoid and in the middle ear were almost with the same frequency (table 2). A relapse has not appeared during the follow-up years.

Literature:

1. GROTE J.J. et al. Middle ear effusion and sinusitis. *Journal of Laryngology and Otology* 94, 177-83, 1980.
2. NIHO M. Chronic non-suppurative otitis media and cholesterol otitis media. In: Tato J.M., Arauz S.A. eds. XI World congress on otorhinolaryngology. Buenos Aires: Club otorhinolaryngologico, 788-91, 1978.
3. NIHO S. et al. Ostitis or osteomyelitis temporalis chronica (otitis media chronica in the broad sense) with cholesterol granuloma. *Jap. J. Otol. Tokyo* 66, 788-803, 1963.
4. NIHO S. et al. Radical surgery on the temporal bone and labyrinth operation for hearing improvement. *Ann. Otol. Rhinol. Laryngol.* 66, 1064-75, 1958.
5. NIHO M. Sinus irrigation therapy for children with chronic sinusitis. *Jap. J. Otol. Tokyo* 83, 424-33, 1980.

Pathohistology of otosclerosis

O. Ribári, I. Sziklai, J.G. Kiss

Spongiotic disease of the labyrinthine capsule, which causes stapes fixation in the area of the fenestra ovalis, was first described by Valsalva in the 18th century (1742)[1]. After dissecting 1,659 ears, Toynbee reported in 1824[2] that osseous ankylosis of the stapes has been the most frequent cause of hearing impairment. The histological examinations by Politzer led him to give the name "otosclerosis" to the disease in 1894.[3]

However, the word otosclerosis does not conform to the actual pathological process. The diseased bone is rather porous or spongiotic, and contains less Ca than the bone of the normal labyrinth, and for this reason the disease has recently been referred to as otospongiosis.

Otosclerosis in some cases begins in childhood, but its first symptoms mostly appear in adults, with stapes fixation in the area of the labyrinthine windows.

The studies of Guild (1944)[4] indicated that otosclerotic foci are found in 10 % of temporal bones, while stapes fixation occurs in only 1 % of histologically proved otosclerosis.

In the aetiology of otosclerosis, constitutional factors undoubtedly play a rôle. Genetic examinations point to the hereditary character of the disease; auto-immunity and/or metabolic changes may contribute to its origin. Among the local factors, cartilage remnants persisting in the bone during development are predisposed areas for the occurrence of otosclerotic foci. Gestation increases the progression of the pathological process, when the lysosomal hydrolases of the osteoclasts are activated, causing resorption of the bone. It seems evident that the metabolism of the bone undergoes cellular and enzymatic changes. Histologically, destruction by osteoclasts and also resorption and remodelling of the bone may be found. In the otosclerotic foci a fibrous tissue develops at the site of the degenerated bone and a new embryonal type of osseous tissue is to be seen.[5]

Consequently, otosclerosis is a complex patholocical process in the bony capsule of the labyrinth, which causes focal morphological changes in the bone and alters the activity of some of the proteolytic enzymes indirectly damaging the nerve cells and/or the sensory epithelia of the inner ear. Otosclerosis involves a chronic development with a focal process. It has two different phases: a destructive, lytic phase and a reconstructive phase. The two phases are present simultaneously, either one being dominant.

Though the aetiology of otosclerosis is not yet known, the results of its surgical treatment in the past 25 years have shown a great improvement. In 95 % of the cases, patients acquire a lasting hearing improvement from stapedectomy, with decreasing progression of the disease in most cases.[6]

Otologists have recently shown a great deal of interest in the pathology of the auditory ossicles, among the ossicles the structure of the stapes being the most interesting. Normally, cartilage is present in both the head and the footplates of the stapes. The bone of the stapes is covered by mucous membrane and its blood supply comes from submucosal veins. Histologically, the stapes is composed of primitive osseous substance. The head and crus contain branchial fibrillae. The crus displays a lamellar osseous structure, while the osseous fibrillae in the footplate are unorganized and closely correlated. The structure of the stapes exhibits great variability. While the other bones of the osseous system grow until the age of 20 years, there is no significant change in the stapes from the moment of birth on, either in thickness or in length. In cases of otoslerosis, different histological changes appear in the footplate and in the superstructure of the stapes.

In the process of remodelling of the bone, the substances of the bone are continuously absorbed and reproduced. This process is accompanied by a constant structural change. Earlier, it was thought that the middle layer of the bony capsule of the cochlea remains unchanged throughout life, but it was later demonstrated that the labyrinth also undergoes remodelling. Remodelling proceeds partly in the surface of the bone, periosteally, and perivascularly beside the veins. Reorganization in the bone of the labyrinth and the perivascular remodelling are unique and occur in a different way than in the other bones of the body.

Microscopically, four phases of otosclerosis have been described[7]:
— through the activity of the otosclerotic focus, lacunae appear in the bone;
— resorbed bone is replaced by fibrous connective tissue with a porous structure;
— the connective tissue is reformed and the regenerated bone is interwoven by fibrillae;
— lamellar bone is deposited around the veins.

The structure of the newly-developed bone at the end of the remodelling is spongiotic; compact bony structures alternate with vacuolae and lacunae, which are filled either with the network of the connective tissue of blood vessels or with accumulated amorphous substance. Formerly, histological and histochemical examinations of otosclerosis were carried out by means of light microscopy, but electron microscopic examinations later made further observations of the fine structural changes possible. Scanning electron microscopic studies reveal the spatial structure of the diseased bone.

At the ENT Clinic of Szeged University Medical School we perform operations on some 130-150 patients with otosclerosis yearly. In spite of the lasting hearing improvement achieved by surgery and the slowing-down in the progression of the disease postoperatively, the causes of the pathological changes in the otosclerotic bone remain unknown.

The otosclerotic process causes hearing impairment when it invades the footplate of the stapes. The otosclerotic focus appears mostly in the forepart of the foot-

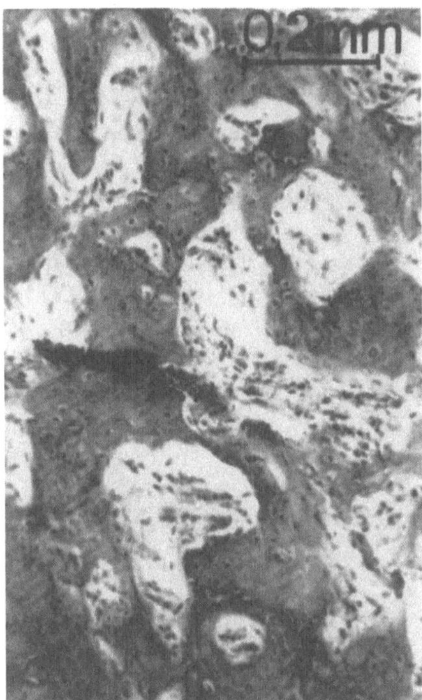

Fig. 1. Typical otospongiosis of the stapes footplate in the active phase. Magnification: 80 x. Haematoxylin-Eosin. Cut: parallel with the plain of the footplate.

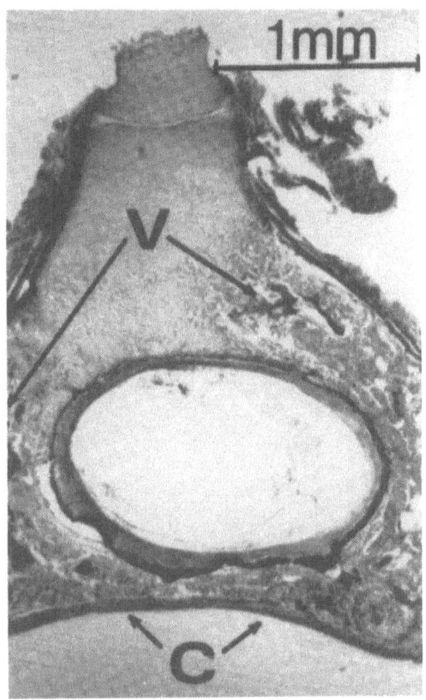

Fig. 2. Whole stapes from 6 month old human fœtus. Large vascular spaces (V) and cartilage (C). Magnification: 25 x, Mallory staining.

plate and gradually extends to the bone tissue around the footplate. In certain cases part of the footplate is involved, and in extremely active otosclerosis it may fill the entire foramen ovale.

The focus in the otosclerotic bone appears in a mosaic-like formation (figures 1 and 2); in some areas the bone is manifestly vascularized, while in other areas deposited connective tissue may be seen. The deposited Ca is irregular in the matrix and results in a web-like bone. The otosclerotic focus is either active or inactive; the active lesion is spongiotic in appearance with numerous cells and osteoclasts and extensive vascularization. The inactive otosclerotic focus contains few cells, but rather compact bone, and is slightly vascularized. Different stages of the otosclerotic activity may be seen at the same time in both the temporal bone and the footplate. Electron microscopic examinations of the crus and head of the stapes revealed that, besides the large otosclerotic foci, micro-foci occur which later unite with the macro-foci. Electron microscopy may demonstrate pathological processes not only in the footplate

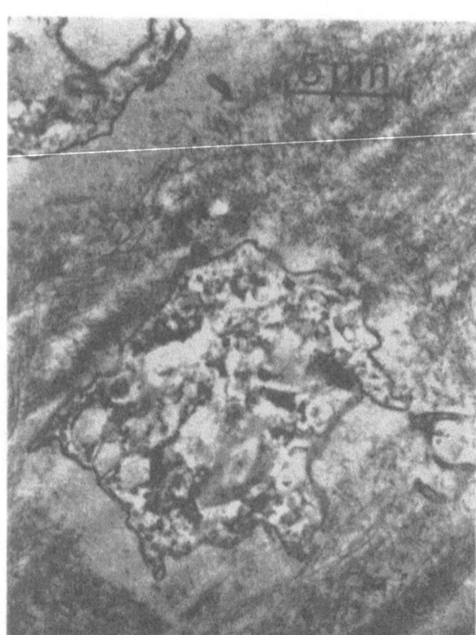

Fig. 3. Transmission electron microscopic picture of the stapes superstructure in otosclerosis (4,500 x). A degenerated osteocyte can be seen in the center surrounded by collagen fibrillar network.

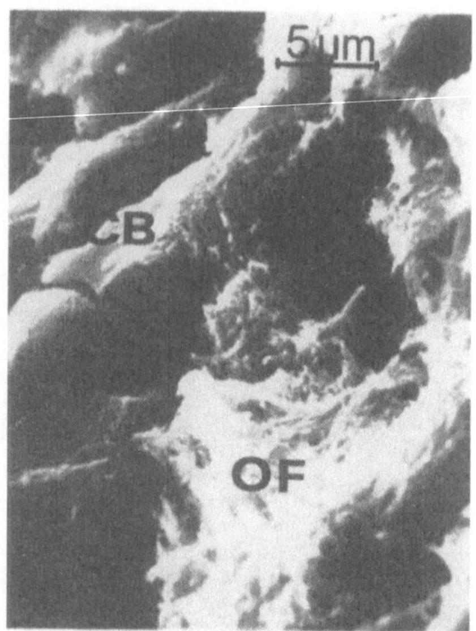

Fig. 4. Invasion border-line between the compact bone (CB) and the otosclerotic focus (OF) on the cross-edged surface of the stapes footplate by scanning ELMI. Magnification: 3,000 x.

but also in the crus and in the head of the stapes, though this is not typically otosclerosis, but cellular degeneration of different degrees (figure 3).

Mostly, degenerated osteocytes may be detected in the otosclerotic crus and head. Clinically, this means that the crus and head are not healthy, and it is therefore preferable to remove them surgically, for reimplanted superstructures are sooner or later absorbed and become degenerated in most cases.

A greater extent of degeneration may be found, especially in the superstructure of stapes where partial stapedectomy was previously performed, the footplate of the stapes was removed, but the other parts of the superstructure were put back.

Scanning electron microscopy allows good examination of the surface of the otosclerotic bone, and cross-edge surface examinations yield further information on the location of the pathological bony tissue (figure 4). The collagen structure is seen to be damaged and the perilymphatic surface, e.g. that of the footplate of the stapes, becomes connected to the otospongiotic lacunae. This is especially noticeable in florid, active otosclerosis, when damage of the inner ear is more definite. It may be assumed that in active otosclerosis substances entering the perilymph from the focus are responsible for the damage of the inner ear. Sensorineural hearing loss caused by vascular otosclerosis at a young age is more severe than in cases of slowly progressing otosclerosis. A large and active otosclerotic focus causes sensorineural hearing impairment more often. Cochlear otosclerosis may occur without conductive hearing loss, but Schuknecht (1983)[8] states that this accounts for only 1% of the cases of progressive sensorineural hearing impairment.

We have examined the changes in the patterns of the non-collagen proteins in the otosclerotic bone.[9] The non-collagen proteins are loosely bound to the matrix of the bone and are released in all processes of demineralization. Low molecular mass non-collagen proteins may be found mainly in the otosclerotic process. This supports the hypothesis that the otosclerotic bone produces newly synthesized protein molecules which have definitive biological effects. It is likely that the constructional disorder of the otosclerotic bone is caused by the qualitative and quantitative changes in the organic matrix of the bone. Quantitatively, we could find only small changes in the collagen substances, whereas the changes in the non-collagen proteins were significant. The components responsible for the emergence of the process are not yet known, but it is evident that through the remodelling of the bone the balance is upset and different enzymes become released.[10]

The release of the hydrolytic enzymes is accompanied by an increased depolymerization of the bone matrix. The activity of Cathepsin-B is much higher in the area of otosclerotic bone than in the normal cortical bone and superstructure. The activities of collagenolytic enzymes are much greater in the otosclerotic bone than in other bony structures.[11] The increased collagenase activity is probably a result of the activity of the accumulated mononuclear cells around the otosclerotic focus. Besides the evident histological changes, therefore, increased proteolytic enzyme activity and altered protein composition are to be found. Consequently, the change in biochemical structure of the bone gives rise to the discussed histological and morphological picture. It has been proved that peptides may enter the perilymph. Isotachophoresis of the perilymph revealed middle molecular mass peptide only in the otosclerotic bone and otosclerotic perilymph, but not in the serum or in healthy perilymph.[12]

Different conditions, e.g. pregnancy or taking of contraceptive pills, can increase the activity of the otosclerotic focus. Certain hereditary factors also promote the progression of otosclerosis. It may be assumed that in some cases NaF treatment may decrease the pathologic activity of the enzymes in the bone, thereby slowing down the progression of the process. We did not find the diminutive effect of fluoride to be significant in our material, but the oral administration of Iprifla-von for 1 to 2 years resulted in a decrease in the progression of the process.

In our view the pharmaceutical treatment of otosclerosis must be investigated further in the hope that the progression of the otosclerotic process causing sensorineural hearing impairment may be successfully controlled other than by surgical treatment.

References:

1. VALSALVA A.M. Tractus de aure humano. Cap. II., X., Lugduna, 24, 1742.
2. TOYNBEZ J. Pathological and surgical observations on the diseases of the ear. *Med. Chir. Trans.* 24: 190-205, 1824.
3. POLITZER Á. Die Otosclerose, in: *Lehrbuch der Ohrenheilkunde für Praktische Ärzte und Studierende.* ed. 2 Stuttgart. Ferdinand Enke Verlag, 1899.
4. GUILD S.R. Histologic Otosclerosis. *Ann. Otol.* 53: 246-266, 1944.
5. CHEVANCE L.G., BRETLAU P., BALSKO M., JÖRGENSEN M.B., CAUSSE, J. Otosclerosis. an electron microscopic study. *Acta Otolaryngol.*, Suppl. 272, 1970.
6. MARQUET J. Otosclerosis: Small hole teKhnique. *J. Laryng. Otol.*, Suppl. No. 8, 78-80, 1983.
7. ALTMANN F. Histopathology and etiology of otosclerosis: a critical review. *Henry Ford Hosp. Int. Symp. Otosclerosis.* Little, Brown and Comp., Boston. 15-42, 1962.
8. SCHUKNECHT H.F. Cochlear Otosclerosis. *J. Laryng. Otol.*, Suppl. No. 8, 81-83, 1983.
9. RIBÁRI O., SZIKLAI I. Examination of non-collagen protein composition of the footplate and superstructure of the otosclerotic stapes. *Acta Otolar.* 95: 580-584, 1983.
10. RIBÁRI O., SZIKLAI I., KISS J.G., SOHÁR I. Cathepsin-B activity in otosclerosis. *Arch. Otorhinolaryngol., 238: 123-125, 1983.*
11. RIBÁRI O., SZIKLAI I. Biochemische Veränderung in otosklerotischen Gehörknochen und der Perilymphe, in: Aktuelles in der Otorhinolaryngologie. Georg Thieme Verlag, Stuttgart, New York, pp. 28-31, 1984.
12. SZIKLAI I., GRÓF J., RIBÁRI O., MENYHÁRT J., PIFFKÓ P. Peptides of the otosclerotic perilymph examined by analytical isotachophoresis. *Acta Otolar.*, in press, 1984.

Evaluation of middle ear biopsies after tympanoplasties

H. Hildmann, E. Steinbach

This paper examines the findings in 200 biopsies removed from the middle ear during revision surgery in apparently inflammation free ears. The surgery was carried out for preplanned two-stage procedures or for restoration of hearing in cases of ossicular displacement or ankylosis after the first intervention.

Normal middle ear mucosa consists of a stroma, a wide net of capillaries covered with the basilar membranes and an epithelium consisting of flat columnar or cuboidal cells. An excellent review of the literature has been given by Arnold.[1] The presence and importance of functional cells, goblet cells and ciliated cells has been discussed by Sadé.[2] Ilberg, Arnold and Steinbach[3] found 90 % ciliated cells in their biopsies after tympanoplasty and an increase of subepithelial collagen. In their short term observations on rather small numbers they did not observe a normalization. These investigations are in contrast to Schoendorf's findings (1974) who saw normal epithelium after tympanoplasty. Our observations in animals indicate an increase of goblet and ciliated cells with a maximum between 10 to 16 weeks after tympanoplasties in rabbits. According to these observations, the differentiation of middle ear mucosa cells seems reversible.

In this paper the biopsies are examined for the reversibility of inflammatory changes and the amount of scar formation to find a suitable time for plannable second interventions.

Materials and methods

200 biopsies from apparently non-inflamed ears were removed at revision surgery from ears with successfully reconstructed tympanic membranes at first intervention. Second stage surgery was done as preplanned procedure for hearing improvement in cases of postoperative ossicular displacement or ankylosis between 2 and 6 years after the first intervention.

Results

Among the 200 biopsies, 112 were covered with epithelium suitable for histological examination. Seventy showed normal monolayer cellular covering, 34 two cell layers and 8 epithelial hyperplasia. In 138 specimens the submucous connective tissue could be evaluated, tender structure in 30 cases, 86 cases markedly thickened including concentrations of connective tissue fibres, some containing round cells, 22 showed pronounced thickening of the submucosa in form of fibrous scar tissue. Eighty-eight specimens contained gland-like structures with cystes and ducts.

Discussion

In contrast to our findings in animals and to Schoendorf's observation in man we saw a middle ear lining, epithelium and subepithelium of normal appearance in only one third of our material. There seemed to be a correlation between time after first intervention and inflammatory changes indicating an extremely slow recovery of the middle ear lining. For practical otosurgery this would mean postponing a second stage operation as long as possible.

The amazing tendency for scar formation not observed in animals might endanger middle ear aeration if it occurs at strategic areas and calls for tender surgery and removal of thick granulation cushions. The histological pictures with long time persisting changes might explain some cases of reperforations in so-called easy cases.

References:

1. ARNOLD W. Reaktionsformen der Mittelohrschleimhaut. *Arch. Ohr.-Nas.-Kehlkopfheilk.* 216, 369-473, 1977.

2. SADE J. The middle ear mucosa. In: J. Sadé, Secretory otitis media and its sequelae. Churchill Livingstone, Edinburgh, London, 23-55, 1977.

3. v. ILBERG Ch., ARNOLD W., STEINBACH E. Die menschliche Mittelohrschleimhaut und Tympanoplastik. *Laryng. Rhinol. Otol.* 53, 795, 1974.

The cholesteatomatous ear one year after intact canal wall tympanoplasty

U. Mercke

When the technique of intact canal wall tympanoplasty (ICWT) was described in 1958[1], it seemed very promising that this technique would fulfil the two main goals set up for cholesteatoma surgery, namely
— to eradicate the lesion so thoroughly as to prevent recurrences, and
— to reconstruct the sound-conducting mechanism in such a way as to achieve maximum possible recovery of hearing.

During the latter half of the 1970s an increasing number of adverse reports began to appear, revealing alarmingly high frequencies of both residual and recurrent cholesteatomas after the application of this technique in cholesteatoma cases.[2]

To help clarify the value of ICWT surgery cases of cholesteatoma that were treated with this technique at the Department of Oto-Rhino-Laryngology in Lund have been systematically investigated.

During the investigation period we operated a total of 80 patients with a newly discovered cholesteatoma, i.e. the diseased ear had not been surgically treated for this diagnosis earlier. It was a basic principle that patients for ICWT would have this performed as a two-stage procedure, with the eradicating operation followed by a second look after one year.

ICWT was not used when the diseased ear was deaf preoperatively, when it was the only hearing ear and when the patient constituted such an anaesthetic risk that repeated surgical interventions were not medically justifiable. The technique was also abandoned if the surgeon had any doubts about the radical elimination of the cholesteatoma. For these reasons the two-stage procedure was not applied in 22 patients. The remaining 58 patients underwent ICWT surgery, 56 of these 58 also underwent the second look, i.e. 96,6 %. Second look could not be performed on 2 patients because of psychic problems in the one case and death in intercurrent cardiovascular disease in the other. These 56 patients had a mean age of 34,8 years.

At the eradicating operation, the middle ear and mastoid were explored through a retroauricular incision and the extent of the cholesteatoma determined. Following the ICWT principles stated by Claus Jansen, among others[1], the cholesteatoma was then removed, together with the diseased ossicles and the diseased parts of the tympanic membrane. Defects in the tympanic sulcus were repaired with autologous tragal cartilage and attached perichondrium[3], the drum head with temporalis fascia. All denuded surfaces within the middle ear, cell system and epitympanic space, together with the walls of the posterior tympanotomy were covered with Gelfilm before closure. No ossiculoplasty was included in this first stage. The second look was scheduled for 12 months later. This interval in fact averaged 13,2 months (range 10-26 months). In the period between the two operations the ear was checked at 3, 6 and 12 months and the occurrence of a posterosuperior retraction pocket recorded. All the patients underwent all these checks.

At the second look, the middle ear and mastoid were reexplored via a retroauricular incision. The following were recorded:
— recurrent or residual cholesteatoma,
— open or spontaneously closed posterior tympanotomy opening, and
— open or spontaneously obliterated mastoid cavity.

Results

Recurrent cholesteatoma. Recurrent cholesteatoma implies that the cholesteatoma disease still persists. Recurrent cholesteatoma, here defined as a retraction pocket with a non-visible bottom and containing debris of squamous epithelium, was found in 12 of the 56 patients. This amounts to 21,4 %.

Residual cholesteatoma. Residual cholesteatoma is defined as a new cholesteatoma arising from diseased tissue remaining after the eradicating operation. Residual cholesteatoma was found in 14 of the 56 patients. This amounts to 25 %. In all these 14 cases the residual cholesteatoma had begun to emerge from the middle ear cavity.

Spontaneously closed posterior tympanotomy opening. The posterior tympanotomy opening cre-

Table 1. The number of retraction pockets found at each postoperative check and the number of recurrent cholesteatomas developed from these pockets.

	Postoperative check			
	3 m	6 m	12 m	Total
Retraction pockets	1	8	12	21
Recurrent cholesteatomas developed from retraction pockets	1	5	6	12

ated at the first eradicating stage was found to be closed in 31 cases, 55,4 %. In all these cases the closure was caused by a mucosal fold. There was no case of bony narrowing.

Spontaneously obliterated mastoid cavity. In 22 cases (or 39,4 %) the mastoid cavity created at the ICWT operation was found to be spontaneously obliterated and closed, mainly by fibrous tissue.

Retraction pockets. At each of the postoperative checks, i.e. 3, 6 and 12 months after the first stage operation, the occurrence of a postero-superior retraction pocket was recorded. Table 1 shows the number of new retraction pockets found at each of these postoperative checks. This includes only those retraction pockets that have continued (or grown and become deeper) until the second look operation. As the table specifies the postoperative check at which the retraction pocket was recorded for the first time, it also shows that the frequency of retraction pockets increases in proportion to the time that elapses after the first, eradicating operation.

Out of the 56 patients a total of 21 cases of retraction pocket was found, i.e. 37,5 %. In 12 of these 21 cases, the retraction pocket was so deep that it was classified as a suspected recurrent cholesteatoma. All such suspected cholesteatomas were confirmed by the second look. The table also shows that the number of recurrent cholesteatomas developing from these pockets increases in proportion to the time that elapses after the ICWT operation.

Conclusions

— There were definite pathological findings in 62,5 % of the patients one year after the ICWT operation. These findings consisted of recurrent cholesteatoma, residual cholesteatoma and po-

tential cholesteatoma (= retraction pocket).
— The number of permanent retraction pockets increases with the time that elapses after the ICWT operation.
— A retraction pocket with a non-visible bottom appearing after an ICWT operation must be regarded as a recurrent cholesteatoma until proven otherwise.
— The posterior tympanotomy probably plays no rôle for the aeration of the mastoidectomy cavity. Nor does it help prevent recurrent cholesteatoma.
— When describing results after cholesteatoma surgery, the postoperative point of time to which these results refer must be clearly and exactly stated.

References:

1. JANSEN C. Cartilage-Tympanoplasty. *Laryngoscope* 73, 1288-1302, 1963.
2. SHEEHY J.L., BRACKMANN D.E., GRAHAM M.D. Cholesteatoma surgery: residual and recurrent disease. A review of 1024 cases. *Ann. Otol. Rhinol. Laryngol. 86, 451-462, 1977.*
3. LINDE R.E. The cartilage-perichondrium graft in the treatment of posterior tympanic membrane retraction pockets. *Laryngoscope* 83, 747-753, 1973.

Bone tissue in otitis media

B. Ars, L. Moeneclaey, J.F.E. Marquet

Although an apparently limited subject, bone tissue in the middle ear, its structure and development, is a relatively vast one and there is no question of discussing it in detail here. On the other hand, many points still remain obscure and research workers find it sometimes difficult to understand each other clearly. We shall therefore dwell on a few points which deserve both emphasis and clarification.

In the first place, bone in the middle ear, as in the rest of the body, is an essentially living tissue, and as such it keeps changing and renewing itself all through life. Moreover, it responds to external influences in a dynamic manner, and this may deeply affect its morphology.

In the second place, otitis media is a very common condition, which may assume many aspects; it may present itself in several different forms and is related to various otological syndromes.

For these reasons we shall restrict our communication to the morphological study of bone cells, with the hope that a better understanding of their origin and relationship will lead to a clearer view of bone physiology and pathology.

This study has led us to advocate a classification of bone pathology in the various forms of otitis media.

Four kinds of bone cells are to be distinguished: osteoblasts, osteocytes, osteoclasts and osteoprogenitor cells.

The **osteoblasts** are responsible for the formation of bone matrix. Lying in the superficial layer of the osteoid, these cells vary in shape from "columnar" to "pavement". Active cells are columnar. Their cytoplasm is abundant with a peripherally located nucleus containing prominent nucleoli. They are usually located on osteoid seams. The other cells are flat with a thin dark nucleus and elongated cytoplasm and are thought not to produce matrix. They are refered to as "inactive osteoblasts".

The principal cells of fully formed bone are the **osteocytes,** which lie in lacunae within the calcified interstitial substance. In its development, an osteocyte is essentially an osteoblast that has become embedded in bone matrix. The cell body is flattened, shaped like the lenticular cavity it occupies, but with many fine processes extending some distance into canaliculi in the surrounding matrix. The processes of neighboring osteocytes are in contact with one another at their ends. Thus the bone cells are not completely isolated in their lacunae but in communication with one another and ultimately with the cells at the surface through a series of cell-to-cell junctions. This fact is very important because it may explain how cells deep within the calcified matrix can respond to stimuli. The osteocyte exerts an important influence on the surrounding osseous matrix: the bone matrix immediately surrounding the osteocytes is thus modified and bone salts are resorbed. Osteocytes play an active rôle in the release of calcium from bone into blood. They can cause demineralization and organic matrix degradation around them, a phenomenon known as "osteolysis"; they can also deposit new layers of mineralized matrix on the perilacunar surfaces, a process called "osteoplasis".

Osteoclasts are large multinucleated cells that are easily distinguished from other cells by their fine structure - their "ruffled border", endoplasmic reticulum, vacuoled cytoplasm and numerous mitochondria. These peculiarities of osteoclasts are in keeping with their function; as they are directly involved in the removal of calcified tissue. The exact mechanisms by which they achieve simultaneous degradation of the organic matrix and dissolution of bone mineral still elude us, but there are rather clear indications that they secrete hydrolytic enzymes, which may be largely responsible for digestion of matrix components. Lysosomal acid hydrolases released by osteoclasts are active in resorption of the organic matrix of bone; the stimulated local acid production solubilizes bone mineral and at the same time creates a pH favorable to the action of acid hydrolases.

The **osteoprogenitor** cells have pale-staining, oval or elongated nuclei. They are found on or near all the free surfaces of bone: in the endosteum, the innermost layers of the periosteum; the lining of Haversian canals,... They are relatively undifferentiated cells but very active and with a considerable potential for differentiation into all the other functional specialized cells. The mechanisms and triggering factors of this differentiation are, however, still obscure.

Here they are: the actors with their classical function. That is all well and good but almost too simple. Although they are usually described as distinct cell types, there is clear evidence of transformation from one into the other, and it is evidently more reasonable to regard them as different functional states of the same cell type.

The osteocyte is, indeed, believed to be capable of modulation into other cell types. When its lacuna is destroyed during bone resorption, it is thus released and may revert to a quiescent osteoprogenitor cell, and later undergo modulation into an osteoblast. Osteocytes liberated from bone matrix may incorporate into multinucleate osteoclasts.

Osteoclasts develop usually by coalescence of mononuclear cells.

Fusion of osteoprogenitor cells is the principal source of osteoclasts. But in addition there is new evidence that they may develop by coalescence of mononuclear cells migrating from the blood - presumably monocytes.

In certain conditions, the osteoprogenitor cells undergo division and transform into the bone forming cells: osteoblasts; or coalesce to give rise to bone destroying cells: the osteoclasts. It is believed that the more specialized bone cells, osteoblasts and osteoclasts can also revert to osteoprogenitor cells. The osteoprogenitor cells are active during normal bone growth and may be activated in adult life during internal reorganization of bone, or in the healing of fractures and repair of the other forms of injury.

Such reversible changes in aspect are examples of cell modulation in contrast to differentiation. Thus all the bone cells are seen as interchangeable, requiring only dedifferentiation prior to their modulation. Their rôle depends only on the influence they undergo.

For this reason, we advocate a classification of bone tissue in otitis media based on two opposite and complementary functional processes:

— bone production: osteogenesis and induction,

— bone destruction: osteoclasis and resorption.

A bone production disorder might even originate in the temporal bone itself or in an adjacent area or might be also a local expression of a systemic problem.

Locally, in the healing of fractures, cells in the deepest layers of the periosteum and endosteum, under stimulus of trauma, reassume the form and function of osteoblasts and are, once again, actively engaged in osteogenesis.

Many attempts have been made to utilize the osteogenic potential of the periosteum and bone by transplanting these tissues to areas where bone is wanted. Devitalized homograft may favor induction of new bone formation by the cells of the host. In fact, many types of connective tissue have latent osteogenic potentials that are exhibited only rarely.

The presence of bone itself may be an important factor in activating osteogenic potentials. There is thus histological evidence in favor of induction of bone formation although attempts to isolate a specific inductor substance have, so far, given unconclusive results.

The histological changes occurring in bone inflammation depend entirely upon the stage and its duration. Basically, two elements can be identified, suppurative and destructive reaction, at first, followed by fibrous and bony repair. Considerable new bone formation may be observed also. The osteogenesis is expressed by an increased number of osteoblasts, their hypertrophy and recent deposits of new lamellae. This exuberant proliferation may lead, for example, to fixation of the ossicular chain into the wall of the tympanic cavity, postoperative ankylosis or sclerosis of the mastoid.

This stimulation of bone production in the middle ear may, of course, also be seen in systemic disease: exostoses, fibrous dysplasia, osteogenesis imperfecta, osteopetrosis, osteomalcia, Paget's disease, osteoma, osteosarcoma or metastatic lesion from a distant malignancy,...

Discussing bone destruction; both organic (collagen, water, protein,...) and inorganic (calcium,...) parts of bone have to be resorbed, and such resorption requires enzymatic activity derived from the living cells: osteoclasts, together with osteocytes and osteoprogenitor cells take an active part in resorption. It has been demonstrated that inflammation, with or without infection is the major factor in resorption. But inflammation is not in itself a sufficient cause of destruction.

Various theories have been put forward, they include pressure, ischemia, enzyme activity, hyperemia... The classical explanation is that the inflammatory process causes thrombosis and the resultant anoxia leads to bone destruction. This is the case, for example, in destruction of the lenticular process of the incus.

When inflammation is accompanied by infection, destructive necrosis occurs: with acute suppurative neutrophilic infiltration, edema, vascular congestion and thrombosis of small vessels. The death of such bone is usually seen by disappearance of the bone cells. There are many circumstances leading to such necrosis:
— biochemical disorders due to radiotherapy,
— physical agents: pressure (neuroma compression, tumor,...),
— inflammatory processes: mucosal disease or cholesteatoma...

There remains much to be said and much to be done to clarify this problem. Our purpose was not to solve it but, more humbly, to express it in clearer terms.

In conclusion, we would like to say that the development and preservation of bone is dependent upon the vitality and the optimal function of the bone cells. Cell specialization is controlled by the interaction of the cell with its microenvironment which consists of a whole complex of chemical and physical factors that impinge on the cells.

We hope to have shown, in this paper, that the work done so far is only a beginning and many problems still remain to be solved.

Literature:

1. BASSET C.A.L. Current concepts of bone formation. Instruct. Lect. Am. Acad. Orthop. Surg. *J. Bone Joint Surg.* 44A. 1217, 1962.
2. BELANGER L.F. Osteocytic Osteolysis. *Calc. Tissue Res.* 4,1-12, 1969.
3. ENGSTROM A. Structure of bone from the anatomical to the molecular level. In: Bone structure and metabolism, London, J. and A. Churchill, Ltd, 1956.
4. GLIMCHER M.J., KRANE, G.M. The organization and structure of bone and the mechanism of calcification. In Ramachandan, G.N. and Gould, B.S., eds: Treatise on collagen. London, Academic Press, 1968.
5. HANCOX N.M., BOOTHROYD, B. The osteoclast in resorption. In Sognnaes, R.F., ed: Mechanisms of Hard tissue Destruction. Washington, D.C., American Association for the Advancement of Science, 1963.
6. LUCHT U. Osteoclasts and their relationship to bone as studied by electron microscopy. *Z. Zellforsch.* 135: 211, 1972.
7. YOUNG R.W. Specialization of bone cells. In: Frost, H., ed: Bone Biodynamics. Boston, Little, Brown and Co., 1964.

Middle ear tumours, contribution to classification and diagnosis

J.J. Manni

Introduction

Middle ear tumours are rare and a precise determination of their incidence is difficult. Figures range from one in 6 000 to one in 20 000 patients with ear diseases.[1] The middle ear is the least common site of malignancy in the hearing organ with an incidence varying from 9-12 %.[2] The chance of developing a middle ear malignancy in comparison with other sites is about one in 1 500.[3] Reports have also established that malignant tumours of the middle ear are more frequently encountered than benign ones.[1] Tumours may involve the middle ear cleft primarily, metastatically or by extension from a contiguous area. Occasionally, anomalous conditions such as intrapetrosal carotid aneurysma, aberrant carotid artery or jugular bulb and manifestations of systemic disease such as leukaemia or multiple myeloma, may mimic middle ear neoplasms. This paper is restricted to primary tumours of the middle ear and mastoid.

Classification of primary tumours of the middle ear cleft

Figure 1 presents a classification of benign and malignant primary tumours of the middle ear and mastoid, each with subdivisions into epithelial, non-epithelial and miscellaneous lesions.

An attempt is made to indicate the total number of cases of each histopathological entity reported in the literature. However, since a substantial number of cases do not reach the literature, figure 1 does not present an exact determination of the incidence of the various middle ear tumours. One of the problems not solved in middle ear tumours is the determination of the site of origin, when the partition between middle ear and external ear canal is unrecognisable or the tympanic membrane is perforated.

Squamous cell carcinoma is the most common neoplasm in the adult middle ear and mastoid. It is well-established that this tumour, as well as other malignant tumours, has an associated incidence of pre-existing chronic suppurative otitis media of 60-80 %.[4] Fifty per cent of patients give a history of chronic, and twenty per cent a history of intermittent infections.[2] One may only be alerted to the possibility of a malignancy if unusual symptoms such as pain, bleeding and facial paralysis develop. The correct diagnosis will be made early

Fig. 1. Primary middle ear tumours - **Malignant neoplasms**

Classification of tumours of the middle ear cleft, with the approximate number of cases reported in the literature.

Epithelial	**Approximate Number**
squamous cell carcinoma	450
adeno carcinoma	17-30*
adenocystic carcinoma	15
ceruminoma	7
malignant melanoma	10
undifferentiated carcinoma	10
Non-epithelial	
sarcoma, including subclassification	50
rhabdomyosarcoma	70
Miscellaneous	
lymphangioendothelioma	1

* related to classification of adenomatous tumours

Primary middle ear tumours - **Benign neoplasms**

Epithelial	**Approximate Number**
adenoma (adenomatous tumours)	-40
choristoma	14
pleomorph adenoma	5
melanoma	10
carcinoid apudoma	4
Non-epithelial	
chemodectoma	400
meningioma	18
haemangioma	10
lymphangioma	10
giant cell tumour	5
osteoma	10
ossifying fibroma	1
odontoma	1
neuroma/fibroma (excl. N VIII)	130
myxoma	10
solit-plasmocytoma	10
teratoma, dermoid (epidermoid?)	40
Miscellaneous	
blue nevus	1

* rarely metastasize

if polyps, persistent granulations associated with chronic suppuration of the middle ear, are examined histopathologically. Bradley and Maxwell[5] suggested that any patient with middle ear discharge of more than 20 years duration should be under regular otologic supervision and routinely examined by Papanicolaou smears. Lewis[6] found that 10 out of 28 cases of carcinoma of the middle ear and mastoid operated upon were associated with cholesteatoma. However, primary middle ear squamous cell carcinoma behind an intact tympanic membrane has been reported.[7,8] Kleinsasser[9] observed two cases of squamous cell carcinoma which occurred 8 and 9 years after tympanoplasties. Histological grading is not important in determining the prognosis in squamous cell carcinomas of the middle ear cleft.

Glomus jugular tumours are next in frequency to squamous cell carcinoma of the middle ear. In the great majority of cases these tumours have a benign histology and clinical course. Some consider this tumour to be of low grade malignancy since it invades bone, recurs and occasionally metastasizes.

Rhabdomyosarcoma is the most common neoplasm in children and usually manifests itself after the age of five.

Adenomatous tumours of the middle ear and mastoid have only recently been recognised as a distinct pathological entity by Derlacki and Barney in 1976.[10] Two of Derlacki and Barney's three cases showed microscopic infiltration, which initially prompted the diagnosis of adenocarcinoma. The biological behaviour and prognosis were not reflected by the histological appearance and this tumour was later referred to as adenomatous tumour. In the same year Hyams and Michaels[11] reported another twenty cases under the same name. In their report, the following diagnostic criteria were recorded: absence of bone destruction, tumour confined to the middle ear cleft and no evidence of invasion or metastasis.

Precise classification of these adenomatous tumours as either benign or low-grade malignant neoplasms remains controversial. Terminology, classification and pathological criteria are not uniform in recent papers.[12,13,14] Although the collective term "ceruminoma" has been used in the past, four distinct patterns are now recognized for the middle ear cleft: adenoma, pleomorph adenoma, adenocarcinoma, adenoid cystic carcinoma.[15] Choristoma consists of heterotopic remnants of histologically normal salivary gland tissue, first described in the middle ear by Taylor and Martin.[16] The frequency of ossicular chain and facial nerve anomalies accompanying all except one of the 14 reported cases of choristoma has suggested a syndrome with unilateral conductive hearing loss as the presenting symptom. The few pleomorph adenomas of the middle ear were not associated with middle ear anomalies.

Recently developed histochemical and histo-immune assays may be of value in resolving the controversies in the classification of middle ear tumours. The proper application of these diagnostic techniques usually requires fresh, i.e. unpreserved specimens which should be sent immediately to the pathologist. *"Oncological surgeons do it without formaldehyde, but if you must, do it with plenty of it (20:1)."*

Antibodies to intermediate filament proteins allow the immunohistochemical identification of the cellular origin of tumours.[17] Intermediate-sized filament proteins (IFP) are tissue-specific in that antibodies to keratin, vimentin, desmin, glial fibrillary acidic protein (GFAP) and the neurofilament proteins can distinguish between cells of epithelial and mesenchymal origin, as well as of myogenic and neural origin (figure 2). Malignant cells retain their tissue-specific IFP, which makes it possible to use these antibodies in tumour diagnosis. Carcinomas, for instance, are exclusively identified by antibodies to keratin. Monoclonal antibodies to keratin have allowed the differentiation between subgroups of epithelial tumours, usually between adenocarcinomas and squamous cell carcinomas.[17]

Recent developments in immunohistochemical visualisation of basal membranes could be of eminent value in the detection of micro-invasive growth of malignant tumours. Basal membranes are found at any side of the body as a continuous boundary between epithelial cells, capillaries, muscle- and nerve fibres respectively and the surrounding connective tissue. Collagen type IV and laminine are the most important and exclusive basal membrane biochemical constituents. It was found that polyclonal antisera against collagen type IV and laminine showed evidence of interruption and fragmentation of the basal membrane in the pres-

Fig. 2. Tissue specifity of intermediate-sized filament proteins (IFP). Malignant cells retain their tissue-specific IFP.

Cell type	Intermediate filament protein
Epithelial cells	Keratin
Mesenchymal cells	Vimentin
Muscle cells	Desmin
Neuronal cells	Neurofilament proteins (NF)
Astrocytes	Glial fibrillary acidic protein (GFAP)

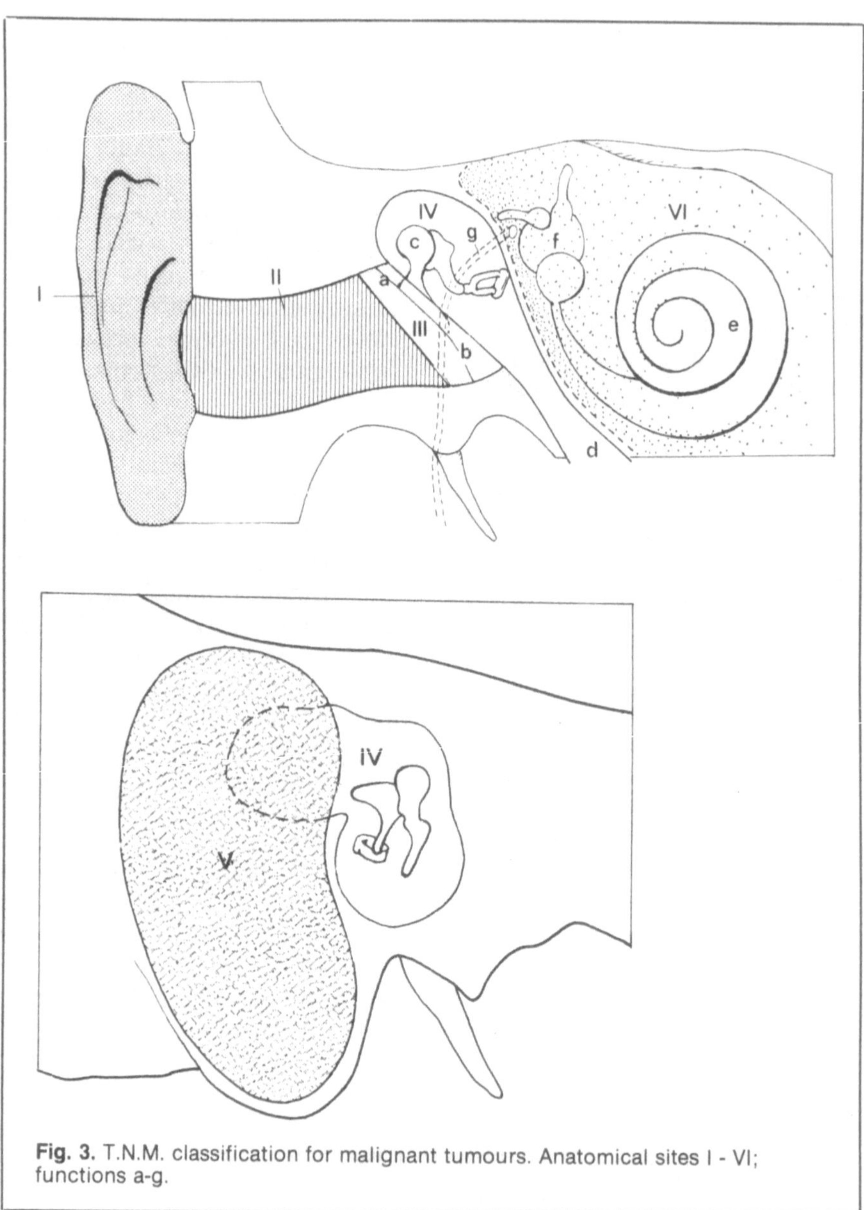

Fig. 3. T.N.M. classification for malignant tumours. Anatomical sites I - VI; functions a-g.

ence of micro-invasive growth, one of the characteristics of malignancy.[18] The histopathological differentiation of glomus tumours, with or without a tendency to malignant growth, or of adenomatous tumours and low grade malignant adenocarcinomas could benefit from the application of this new technique.

Frozen sections of tumours of the middle ear cleft are often difficult to diagnose when inflammatory lesions are encountered. Definite surgery should be deferred pending a final histopathological diagnosis.

Electron microscopy should be routinely performed for middle ear tumours. In the differentiation between adenoma, "adenomatous tumours", adenocarcinoma, adenoid cystic carcinoma, rhabdomyosarcoma and carcinoid, electron microscopy could lead to the ultimate diagnosis.

The most recently described middle ear tumour is the carcinoid Apudoma.[19,20] The presence of intracellular membrane-bound neurosecretory granules varying in size from 120-300 nm demonstrated by electron microscopy, and argyrophily in the Grimelius stain are characteristic. The carcinoid tumours of the middle ear reported until now have behaved clinically benign.

All neoplasms of the hearing organ are rare. This precludes anyone from acquiring sufficient experience to reach meaningful conclusions regarding natural history, diagnosis and treatment. Centralized registration of tumours at this anatomical site and the use of the TNM classification of malignant disease are therefore advisable. We propose the TNM classification as is shown in figure 3.

The sites and functions include: I earlobe, II external auditory canal, III a.b. deep external auditory canal, middle ear adjacent to tympanic membrane, a. eardrum intact, b. eardrum perforated, IV C.D. middle ear, c. destruction of ossicular chain, d. dysfunction of Eustachian tube, V mastoid cavity, VI e.f.g. petrosal bone, e. cochlear involvement f. vestibular involvement, g. facial nerve impairment.

For staging of the disease we suggest: T_1 malignancy is confined to the epithelium or mucosa; T_2 lesions include involvement of cartilage or radiologically confirmed bone destruction; T_3 reveals disease at sites other than defined for the middle ear.

Minimal requirements for assessing TNM category could be defined as follows: T category: clinical examination, tomography/CT scanning, audiometry, vestibulography, facial nerve topodiagnostic and electrical test; N and M category according to the regulations of UJCC or AM.J.C.

Example: $T_2N_0M_0$ III b IV cg. Primary cancer of the middle ear with bone destruction and extension to the external ear canal. The eardrum is perforated, the ossicular chain destructed, the facial nerve function impaired.

References:

1. GOODMAN M.Z. Middle ear and mastoid neoplasms. *Ann. Otol.* 80, 419-424, 1971.
2. MARAN A.G.D., JACOBSON J. in: Clinical Otolaryngology, Maran, Blackwell, Oxford, 1979.

3. MAWSON S.R. Diseases of the ear. Edward Arnold Ltd. London, 1974.

4. FAIRMAN H.D. Radical surgery for carcinoma of the middle ear. *Proc. Roy. Soc. Med.* 65, 274-251, 1972.

5. BRADLEY W.H., MAXWELL J.H. Neoplasms of the middle ear and mastoid. *Laryngoscope* 64, 533-556, 1954.

6. LEWIS J.S. Surgical management of tumours of the middle ear and mastoid. *J. Laryngol. Otol.* 97, 299-311, 1983.

7. BERENDES J. Zur Entstehung des primären Mittelohrkarzinoms. *Arch. Ohr, Nas.u. Kehlk.-Heilk.* 43, 137-143, 1938.

8. MEANS R.G. GERSTEN J. Primary carcinoma of the mastoid process. *Ann. Otol.* 62, 93-101, 1953.

9. KLEINSASSER O., GLANZ H., SCHULZE W. Mittelohrkarzinome nach Tympanoplastik. *Arch. Otorhinolaryngol.* 235, 700, 1982.

10. DERLACKI E.L., BARNEY Ph.L. Adenomatous tumours of the middle ear and mastoid. *Laryngoscope* 86, 1123-1135, 1976.

11. HYMANS V.J., MICHAELS L. Benign adenomatous neoplasm (adenoma) of the middle ear. *Clin. Otolaryngol.* 1, 17-26, 1976.

12. PALLANCH J.F., WEILAND L.H., Mc DONALD T.J., FACER, G.W. Adenocarcinoma and adenoma of the middle ear. *Laryngoscope* 92, 47-53, 1982.

13. JAHRSDOERFER R.A., FECHNER R.E., SELMAN J.W. et al. Adenoma of the middle ear. *Laryngoscope* 93, 1041-1044, 1983.

14. EDEN A.R., PINCUS R.L., PARISIER S.C., SOM P.M. Primary adenomatous neoplams of the middle ear. *Laryngoscope* 94, 63-66, 1984.

15. DEHNER L.P., CHEN K.T.K. Primary tumours of the external and middle ear. *Arch. Otolaryngol.* 106, 13-19, 1980.

16. TAYLOR G.D., MARTIN H.F. Salivary gland tissue in the middle ear. *Arch. Otolaryngol.* 73, 651-653, 1961.

17. RAMAEKERS F.C.S., PUTS J.J.G., MOESKER O. et al. Antibodies to intermediate filament proteins in the immunohistochemical identification of human tumours: an overview. *Histochem. J.* 15, 691-713, 1983.

18. VISSER R., BEEK, J.M.H. van der, BOSMAN F.T. Immunochemical identification of basal membranes: a diagnostic tool to detect (micro) invasional growth of the laryngeal carcinoma. *Clin. Otolaryngol.* (to be published).

19. MURPHY G.F., PILCH B.Z., DICKERSON G.R. et al. Carcinoid tumour of the middle ear. *Am. J. Clin. Path.* 73, 816-819, 1980.

20. MANNI J.J., VAN HAELST H.J.G.M., KUBAT K., MARRES E.H.M.A. Carcinoid of the middle ear. In this publication.

SYMPOSIUM VI
Pathophysiology

Chairman: M. Sakai

The behaviour of the squamous tympanic epithelium

D. Boedts

On the squamous epithelium of the tympanic membrane a migrational movement takes place in man from the centre towards the periphery. This phenomenon has been described a long time ago, as early as 1877 by Burnett, and confirmed by Buck (1880) and Bezold (1908). Several mechanisms underlying this centrifugal migration have been postulated, such as the vibration of the tympanic membrane or the blood flow in the vessels of the membrane. This movement is suggested to occur in the upper layers of the stratum corneum.[1]

The migration of the upper layer of the squamous epithelium, a finely regulated physiological mechanism well adapted to the necessity of cleaning the ear cavity and to the removal of keratin and cerumen, might be responsible, at least partly, for the extrusion and removal of foreign bodies from the drum head e.g. ear grommets. Keratin accumulation and scab formation, for exemple in atelectatic ears, can also be explained by a dysfunction of this migration phenomenon.

This migrational keratin movement has to be differentiated from the epithelialization process which occurs in healing tympanic perforations and in tympanoplasties. In this latter situation a centripetal movement of the whole squamous epithelial layer occurs, from the periphery, often from the external auditory canal. This epithelialization process, a migration of dividing and also differentiating epidermal cells over a wound surface, is influenced by several general and local factors such as age and condition of the patient, infection in loco and so on. The squamous epithelium plays an important rôle in the closure of tympanic perforations. As a matter of fact, the healing of a tympanic membrane differs from the normal healing process of skin wounds where the squamous epithelium can migrate over a newly formed granulation tissue layer (figure 1).

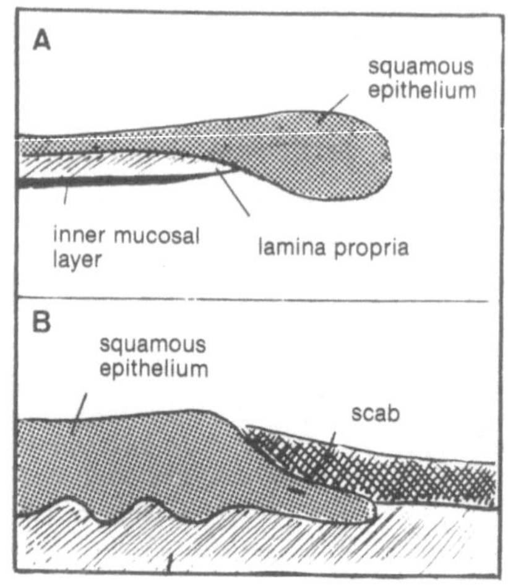

Fig. 1. Diagram of the healing mechanism
A of a tympanic perforation
B of a skin wound

In tympanic perforations, where there is no such underlying tissue, the closure of the connective tissue defect has always a tendency to lie behind the healing of the epithelial layer (figure 2). This phenomenon explains the failure to close large perforations and also the misrouting of the squamous epithelium towards the middle ear cleft (figure 3).

In small perforations, the keratinizing epithelium does not wait for the healing of the underlying connective tissue. It seeks contact with the epithelial margins of the other side over the deficiency, and a thin "replacement membrane" is formed, consisting of an outer epithelial and an inner mucosal layer. Thus, to close large tympanic defects, a support layer is necessary.

Two important, although contradictory, mechanisms influence the epithelial extension over a substratum; on the one hand the cell movement, and on the other hand the cell adhesion to this substratum.[2] Concerning the adhesion, much depends upon the nature of the substratum, e.g. ectoderm shows good adhesion to mesoderm but not to entoderm. Cell movement is contrary to adhesion to the substratum.

The first condition necessary for cell migration is the presence of free edges. Well known is the slogan of Trinkaus[3] "an epithelium will not tolerate a free edge" and also "marginal cells are the

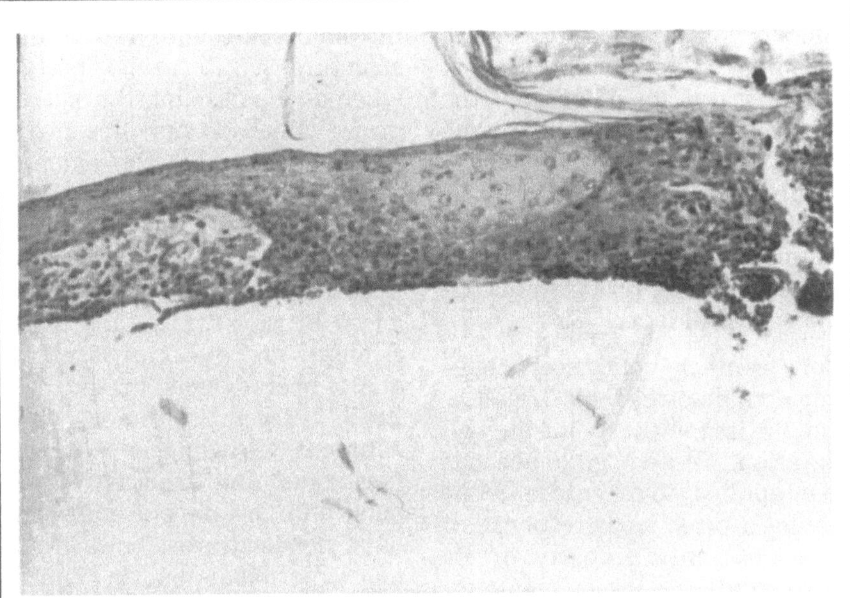

Fig. 2. Hypertrophia and hyperplasia of the healing squamous tympanic epithelium. "Snake head" appearance

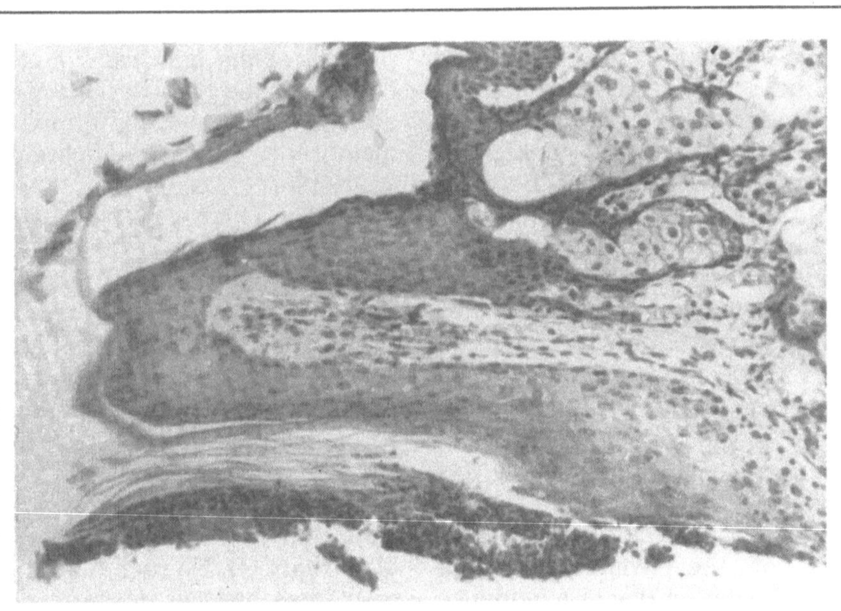

Fig 3. Misrouting of the squamous epithelium towards the middle ear cleft

prime movers". Therefore, in order to obtain a good epithelial spreading in tympanoplasties, it is necessary to interrupt the "mucocutaneous junction" at the rim of the perforation. The cleaning up of perforation margins is based on this principle; thus, the squamous epithelium is lifted from the lamina propria and the inner mucosal layer.

The "contact guidance" phenomenon described by Weiss[4] is another important point in cell migration. Contact guidance has been applied to phenomena involving a directional response of a cell to some property of its substratum.

It is interesting to mention here the experiments of Yoshizato et al.[5] In their in vitro experiments human dermal fibroblasts and chicken embryo myoblasts were cultured both on non-oriented and aligned collagen film. There was a close relationship of structural interaction between cells and collagen fibres. Nearly all innoculated cells, fibroblasts and myoblasts were oriented in the direction of the aligned collagen bundles. It was suggested that a three-dimensional collagen fibre structure is required in order to elicit a contact guiding response to cells. Concerning this phenomenon, we may assume that the outer radial fibre structure of the tympanic lamina propria plays a rôle as a guidance system for the migrating epithelium. There is some clinical evidence that the epithelial and vascular expansion over a tympanic homograft with radial fibre structure has a radial pattern, whereas this is not the case in grafts which do not present this radial pattern as, for example, fascia grafts or moulded dural homografts.

Epithelial spreading is also influenced by the stiffness and tensile strength of the graft and by anatomical defects in the graft itself.[6,7] Several authors such as Albrecht,[8] Friedmann,[9,10] Rüedi,[11] Fernandez and Lindsay,[12] Steinbach and Gruninger,[13] Marquet,[14] have demonstrated, both in animal experiments and in humans, proliferation of stimulated basal epithelial cells of the tympanic membrane and the external auditory meatus towards the middle ear cleft, provided the membrane propria of the pars tensa and/or corium of the pars flaccida were damaged, although the tympanic membrane seemed apparently "intact".

In this respect, in a histological review of unsuccessful "fresh" fascia grafts and "preserved" dura and tympanic homograft specimens we were able to demonstrate epithelial spreading through the loose connective tissue layer in so-called "vital grafts" in which apparently autolysis and necrosis had occurred also (figure 4). No such migration could be observed in grafts preserved and fixed in formaldehyde. This fixative increases the tensile strength and hardens the

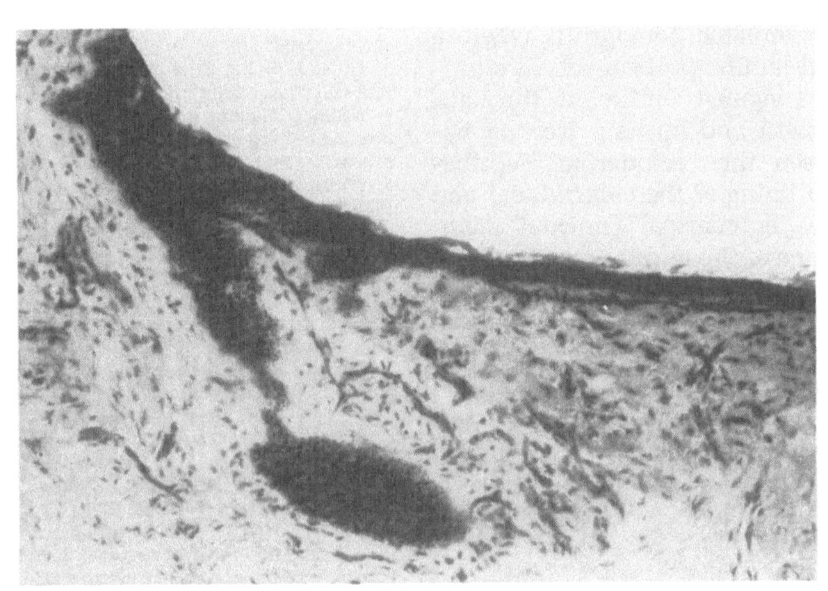

Fig. 4. Epithelial spreading through the connective tissue in a non-preserved "fresh" fascia graft

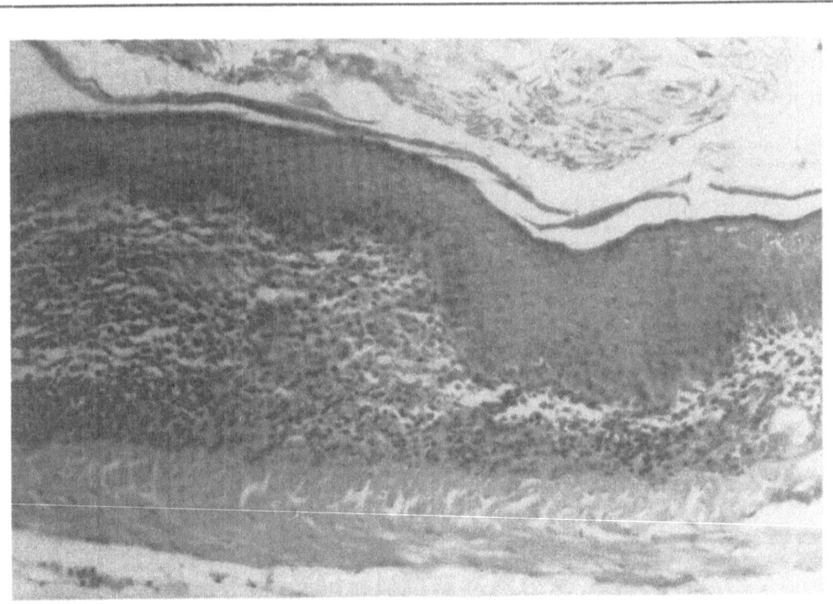

Fig. 5. Lamina propria homograft acts as a barrier against epithelial migration

graft. This is particularly the case in tympanic homografts where a real lamina propria acts as a barrier against epithelial throughgrowth and forms a frontier between the "ectodermal" epithelial lining of the external ear and the "entodermal" mucous membrane of the middle ear (figure 5).

We feel that some of the above mentioned factors concerning tympanic epithelial migration and differentiation are most important in the search and development of a suitable tympanic graft and in tympanoplasty surgery.

Acknowledgement
I would like to thank Prof. J. Marquet for his guidance and stimulation in otologic research and Mrs. L. Moeneclaey for the histological preparation.

References:

1. BOEDTS D. Tympanic epithelial migration. *Clin. Otolaryngol.* 3, 249-253, 1978.
2. VAUGHAN R.B., TRINKAUS J.P. Movement of epithelial cell sheets in vitro. *J. cell. Sci.* I, 407-413, 1966.
3. TRINKAUS J.P. Cells into organs. Prentice Hall Inc., Englewood Cliffs, New Jersey, 1969.
4. WEISS P. Guiding principles in cell locomation and cell aggregation. *Exp. Cell Res.*, suppl. 8, 260-281, 1961.
5. YOSHIZATO K., OBINATA T., HUANG H.Y., MATSUDA R., SHIOYA N., MIYATA T. In vitro orientation of fibroblasts and myoblasts on aligned collagen film. *Develop. Growth and Differ.* 23(2), 175-184, 1981.
6. BOEDTS D. L'épithélialisation tympanique des autogreffes et des implants préservés. *Rev. Laryng.* 102, 9-10, 367-371, 1981.
7. BOEDTS D. The behaviour of the keratinizing epithelium in tympanoplasty. *J. Laryng. Otol.* 98, 1984 (in press).
8. ALBRECHT W. Die Bedeutung des lockeren Bindegewebes für die Entstehung des Cholesteatoms. *Arch. Ohren, Nasen- und Kehlk., Heilk.*, 157, 341, 1950.
9. FRIEDMANN I. The histopathology of experimental otitis of the guinea-pig with particular reference to experimental cholesteatoma. *J. Laryng. Otol.* 69, 588, 1955.
10. FRIEDMANN I. The pathology of the ear. Blackwell, Oxford, England, 1974.
11. RÜEDI L. Cholesteatoma formation in the middle ear in animal experiments. *Acta Otolaryng.* 50, 233, 1959.
12. FERNANDEZ C., LINDSAY J.R. Aural cholesteatoma. Experimental observations. *Laryngoscope*, 70, 1119-1141, 1960.
13. STEINBACH E., GRUNINGER G. Experimental production of cholesteatoma in rabbits by using non-irritants (skin tolerants). *J. Laryng. Otol.* 94, 269-279, 1980.
14. MARQUET J. Cholesteatoma or Keratoma - A pathological approach. *Acta ORL Belg.* 34, 5-11, 1980.

Postoperative long-term ventilation of the middle ear and mastoid cavities

I. Eliachar

Introduction

Malfunction of the Eustachian tube (ET) contributes to many disorders of the middle ear (ME). Assertive management of ears with persistent malfunctioning ET is important in preventing imminent sequelae.[1,2]

Experience in applying long-term ventilating tubes (LTVTs) of various forms and modes in order to prevent the sequelae of persistent ET malfunction has been widely reported.[3-7] Effective prolonged ME ventilation may readily postpone the need for surgery or reduce the extent of the operation. Employment of the LTVT ought to be attempted in selected conditions, recognizing that ME and mastoid surgery may not reestablish effective ET function.

Long-term ventilating tubes may extend reconstructive surgery to selected patients with poorly functioning ETs. Ventilating tubes (VT) inserted in tympanoplasty might save more ears and preserve more hearing than any other conservative surgical measure.[8,9]

Several studies describe methods of overcoming postoperative complications, using short and LTVTs in operations performed on atelectatic ears.[10-14]

Material and methods

Over an 8-year period (1976-1984), 54 patients (58 ears) with chronic otitis media, had inadequate ME ventilation preoperatively or in the immediate postoperative period. These ears were managed by LTVTs and made up 11% of the operations for chronic otitis media during that period.

The LTVTs were placed either through the healthy remnants of the tympanic membrane (TM) in the anterior hemitympanum, or introduced into the antrum or mastoid cavity through the posterior bony canal wall (figures 1 and 2). The T-shaped silicone tube was used throughout this study.[15] This tube has a long shaft that rises above the Gelfoam used for packing the external ear canal to provide immediate ventilation. The intratympanic wings of the Goode tube may be positioned under surgically released sections of the retracted tympanic membrane. They may maintain the drum or graft in position, promote drainage and prevent recurrence of intratympanic postoperative adhesions (figure 3). Table 1 summarizes the types of

Fig. 1. A typical atelectatic ear with relatively spared anterior hemitympanum into which a LTVT may be introduced at surgery.

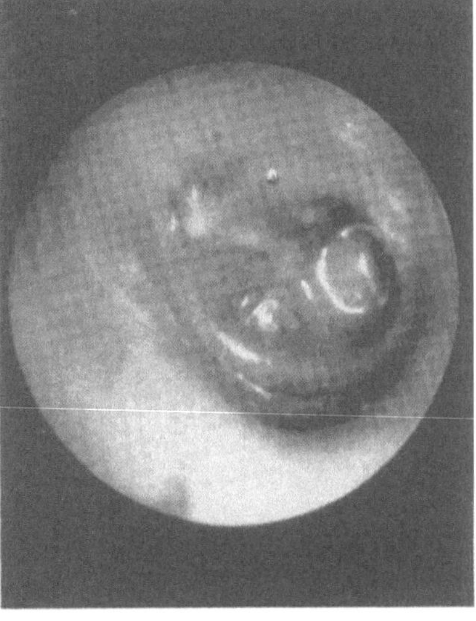

procedures performed, lesions encountered and indications to insert the tubes.

Twenty-seven patients suffered from bilateral ME disease. Many had to be periodically ventilated, usually in the winter. Five of the poorly ventilated contralateral ears were simultaneously managed by LTVTs, delaying or negating the need for major surgery.

Patients were repeatedly encouraged to keep their follow-up appointments. The ears were examined and managed under the microscope. Audiometry was performed routinely every six months.

Eight tubes were removed deliberately and ten tubes extruded spontaneously; of these, eleven had to be reinserted. Only 7 ears remained electively extubated by the end of the study period.

One case was lost to follow-up at 9 months. Five ears had second or revison surgery.

Management and course

Seventy of the postsurgical problems over the eight-year period were trivial and could be managed in the office. Eight necessitated general anesthesia. It is noteworthy that the problems tended to concentrate in selected susceptible ears (tables 2 and 3). Ceruminous plugs, blood clots

Fig. 2. Anterior superior tympanic retraction pocket. The posterior mesotympanum is relatively spared. In this case the LTVT may be inserted through the posterior external ear canal into the antrum to obtain immediate postoperative ventilation, avoiding disruption of the graft.

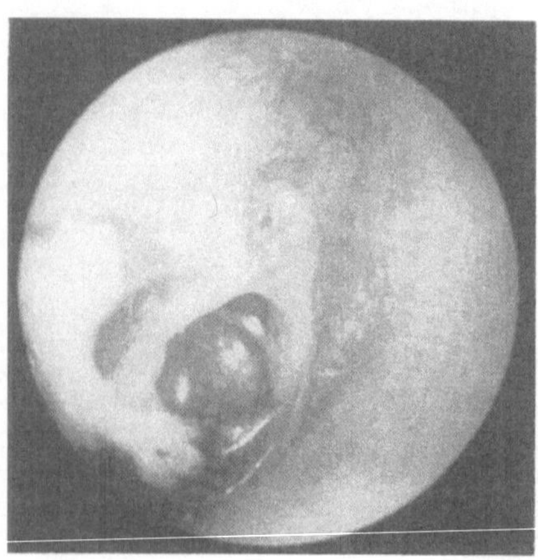

Fig. 3. A long-term ventilating tube in an ear following modified radical mastoidectomy.

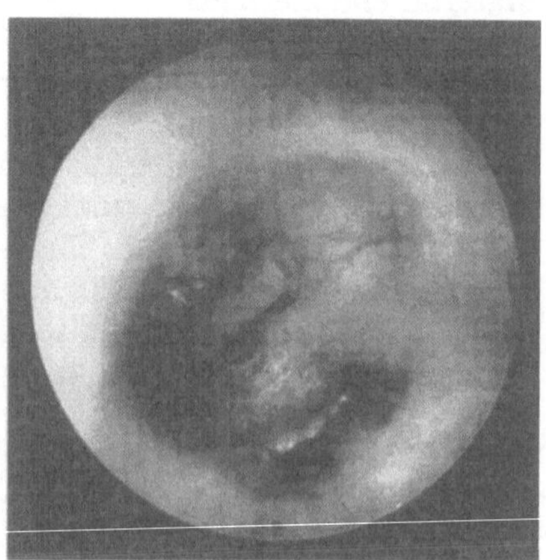

Table 1. Types of surgery performed

	In-surgery insertions of LTVTs	Postoperative insertions of LTVTs
Tympanoplasty types I & II, fascial graft repair of perforation	11	8
Atticotomy with tympanoplasty	5	2
Tympanomastoidectomy (ICW)	7	6
Modified radical mastoidectomy with tympanoplasty	9	4
Ossiculoplasty, ICW		
— ossicular interposition	1	3
— TORP	1	1
Total ears	34	24

LTVT - Long-term ventilating tubes
ICW - Intact canal wall
TORP - Total ossicular replacement prosthesis

Table 2. Developments and complications

27 (46%) ears had uneventful follow-up)
31 ears had 78 developments or complications that required specific interventions.
(64 directly related to the LTVT
14 not related to the LTVT)

Susceptibility:

7 ears had one intervention	(25%)
6 ears had two interventions	(18%)
13 ears had three interventions	(42%)
5 ears had four interventions	(15%)

and crusted secretions (N=22) were extracted from within the tubes with the aid of curved alligator forceps.

Peritubal keratinizations (N=22) were removed by microscopic debridement, occasionally removing the LTVT together with the surrounding keratin layers and

Table 3. Breakdown of developments and complications that required interventions in 31 ears

Descriptions	Total No.	Details	LTVT related
Occlusion of the LTVT	22		X
Spontaneous tubal extrusion	10		X
Peritubal keratinization	22		X
— with secondary infection		7	
— with granuloma		4	
— with bleeding		3	
— with invasion into ME		1	
Migration of the LTVT	2		X
Recurrent ME infections:	15		
— due to extrinsic contamination		5	X
— incidental to upper resp. inf.		4	
— incidental to allergy		6	
Persistent perforations following:			
— extrusion or removal	3		X
Recurrent cholesteatoma	1		
Persistent or recurrent ME			
— disease unrelated to the VT	3		
Total Complications	78	—	64

Comp. = Complications
Inf. = Infections
Resp. = Respiratory
LTVT = Long-Term Ventilating Tube
ME = Middle Ear

promptly replacing it (figure 4). Granulation tissue (N=9) was removed with alligator cup forceps. Bleeding (N=3) was controlled by 2-3 drops of 1% ephedrine. Whenever infection was encountered, (N=5) topical treatment with dexamethasone and neomycin drops was administered for several days. Mycotic growth was removed and irrigated with antimycotic solutions. Two tubes migrated from their original point of insertion. Both were removed, and reinserted.

Invasion of the middle ear cavity by squamous epithelium was observed in one ear. It was surgically removed and the drum regrafted.

Three small dry perforations, 2 mm in diameter, persisted following the intentional removal of the tubes. The air bone gap was under 15 and 10 dB throughout the speech frequencies. These ears were kept under observation with no plans for further surgical intervention.

Fig. 4. Peritubal keratinization. Note dissociated myringosclerotic distribution.

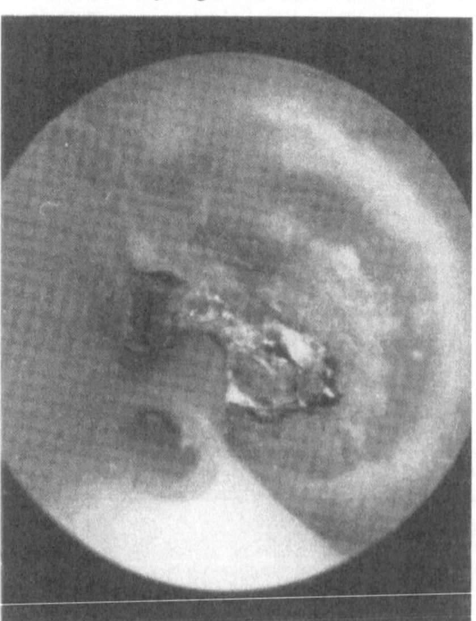

Fourteen complications were not related to the LTVTs. These included 10 middle ear infections that occurred in correlation with upper respiratory diseases and bouts of allergy; removal of the LTVTs was not indicated. Myringosclerosis was noted in 4 TMs. Three ears had persistent mucopurulent discharge that did not abate following intentional removal of their tubes and had to be reoperated. Cholesterol granuloma was found in two, and subacute mucosal disease in the third ear. Radical mastoidectomy was performed in the first two ears and revision tympanomastoidectomy in the third. One case with persistent facial recess cholesteatoma was unrelated to the LTVT. The ear was reoperated.

Audiometric findings and results

Late postoperative changes lead to deterioration in hearing thresholds.[16] Effective measures should be persued to improve ME ventilation whenever it contributes to late hearing loss.

Table 4 compares the preoperative audiometric findings with the results obtained two months postoperatively and one year postoperatively. Pure-tone averages (500, 1 000 and 2 000 Hz)

Table 4. Pure-tone averages AC & BC in dB in 58 long-term ventilated ears

	AC	Air bone gap	BC
Pre-op thresholds	44	31	12
2 months post-op thresholds	34	26	11
1 year post-op thresholds	30	20	13

were computed for both air conduction (AC) and bone conduction (BC). The individual averaged thresholds were reaveraged for the group as a whole.

It is noteworthy that hearing thresholds remained stable throughout the first postoperative year. Furthermore, there was a marked improvement in hearing after insertion of the LTVTs in the postoperatively ventilated subgroup. Once achieved, these thresholds remained stable.

Attempts to manometrically determine ET function through the LTVTs demonstrated inability to equalize or reduce negative intratympanic gradients in almost all the cases, indicating continuation of ventilation.

Discussion

Chronic otitis media with atelectasis can be managed conservatively with interrupted periodic or prolonged introductions of VTs. ET functions may not be expected to improve in patients with allergy, hypoimmunity, cleft palate, cranio-facial anomaly, head trauma, nasopharyngeal tumors and following radiotherapy. Detection of persistent negative ME air pressures, ME effusion, conductive hearing loss, progression of the atelectatic condition with ingrowth, deepening and widening of retraction pockets, are definite indications for active intervention.

It is our policy to restrain the atelectatic process by establishing effective long-term ventilation of the ME and/or the mastoid cavity. This may be achieved when the retracting pocket is mobile and not adherent to the underlying structures; its fundus shiny, clearly observed throughout its circumference, self-cleansing and not perforated.[6]

The cases included in this study presented for treatment with either overt neglected cholesteatoma, or demonstrated progressive otoscopic and tympanometric deterioration in conjunction with hearing loss. Over 50% had been treated bilaterally in the past with VTs; four had indwelling LTVTs preoperatively. VT insertion may be impossible in surgery due to absence of adequate healthy tympanic membrane remnants. Attempts should be made to avoid placement of the VT through the graft. This may lead to premature extrusion after surgery or to non-healing perforations. In such cases postoperative insertion of the LTVT or ventilation by route of the mastoid cavity are opted for.

The single case of persistent cholesteatoma in this series was related to surgical failure rather than to the LTVT. The case with ingrowth of squamous epithelium into the ME was detected in time and surgically corrected.

Non-healing small perforations can be considered "welcome" results of prolonged ventilation, provided they are dry and hearing is adequate.[7] It is noteworthy to compare the number of ears adversely affected by recurrent upper respiratory tract infections and allergy before surgery (N=30), with the lower postoperative incidence of this correlation.

The seven successfully extubated ears and the 45 stable ears with prolonged ventilation support the use of perioperative management with LTVTs in poor surgical risk cases. Overall take-rate of the grafts in this series was better than expected. Short and long-term thresholds of hearing also support this form of management.

The Goode tube was widely used in this series. It is suggested, however, that tube type per se was not the dominant factor in achieving prolonged ventilation; rather diligent management was the critical factor that determined the extended efficacy.

Conclusion

Long-term ventilation of the operated middle ear and mastoid cavities contributed to preliminary success in this series. It is effective in by-passing and replacing ET mechanism until it recovers function or better solutions are reached. The results are encouraging, keeping in mind that eradication of disease, together with maintenance and possible improvement of hearing, are the goals of this type of surgery. Complications are either minor or readily overcome in the majority of cases.

References:

1. BLUESTONE C.D., CASSELBRANT M.L., CANTELIN E.I. Eustachian tube function in the pathogenesis of cholesteatoma in children. In: Sadé J. ed., Cholesteatoma and Mastoid Surgery: Proceedings, Second International Conference, Amsterdam: Kugler Publication: 211-224, 1982.
2. BUCKINGHAM R.A., FERRER J.L. Reversibility of chronic adhesive otitis media with polyethylene tube, middle ear air-vent, Kodochrome time-lapse study. *Laryngoscope* 76:993-1014, 1966.
3. ARMSTRONG B.W. Prolonged middle ear ventilation: the right tube in the right place. *Ann. Otol. Rhinol. Laryngol.* 92:582-586, 1983.
4. LUXFORD W.M., SHEEHY J.L. Myringotomy and ventilation tubes: a report of 1568 ears. *Laryngoscope* 92:1297-1298, 1982.
5. SILVERSTEIN H. Permanent middle ear aeration, *Arch. Otolaryngol.* 91:313, 1970.
6. ELIACHAR I., JOACHIMS H.Z., GOLDSHER M., GOLZ A. Assessment of long-term middle ear ventilation. *Acta Otolaryngol.* 96:105-112, 1983.
7. PER-LEE J.H. Long-term middle ear ventilation. *Laryngoscope* 91:1063-1073, 1981.
8. ARMSTRONG B.W. Experience with the ossicular chain. *Ann. Otol. Rhinol. Laryngol.* 78:939-949, 1969.
9. ARMSTRONG B.W. The role of ventilating tubes in tympanoplasty. *Arch. Otolaryngol.* 97:13-14, 1973.
10. WEHRS R.E. Aeration of the middle ear and mastoid in tympanoplasty. *Laryngoscope* 91:1463-1468, 1981.

11. PAPARELLA M.M., JUNG T.T.K. Experience with tympanoplasty for atelectatic ears. *Laryngoscope* 91:1472-1477, 1981.
12. BLATNIK D.S., MILLEN S.J., TOOHILL R.T. Ventilating tube in tympanoplasty. *Laryngoscope* 87: 1847-1852, 1977.
13. GOODHILL V. Unresolved otitis media. *Texas State J. of Med.* 54:579-584, 1958.
14. TOS M. Management of tubal function in reconstructive middle ear surgery. *J. Laryngol. Otol.* 94:25-30, 1980.
15. GOODE R.L. Advantages of the T-tube for short and long-term middle ear ventilation. *Laryngoscope* 93:376-378, 1983.
16. OJOLA K., PALVA A., SORRI M. Late changes in hearing results after mastoid obliteration with tympanoplasty. *Arch. Otolaryngol.* 108:569-573, 1982.

Sensorineural hearing loss after middle ear surgery

D. Nir, I. Eliachar, H.Z. Joachims, M. Goldsher

Postoperative sensorineural (SN) hearing loss is a calculated risk in middle ear surgery.[1] Physical factors like noise and vibration of suction and drill and ossicular manipulation, [2,3,4] and chemical factors like exotoxins and absorbable gelatin sponge, [5,6] inevitably cause SN damage, even in most experienced hands. In our opinion thease losses are unjustifiably overlooked. The following results demonstrate the severity and incidence of postoperative SN dammage, which is much higher than generally expected.

Materials and Methods

Within a period of 5 years, 417 eare were reviewed. They were divided into 7 groups: 1. myringoplasty; 2. tympanoplasty type 2 and 3; 3. atticotomy, atticoantrotomy, tympanomastoidectomy; 4. modified radical mastoidectomy; 5. radical mastoidectomy; 6. stapedectomy; 7. explorative tympanotomy. (Groups 6 and 7 differ from the first five in that surgery was performed on non-infected ears.)

Comparison was made between preoperative and six months postoperative bone conduction thresholds, averaging the results and plotting them for the different surgical procedures. The factors reviewed were postoperative change in bone conduction and the prevalence of loss in bone conduction in relation to severity.

Results

Figure 1 summarizes the postoperative changes in bone conduction for each frequency in the different groups of operations. Note the improvement in bone conduction in stapedectomies at 500 to 2000 Hz. Figure 2 shows the incidence of loss of 10 dB or more in bone conduction, and figure 3 of 20 dB and above.

Discussion

Since the beginning of otologic surgery eradication of chronic in-

Figure 1. Change (dB) in bone conduction following surgery

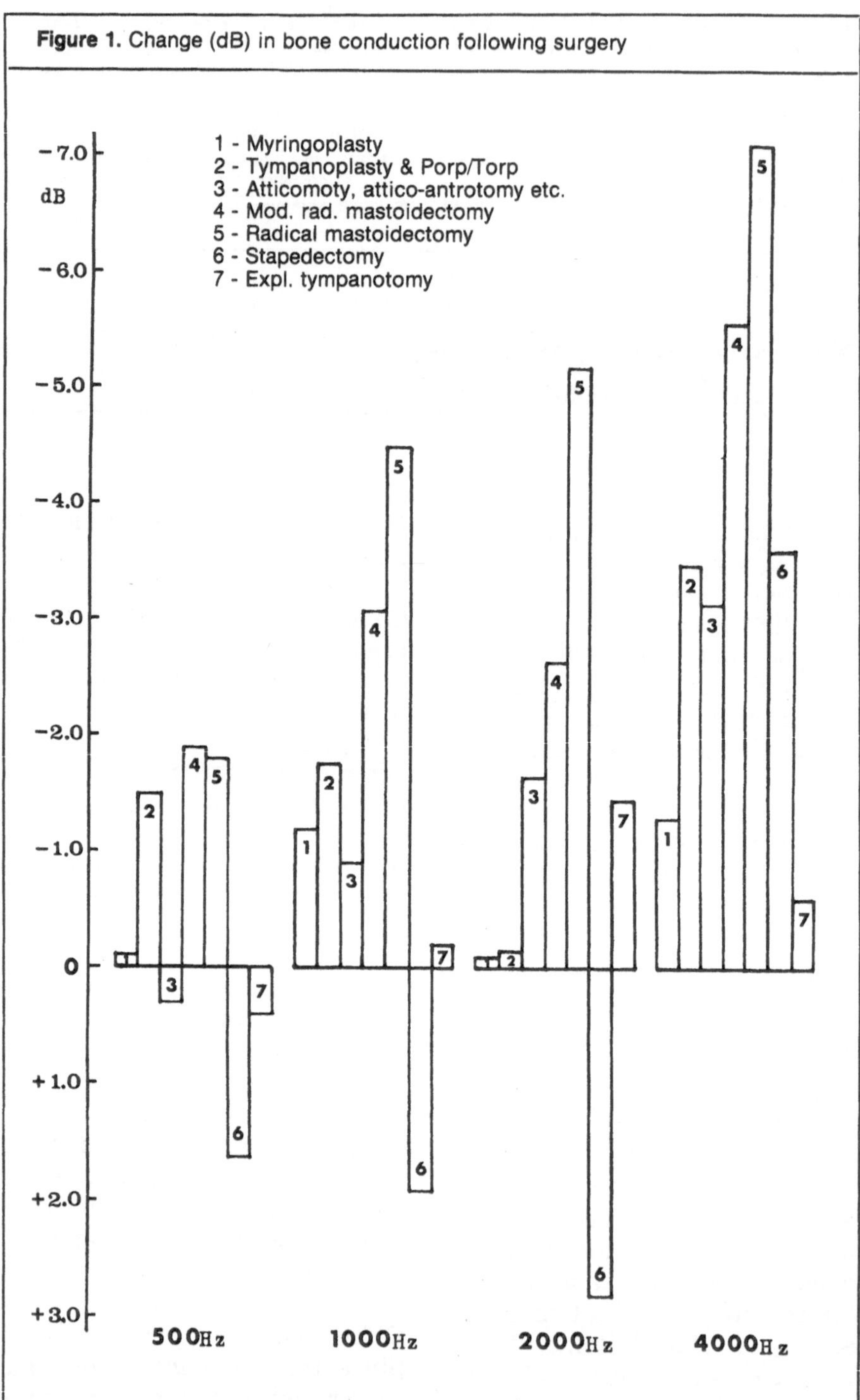

Figure 2. Incidence (%) of above 10 dB sensorineural hearing impairment following surgery

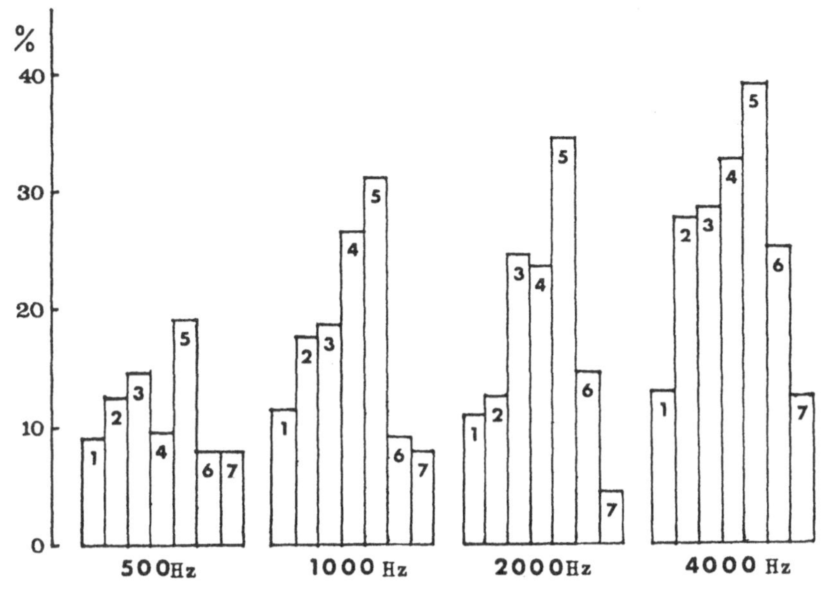

Figure 3. Incidence (%) of above 20 dB sensorineural hearing impairment following surgery

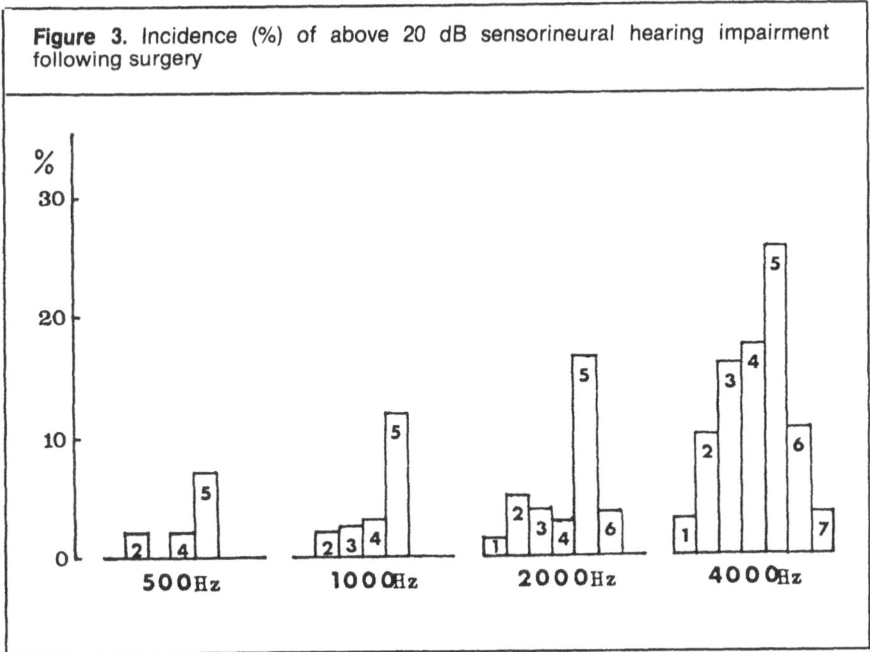

fection was the main objective, even at the expense of hearing loss. Today, with advances in technique and equipment, preservation of hearing plays a more important rôle. Nevertheless, any kind of ear operation has its own inherent risk of hearing damage.

The results presented here demonstrate the average SN hearing loss for different types of operations and its incidence. Figure 1 shows a clear difference between operations for chronically infected ears (groups 1 to 5) and stapedectomies (group 6), performed in a non-infected milieu. While all operations were performed by the same surgeons, the stapedectomy patients demonstrate postoperative improvement in bone conduction in frequencies 500 to 2000 Hz, in contrast to a SN loss in the other patients. Therefore, it appears that chronic infection predisposes to intraoperative SN loss.

A corrolation is also to be found between bone conduction loss and amount of drilling and noise of suction, as shown in figures 1 to 3 in relation to the modified radical and radical mastoidectomies, operations in which drilling is most prolonged. In all types of operations, the high frequencies are more prone to damage, as shown by the average hearing loss (figure 1) and incidence (figures 2 and 3).

The relatively high incidence of postoperative SN damage stresses the importance of this factor which, even if minor, is common and should be considered in every ear surgery.

References:

1. MICHLKE A. Complications in ear surgery. In: Conley J.J. ed. Complications of head and neck surgery. Philadelphia: Saunders, 142-66, 1979.
2. SHEEHY J.L.
ANDERSON R.J. Myringoplasty, a review of 472 cases. *Ann. Otol.* 89: 331-4, 1980.
3. MAWSON S.R., LUDMAN H. Diseases of the ear - textbook of otology. Chicago: Yearbook Medical Publishers, 530-70, 1979.
4. PALVA T., JUHANI K., PALVA A. High tone sensorineural losses following chronic ear surgery. *Arch. Otolaryngol.* 98: 176-8, 1973.
5. SCHUKNECHT H.F., MENDOSA A.M. Cochlear pathology after stapedectomy. *Am. J. Otolaryngol.* 2(3): 173-87, 1981.
6. SHENOI P., BALLANTYNE J. Absorbable gelatine sponge B.P. (Sterispon), and poststapedectomy sensorineural hearing loss. *J. Laryngol, Otol.* 89: 159-68, 1975.

Literature:

1. AVIEL A., OSTFELD E. Aquired sensorineural hearing loss associated with otitis media with effusion. *Am. J. Otolaryngol.* 3: 217-22, 1982.
2. GINSBERG I.A., HOFFMAN S.R., WHITE T.P., STINZIANO G.D. Hearing changes following stapedectomy: a six year follow-up. *Laryngoscope.* 91: 87-92, 1981.
3. GOYCOOLEA M.V., PAPARELLA M.M., GOLDBERG B., CARPENTER A.M. Permeability of the round window membrane in otitis media. *Arch. Otolaryngol.* 106 (7): 430-3, 1980.
4. PRATT L.L. Complications associated with the surgical treatment of cholesteatoma. *Laryngoscope.* 93: 172-4, 1983.
5. SCHACHERN P.A., PAPARELLA M.M., GOYCOOLEA M., GOLDBERG B., SCHLIEVERT P. The round window membrane following application of staphylococcal exotoxin: an electron microscope study. *Laryngoscope.* 91 (12): 2007-17, 1981.
6. SHAMBAUGH G.E. Jr. Cochlear pathology after stapes surgery. *Arch. Otolaryngol.* 72: 1109-23, 1963.

Rôle of Eustachian tube function on the tympanoplasty results

ABSTRACT

J.P. Bebear, M. Bagot d'Arc

While the Eustachian tube constitutes by its functions of equipression, ventilation and drainage one of the determining elements of sound transmission, it is also the one on which it is the most difficult to take effect.
Eustachian tube dysfunctions persistence after tympanoplasty interferes, by negative pression in the tympanic cavity, with good quality of anatomical and functional results.

Valuation of the tubal function, its keeping or its restoration, before, during and after operation, must constitute for the otologist a permanent objective.

The Eustachian tube

ABSTRACT

N.B. Gagnon

The author reviews the methods to assess tubal function. The numerous methods provide some reliable information but their prognostic value is still limited.

Cholesteatoma and benign paroxysmal nystagmus

R. Boniver, R. Hutten

Definition

Benign paroxysmal nystagmus, as shown by Dix and Hallpike, is a form of Type III positional nystagmus in Aschan's classification. For this research it is necessary that the patient keeps his eyes open, gazing at a fixed point. The head is turned by about 30° on a shoulder; then, in a straight line with the trunk, it is tilted laterally on a plane lower by 30° than the horizontal line.

Characteristics

— Often marked latency, sometimes up to 15 sec, sometimes very short and not visible.

— Sensation of distress or of vertigo preceding and accompanying nystagmus.
— Rotatory nystagmus towards the undermost ear, with an intensity which increases from a fraction of one second to 10 sec, according to the cases, then decreases and disappears, the head being maintained in the low position.
— On sitting up, the nystagmus is inversed and is accompanied by vertigo.
— It disappears after a few manœuvres.

It is currently accepted that if one of the characteristics is missing, it is no longer a benign paroxysmal nystagmus and it objectivates a central lesion of the vestibulo-oculomotor pathway. Our findings, described in another publication, demonstrate:
— One of the nystagmus characteristics can be missing although one cannot objectivate a central lesion of the vestibulo-oculomotor pathways, and the evolution is that of benign paroxysmal nystagmus, without any other pathology developing for the patient.
— There is a syndrome in which benign paroxysmal nystagmus, in its typical form, exists for a few days to a few weeks, disappears for a more or less long time, then reappears. This syndrome is frequently observed in hypersympathicotonic individuals, often during a period of tiredness, or in subjects with cervical arthrosis.
— When the nystagmus is very intense, one can sometimes obtain, in Hallpike's heterolateral position, rotatory nystagmus towards the side opposed to the inclination of the head, occurring with a variable latency, lasting a few seconds, and which is sometimes intense.
— In individuals who have had nystagmus for several years, its typical characteristics may vary from one examination to the other, and nystagmus may transitorily lose its rotatory component and become vertical, for instance.
— Benign paroxysmal nystagmus is inhibited when, before the test, with the patient in sitting position, the contralateral ear is irrigated with warm or cold water. This experiment was carried out in 15 individuals with recent benign paroxysmal nystagmus, thus confirming the studies of Ledoux and Devos.

Physiopathology

The aetiology of benign paroxysmal nystagmus is not certain yet. Although some authors (among them Jongkees) have evoked a cervical factor as being responsible for benign paroxysmal nystagmus, most of them admit that it is a lesion of the peripheral organ, of the utricle or a disturbance of the system integrating the nervous influxes issuing from the utricle and the semicircular canals (Mayne, Oosterveld).

Stimulation of the otoliths by themselves does not induce this type of nystagmus (Kornhuber, Fluur).

Destruction of the responsible labyrinth suppresses paroxysmal nystagmus (Citron and Hallpike).

Following a series of physiological experiments and of anatomopathological studies, Schuknecht has shown that the syndrome was due to the deposit of a substance on the cupula of the posterior semicircular canal. He presumes that the substance has a high density and that it makes this organ sensitive to the law of gravity. He thinks that, in most cases, the deposit is due to the otoconia of the utricle.

As aetiologies he suggests: spontaneous degeneration of the utricular otolithic membrane, a labyrinthine commotion, otitis media, surgery on the ear, occlusion of the anterior vestibular artery.

Kornhuber evokes the possibility of mechanical disorders in a semicircular canal, due for instance to a blood clot or to small agglomerations of desquamated cells in the endolymph or in the perilymph. Miehlke has shown the existence of benign paroxysmal nystagmus after a traumatism having induced a small discharge of blood into the perilymph. Stenger has demonstrated benign paroxysmal nystagmus following a labyrinthine fistula.

After a series of experiments, Fluur objectivates the following facts: normal labyrinthine function is necessary to produce nystagmus, since destruction of the labyrinth induces its suppression. According to him, the vestibular system is a differential one: the difference between the left and right influxes induces ocular reactions. The disturbance in the balance system between the two vestibulo-ocular reflex arcs induces nystagmus. Electrical stimulation of different areas of the utricular surface produces distinct ocular movements. In man, these various surfaces cooperate with the semicircular canals in an integrated complex acting on the oculomotor system.

After unilateral labyrinthectomy, horizontal nystagmus is facilitated if the patient is tilted back along a longitudinal axis towards the injured ear, and is inhibited if he is tilted back towards the intact ear. Thus, the utricle and the ipsilateral horizontal semicircular canal function synergically, whereas the utricle is antagonist of the heterolateral semicircular canal.

For this reason, spontaneous nystagmus beating to the right becomes more intense in a left lateral position than in a right lateral position.

The author has also carried out various experiments by cutting the two anterior ampullar nerves, then the posterior, then the vertical ones.

Uemura and Cohen have shown the inhibitory influence on positional nystagmus of rostral lesions of the descending vestibular nucleus, a zone which receives the electrical activity of the otolithic organs.

All this research, therefore, shows the influence of an utricular lesion or at least of a disturbance in the integrated electrical activity of the semicircular canals and of the utricle in the genesis of benign paroxysmal nystagmus.

Our personal studies have shown, besides the above-described variances, the lack of correlation between benign paroxysmal nystagmus and the syndrome of directional preponderance of nystagmus.

These findings, which extend the norms that define benign paroxysmal nystagmus, are in favour of a complex origin of the latter, as proposed by Fluur.

Benign paroxysmal nystagmus and cholesteatoma

We studied 15 cases of benign paroxysmal nystagmus associated with cholesteatoma on a population of 200 cholesteatomas. Their size varied but in all the cases, they reached the round window or they produced cholesterin crystals filling the round window. There was no sign of labyrinthic fistula, nor spontaneous nystagmus, even eyes closed, controlled by electronystagmography and the pendular proofs were symmetrical. There was always a cochlear lesion associated, mild or moderated, on the frequencies above 2 000 Hz.

Discussion

We do not think that the pressure exerted by the mass indirectly on the window disturbs the endolymphatic circulation and produces the benign paroxystic nystagmus in Hallpike's position. Indeed, we never found such a nystagmus in more than 2 000 cases of glue ear where the liquid acts on the window.

A metabolic disturbance of the endolymph induced by the cholesteatoma may be responsible for the symptom. A cochlear lesion in the high frequencies is always associated. When the disturbance is important, the lesion is definitive. When the disturbance is light, the lesion is reversible. This hypothesis is in correlation with the postoperative findings. In some cases, the symptom disappears immediately after the operation (10 cases). In other cases, the symptom remains for a long time and the caloric proofs, after tympanoplasty, reveal an associated labyrinthic paresis (5 cases). In all the cases, however, the auditory lesion remains. Therefore, it seems possible that cells of the first coil of the cochlea are more sensitive to cholesteatoma toxins, perhaps because of their greater concentration, than cells of the labyrinth organs. In this organ, the toxins act on the posterior semicircular cells either directly or indirectly by a modification of the otolith cupula which fragments act on the semicircular macula in the Hallpike's position.

Literature:

1. ASCHAN G. The Pathogenesis of Positional Nystagmus. *Acta Otolaryng.* (Stock.) Suppl. 159, 90-93, 1961.
2. BARANY R. Diagnose von Krankheitserscheinungen im Bereiche des Otolithenapparates. *Acta Otolaryng.* (Stock.) 2, 434, 1921.
3. BARBER H.O. Positional Nystagmus in the Vestibular System, ed. R.E. Naunton. Academic Press New York, 303-319, 1975.
4. BARBER H.O. Positional Vertigo and Nystagmus. *Otolaryngologic Clinics of North America* 6, 169-187, 1976.
5. BARBER H.O., WRIGHT G. Positional Nystagmus in Normals. *Adv. Oto-Rhinolaryng.* 19, 276-285, 1973.
6. BONIVER R. Nystagmus paroxystique bénin et syndrome de prépondérance directionnelle du nystagmus. *J. Franç. ORL* 26, 685-692, 1977.
7. BONIVER R., LEDOUX A. Association d'un nystagmus de position et d'un nystagmus congénital. *Acta Oto-Rhino-Laryngologica Belg.* 26, 249-261, 1972.
8. BONIVER R. Systématisation des nystagmus de position. *J. Franç. ORL* 31, 747-752, 1982.
9. CITRON C., HALLPIKE C.S. Observations upon the mechanism of positional nystagmus of the so-called benign paroxysmal type. *J. Laryng.* 70, 253-259, 1956.
10. COLLARD M., CONRAUX C., WARTER J.M. Les syndromes vestibulaires centraux, ed. Masson et Cie Paris, 1973.
11. DIX M.R., HALLPIKE C.S. The Pathology, Symptomatology and Diagnosis of certain common disorders of the Vestibular System. *Proc. Roy. Soc. Med.* 45, 341-354, 1952.
12. DUMICH P.S., HARNER S.G. Cochlear Function in Chronic Otitis Media. *Laryngoscope* 93, 583-586, 1983.
13. EDWARDS C.H. Benign Paroxysmal Positional Nystagmus in "Neurology of ear, nose and throat diseases", ed. Butterworths London, 149-160, 1973.
14. EDWARDS C.H. Neurology of ear, nose and throat disease, ed. Butterworths London, 109-160, 1973.
15. FLUUR E. Positional and Positioning Nystagmus as a result of utriculocupular integration. *Acta Otolaryng.* (Stock.) 78, 19-27, 1974.
16. FLUUR E. Interaction between the utricles and the horizontal semicircular canals. Four articles in *Acta Otolaryng.* (Stock) 17, 393-485, 1973.
17. FLUUR E., MELLSTROM A. Vestibular Nystagmus, a differential reaction. *Acta Otolaryng.* (Stock.) 71, 299, 1971.
18. FLUUR E., MELLSTROM A. Utricular stimulation and oculomotor reactions. *Laryngoscope* 80, 1701-1712, 1970.
19. FLUUR E. Investigation of Positional and Positioning Nystagmus by using a new type of electrically driven rotative table. *Acta Otolaryng.* (Stock.) 78, 385-390, 1974.
20. JONGKEES D.B.W. Pathology of Vestibular Sensation in Handbook of Sensory Physiology. *Vestibular System,* Springer Verlag, Berlin, New York, VI, 2, 413-450, 1974.
21. KATSARKAS A., OUTERBRIDGE J.S. Nystagmus of Paroxysmal Positional Vertigo. *Ann. Otol. Rhinol. Laryngol.* 92, 146-150, 1983.
22. KORNHUBER H.H. Nystagmus and related phenomena in Man: an outline of otoneurology. *Vestibular System* Handbook of Sensory Physiology Springer Verlag. Berlin, New York, 194-232, 1974.
23. LARMANDE A., GODDE JOLLY D. Nystagmus de position. Les nystagmus. Masson et Cie ed. Paris 2, 1091-1103, 1973.
24. LEDOUX A., DEVOS J. Benign Paroxysmal Positional Vertigo and Rotatory induced Nystagmus. *Adv. Oto-Rhino-Laryng.* 22, 162-168, 1977.
25. LINDSAY J.R., HEMENWAY W.G. Postural Vertigo due to unilateral sudden partial loss of vestibular function. *Ann. Otol.* 65, 692-702, 1956.
26. MAYNE R. A system Concept of the Vestibular Organs. Handbook of Sensory Physiology 2, *Vestibular System.* Springer Verlag, Berlin, New York, 493-580, 1974.
27. MIEHLKE A. Tierexperimentelle Untersuchungen über die Ursache und den Ort der Auslösung des peripheren Lagennystagmus. *Arch. Ohr, Nase u. Kehlk. Heilk.* 166, 327-349, 1955.
28. NORRE M., STEVENS A. Le nystagmus cervical et les troubles fonctionnels de la colonne cervicale. *Acta ORL Belg.* 30, 457-467, 1976.
29. NYLEN C.O. Positional Nystagmus. A review and future prospects *J. Laryng.* 64, 295-318, 1950.
30. OOSTERVELD W.J. et al. Nystagmus de position bénin paroxystique. Les vertiges. Doin ed. Paris, 132-138, 1976.

31. SCHUKNECHT H.F. Cupulolithiasis. *Arch. Otolaryng.* 90, 765-778, 1969.
32. SCHUKNECHT H.F. Positional Nystagmus of the benign paroxysmal type. *The Vestibular System*, ed. R.F. Naunton, Academic Press, Inc., London, 421-428, 1975.
33. SPECTOR M. Positional Nystagmus and ear, nose and throat examination. *Dizziness and vertigo.* Grune & Stratton, New York London, 51-55, 1967.
34. STAHLE J., TERINS J. Paroxysmal Positional Nystagmus. An electro-nystagmographical and clinical study. *Ann. Otol.* 74, 69-83, 1965.
35. STENGER H.H. Über Lagerungsnystagmus unter besonderer Berücksichtigung des gegenläufigen transitorischen Provokationsnystagmus bei Lagewechsel in der Sagittalebene. *Arch. Ohr, Nase u. Kehlk. Heilk.* 168, 220-268, 1955.
36. UEMURA T., COHEN B. Effects of Vestibular Nuclei Lesions on vestibulo-ocular reflexes and position in Monkey. *Acta Otolaryng.* (Stock) Suppl. 315, 1973.

Evaluation of the fistula of the ear

M. Lachman

Fistulas are found in the outer, middle and inner ear much more frequently than we normally imagine.

The diagnosis is easy when there is pus or fluid flowing from the postauricular incision or from the external canal, otherwise the diagnosis is more difficult. The localizations of the fistulas are numerous and can affect the external, middle or inner ear.

In the external ear, fistulas are most often located in the mastoid and very rarely flow out through the mastoid skin. More often, they flow from the postauricular incision or the external canal wall.

In the middle ear, it may be found in the round and oval windows and sometimes the fluid can flow out through the Eustachian tube. It may also affect the semicircular lateral canal. In the inner ear all the semicircular canals, the cochlea, or the internal auditory canal may be affected.

Different types of fluids can be described: pus, cerebro-spinal fluid or perilymph.

The origins of these fistulas are numerous. Most often they are caused by infections and one of the causes is the cholesteatoma. Other tumours may be found (cancer, glomus, etc.). Fistulas can be caused by traumatism or by the surgeon's hand.

Even more rare are congenital malformations of one of the three parts of the ear, or all three, or any combination of the three.

We have to look out for a sensorineural hearing loss, which may appear postoperatively, or dizziness, problems of balance, or tinnitus. These symptoms may be associated and their apparition makes us aware of the possibility of a fistula. These signs lead us to make further tests in order to establish a more precise diagnosis.

Pressure of the tragus is not always significant, neither are Valsalva's, Toynbee's or Hennebert's manœuvres. More value is accorded to the combination of the electromystagmography and impedance bridge described by Daspit and Lithicum at the House Ear Institute. The modifications of the pressure of the impedance bridge modifies the direction of the nystagmus which can be registered by the ENG. The authors report this test to be of value in 90 % of the cases. All these tests are merely suggestive of a fistula but do not give definite proof. This proof can be obtained through tomographies or scannings which are the most accurate tests. The isotopic scintigraphy is often difficult to interpret when CSF is flowing out through the Eustachian tube. It is not always easy to see. Otherwise the diagnosis is made during the operation.

Prevention of the fistulas is first a matter of an early diagnosis of cholesteatomas and their eradication before their growth becomes too big. A good knowledge of the anatomy of the temporal bone and a good practice of drilling prevents iatrogenic fistulas.

In **conclusion**, if we suspect a fistula we can give great value to Daspit's test and even more to tomographies and scanning. Cholesteatomas and other kinds of tumours should be eradicated and the surgeon should have a thorough knowledge of the anatomy of the temporal bone.

Plenary session

ISO standards in audiology

ABSTRACT
P. Hennebert

The ISO (International Standard Organisation) is part of the UNO. Its goal is to establish recommendations concerning all human problems. Most important to us are the electro-acoustics and their diagnostic and therapeutic applications.

The final conclusions of specific items are transmitted to the different countries only after the advice and informed consent of ad hoc committees. These recommendations are regularly revised. The author explains the specific audiological field.

PANEL III

Functional evaluation

Moderator: H. Diamant

Postoperative functional evaluation

ABSTRACT

H. Harder, P. Kylén

Audiological evaluation after middle ear surgery should describe middle ear function and cochlear losses related to surgery. This paper concentrates on the evaluation of the mechanical success of surgery. The air-bone gap is the most direct measure of acoustic middle ear function. However, the bone conduction (BC) thresholds do not only reflect cochlear function, but also abnormalities in the external and middle ear. Depressed BC thresholds improving with surgery are well known in cases of otosclerosis (Cahart notch) but similar phenomena are often recorded after surgery for chronic otitis media. The BC improvement is most pronounced after successful surgery for advanced middle ear pathology, i.e. the cases with the greatest hearing improvement. Therefore, if one wishes to describe postoperative middle ear function with the air-bone gap, the postoperative BC threshold should be the reference. Otherwise, the size of the postoperative air-bone gap would be unduly influenced by preoperative middle ear pathology.

In order to find the most successful surgical procedures, the method chosen for describing the results must allow fine qualitative judgements. Generally speaking, success rate figures are coarse measures and results presented with such methods are to a considerable extent dependent on the choice of criterion and minor variations in audiometric methods can exert a significant influence. Mean values will carry more information and can be compared with more powerful statistical tests. Audiometric methods and complete basal data should always be presented. Results presented as mean values of postoperative air-bone gap can then be accurately evaluated and compared.

Literature:

1. HARDER H., EKVALL L., KYLEN P., ARLINGER S.D. Hearing gain calculations after stapedectomy. *Acta Otolaryngol.* Suppl. 360, 158-160, 1979.
2. HARDER H., JERLVALL L., KYLEN P., EKVALL L. Calculation of hearing results after tympanoplasty. *Clin. Otolaryngol.* 7, 221-229, 1982.

Standards in audiological and in statistical reports

ABSTRACT

G. Flottorp

Audiological data should be valid and relevant.

Validity
Validity is secured when making audiological measurements in rooms satisfying international standards, using ISO standardized methods for measurements.
The presentation should use standardized formats (pure tone audiograms) and symbols.

Relevance
Only relevant data should be reported.

Evaluation of audiological function may be based upon pure tone audiograms, brain stem responses (ERA), impedance data for the middle ear including data of reflex mechanisms changing middle ear impedance, data for supra-threshold hearing, especially speech audiometry data.
Bone conduction data should never be used for evaluation of surgical treatment, since surgery of the middle ear may change the mechanism for bone conduction.

Unfortunately, speech audiometry is not yet standardized. Such standardization shall most probably contain recommendations of speech material, method of performance of test, and of presentation of data. The discrimination curves for at least easy and hard test material are in my opinion the most informative audiological data for functional evaluation.

Statistics
Statistical reports must be based upon sufficiently large material to justify statistical treatment. Omitting and selecting data should as a rule be banned, and when exceptions are justified, reason and amount should be clearly stated.

General rules for statistical treatment and presentation should be followed, such as presentation of standard deviation, level of significance, etc. Usually, threshold data are not suitable for averaging, but for calculation of median and various percentile values.

In order to treat large numbers of pure tone audiograms, it may be advantageous to group them in five categories.

A proposal of such grouping to be standardized by ISO was presented by Denmark a couple of years ago, however, not accepted. A small Nordic group has agreed upon a proposal for five categories of pure tone audiograms. Three of them concern different types of noise inducing hearing loss.

It is of importance that ISO standardized data for hearing as a function of age and sex be used when pure tone audiograms are prepared for such statistical grouping.

Standards in tympanometry

K.J. Van Camp

The International Electrotechnical Commission (IEC) in January 1984 issued a document (29C46) entitled "Aural impedance/admittance instruments". It was distributed for approval under the "six months rule". Although this document contains mainly specifications to be met by the manufacturers, some specifications may be of direct interest to the user and frame in an attempt to standardize the representation of tympanometric results. Of special interest for routine use are the following statements:

— Probe tone frequency: (226±6)Hz. In the document it is recognized that other probe signals may be used.

— Units: S.I. units shall be used.

• ear canal pressure: deca Pascal daPa (=1.02 mm H_2O)

• admittance: at 226 Hz ONLY equivalent volume V_{ea} in cm^3 at all frequencies $10^{-9}m^3/Pa.s$=nano $m^3/Pa.s$ remark that 1 cm^3 equals $10^{-8}m^3/Pa.s$ at 226 Hz ONLY!

• impedance: 10^9 $Pa.s/m^3$ = giga $Pa.s/m^3$ resulting in the conversion relation for the old units to 1 c.g.s.ac. ohm = 10^8 $Pa.s/m^3$ = 0.1 giga $Pa.s/m^3$.

— Rate of pressure change in the ear canal: although no pump speed is mandatory, a rate of pressure change of (50±10) daPa/s is preferred.

— Format of a tympanogram: this specification is mandatory and most useful for a quick comparison of results as it influences the shape of the tympanogram. For a probe tone frequency of 226 Hz ONLY, the scale proportion will be so that the length corresponding to 300 daPa on the horizontal pressure axis equals the length of 1 cm^3V_{ea} (or $10^{-8}m^3/Pa.s$)

on the vertical admittance axis. Both vertical and horizontal scales shall be linear. When the impedance is plotted on the vertical axis, the scale should be inverted and non-linear divided relative to a linear admittance scale. For other probe tone frequencies no specifications are put forward.

The IEC document also contains valuable information on the required temporal characteristics of the instrument when measuring the acoustic reflex. These characteristics must be met by the manufacturers.

It is advisable that researchers designing their own aural admittance meter consult the complete IEC document when the final approved version is available.

Although the IEC document does not exclude higher probe tone frequencies and immittance components other than the admittance, one could conclude erroneously that they are of minor importance. Clinical tympanometry should include other approaches in order to exploit all diagnostic possibilities of tympanometry. Already in 1970, G. Liden[1] pointed out the practical benefits of higher probe tone frequencies. From our own investigations one can conclude that the best impedance/admittance components and probe tone frequency for detecting low impedance pathologies (necrosis luxations etc.) are the admittance and electrical phase angle of the probe set at test frequency of 660 Hz.[2]

References:

1. LIDEN G., PETERSON J.L., BJORKMAN G. Tympanometry. *Arch. Otolaryng.* 92; 248-257, 1970.
2. VAN CAMP K.J., CRETEN W.L., VAN DE HEYNING P.H., DECRAEMER W.F., VANPEPERSTRAETE P.M. A search for the most suitable immittance components and probe tone frequency in tympanometry. *Scand. Audiol.* 12, 27-34, 1983.

SYMPOSIUM VII
Computer processing of data

Chairman: G. Gates

Computerized data processing in middle ear surgery

A. Bismuth, C. Bismuth, L. Vergnon

Computerized data processing in middle ear surgery can be divided in two chapters, closely linked though basically different:
— statistical studies,
— computerized analysis of investigations.

The computer is very helpful for every statistical study as its possibilities regarding memorization and processing are huge.

Therefore, we had first to complete a statistical study in Professor Rouleau's unit. This study has not appeared to be too difficult as the test criteria had been very clearly defined in the protocol.

When we decided to compare this study with those of other teams, particularly ours, we were surprised at the wide range of methods that were used.

— First, the way the results are set out: identical results can look thoroughly different (figures 1 and 2).

— Second, the way the same criteria can be modified by other elements: these first results, which only take into account the air-bone gap, cannot be compared with those, which furthermore integrate the delay which runs between the operation and the investigation.

— Third, the very criteria can be different: in the first diagram, the result of the operation is judged on the pure tone 1000 hertz frequency, on the other it is judged

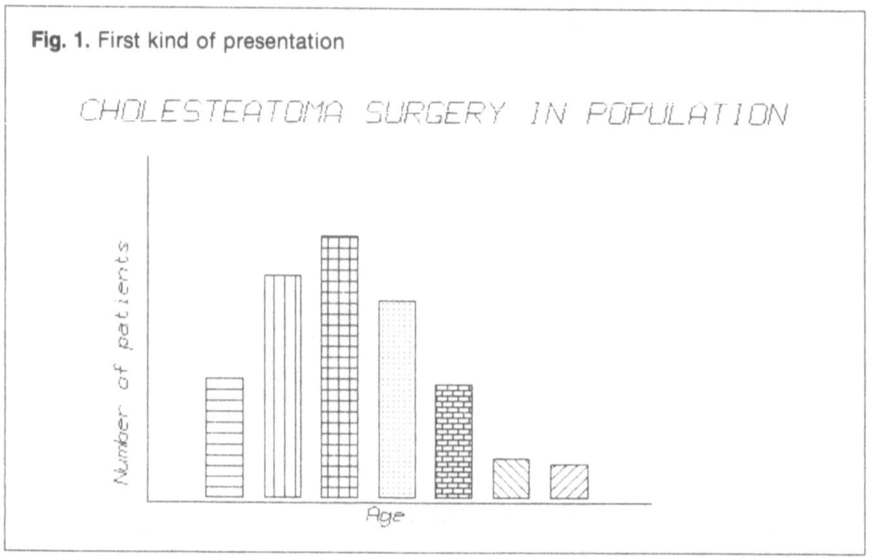

Fig. 1. First kind of presentation

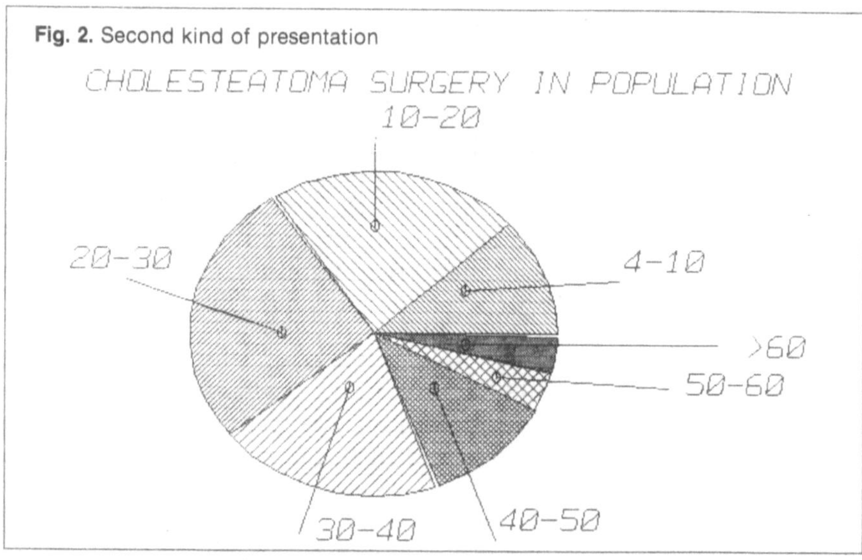

Fig. 2. Second kind of presentation

on the 500 - 1000 and 2000 hertz frequencies, and a last author uses the 500, 1000, 2000 and 4000 hertz frequencies.

Thus, a same audiogram gives different if not contradictory results according to the selected criteria. For instance, in figures 3, 4 and 5 the air-bone gap is 20, 23 and 32 dB respectively.

Furthermore, when a given criteria, such as the air-bone gap,

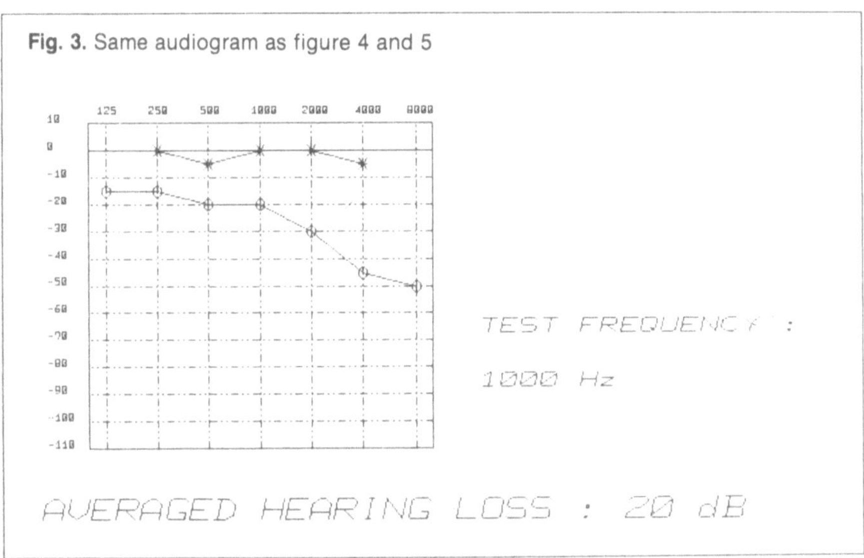

Fig. 3. Same audiogram as figure 4 and 5

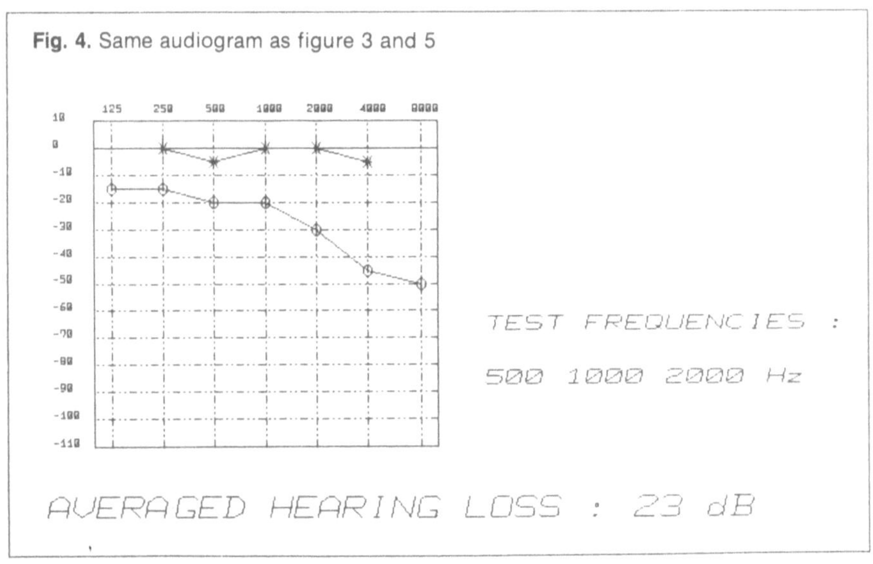

Fig. 4. Same audiogram as figure 3 and 5

is used too narrowly, it can lead to interpretation mistakes. As a matter of fact, if one compares the 10 dB gap of one patient with the same 10 dB of another patient, one completely ignores the discrimination troubles which are far more serious for the latter (figures 6-9).

We have been disturbed not only by these differences, but also by the lack of an internationally

Fig. 5. Same audiogram as figure 3 and 4

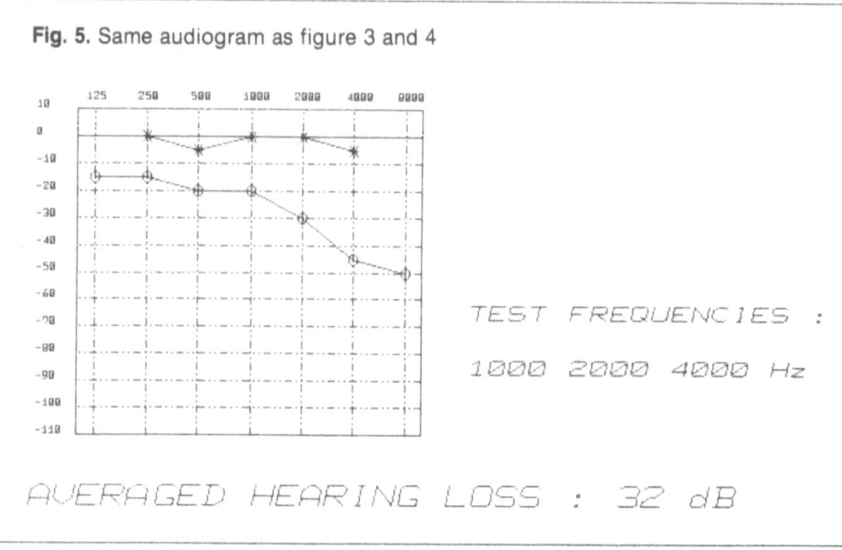

Fig. 6. Same air bone gap as figure 7

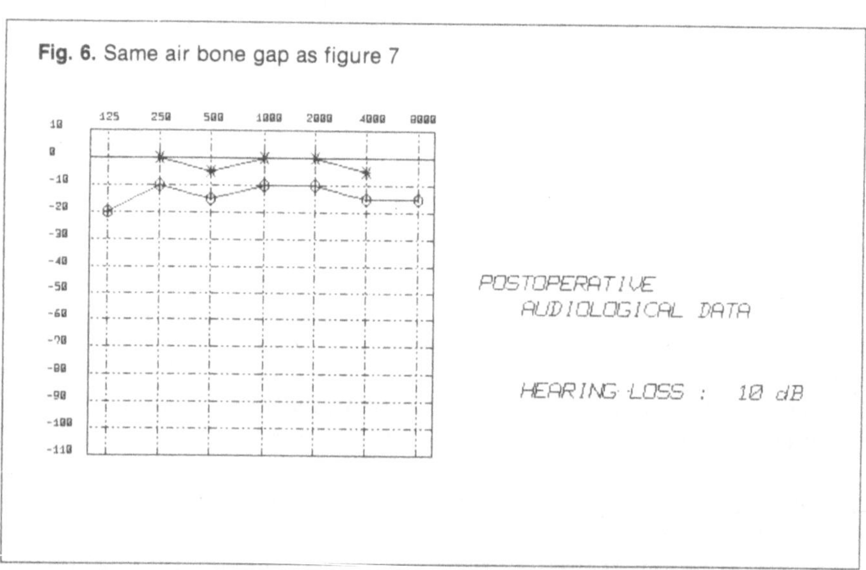

Fig. 7. Same air bone gap as figure 6

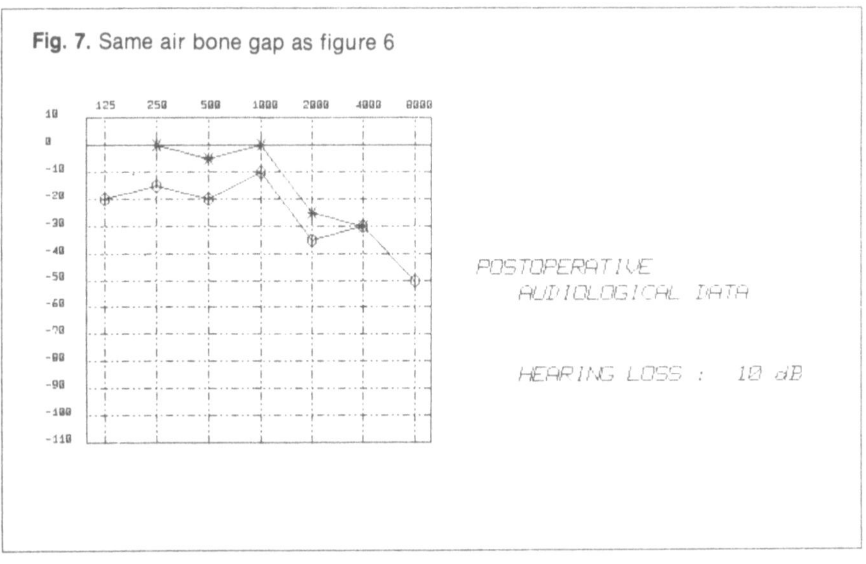

Fig. 8. Speech test for the patient of figure 6

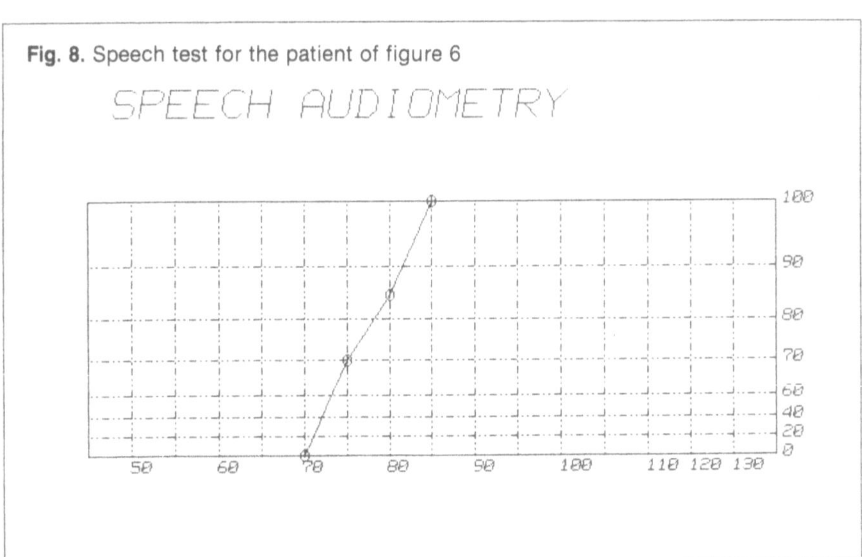

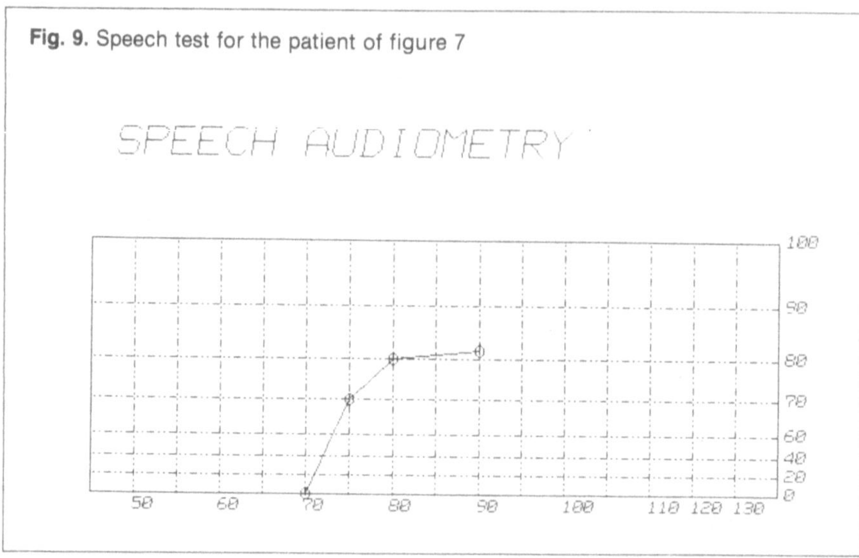

Fig. 9. Speech test for the patient of figure 7

accepted description of diseases and taxonomy of operating techniques.

For instance, the study which has been completed in Professor Roulleau's unit cannot be strictly compared with a similar one completed in a similar unit, as the first used Wullstein's classification and the second Marquet's.

The exactness of the computer implies that operators use strictly comparable criteria for middle ear surgery, which first means a common international language.

It also leads to difficulties when subjective elements are taken into account for the realization and interpretation of audiometrical investigations. These elements can depend on the operator or on the patient.

It is out of question to try to eliminate the subjectivity which is linked to the patient, as this would severely corrupt the interpretation of his auditory function, but we have tried to get rid of the subjectivity of the operator.

The computer manages the whole investigation. First, the best ear of the patient is tested, starting with a pure tone of 1000 hertz and 20 dB. If the patient hears that sound, he presses a switch, and the computer delivers a sound, the loudness of which decreases 5 dB by 5 dB until the patient no longer presses the switch.

This method is used for all the tonal frequencies, for air and bone conduction. The Weber test is logically interpreted by the computer. The loudness of the masking sound is also determined by the computer. For the speech test, the computer compares the phoneme repeated by the patient to the one it delivers.

For brainstem evoked responses auditory, the computer allows total objectivity of the interpretation. Indeed, the brainstem responses are directly conveyed to the computer through an interface, and it analyses, processes and interprets them, taking into account the clinical data.

Furthermore, the computer allows a great amount of statistical studies. It also builds standard graphs for various kinds of diseases, and so on.

The implementation of internationally recognized language and taxonomy in the field of middle ear surgery would increase the productivity of the computer. But one could make the most of its potentialities by designing new approaches to the auditory function, closer to the social authenticity of this complex phenomenon.

In the sequence "Perception, Understanding, Action" which is in all physiological phenomena, we have now to improve the investigations which reflect quality more than quantity.

As long as we use a computer to investigate a human physiological phenomenon as well as the mechanism of a robot, we will be on the wrong road.

Randomized clinical trials in ear surgery

J. Holmquist, T. Rådmark

Introduction
Randomized clinical trials are universally accepted as the most conclusive way to evaluate therapeutic efficiency. Most new drugs are tested on defined groups of patients to gain knowledge of positive and negative effects, and medical trials have proved to be a powerful tool to evaluate various medications. In surgery, prospective clinical trials are few and those published have been met with scepticism as surgical trials contain a number of errors which may bias the study and make the results less reliable.

Despite a tremendous number of reports in ear surgery we still have confusing and conflicting knowledge of the best operative method and technique in a number of common clinical situations. In ear surgery, new achievements are mostly accepted based on comparison with anecdotic references to techniques and materials used by other surgeons. Also, series of patients are analysed retrospectively.

Our attempts to evaluate techniques in cholesteatoma surgery using a prospective randomized trial have been reported earlier (Holmquist et al., 1981, Tjellström et al., 1982). The aim of this communication is to present data from the two years' postoperative assessment and to discuss some of the problems experienced in conducting the study.

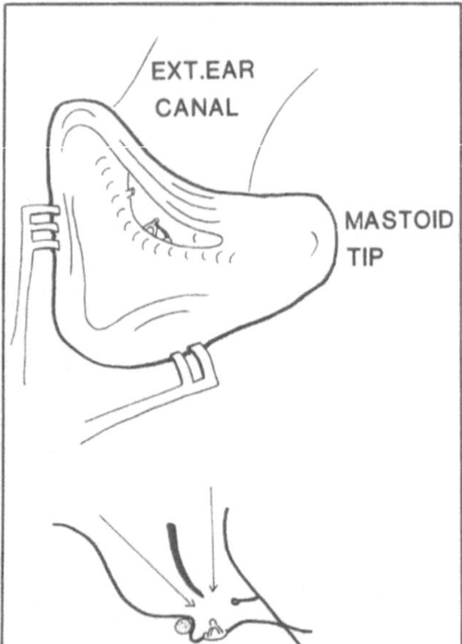

Fig. 1. A schematic drawing of the canal wall up procedure which includes posterior tympanotomy with a wide opening between the tympanic cavity and the mastoid. Incus and head of the malleus are sacrificed. The tensor tympani tendon is cut. A fascia graft is placed under the remnant of the tympanic membrane anteriorly. Silastic sheeting is used to prevent middle ear adhesions and to keep the posterior tympanotomy open. Ossicular reconstruction is done at the second look procedure one year after primary surgery.

Design of the study

The design of our prospective study in cholesteatoma surgery was presented in earlier reports.[1,2] Two well-defined techniques were used, the canal wall up and the canal wall down procedures (figures 1 and 2). After eradication of the disease the middle ear was closed by a fascia graft using the underlay technique. The surgeon had to do the selection of surgical technique in the operating room when he had evidence of a cholesteatoma. A sealed envelope was opened where it was stated whether a canal wall up or canal wall down procedure should be performed.

Follow-up

All ears in this study are checked and registered yearly with as many objective data as possible. All canal wall up ears were scheduled for a second look one year after the primary surgery for possible residual or recurrent cholesteatoma and for ossiculoplasty.

In evaluating the outcome after surgery certain parameters have been defined which should be used as a base for the follow-up assessment. The schema in table 1

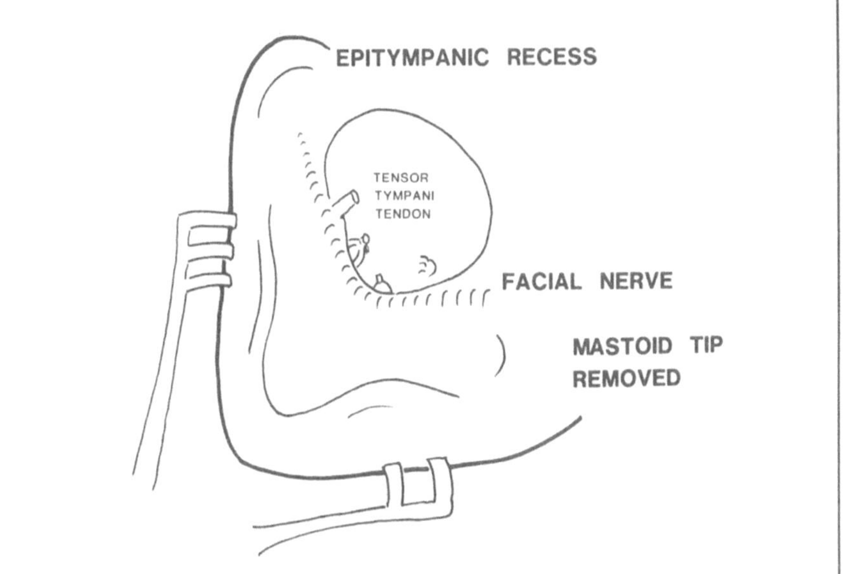

Fig. 2. A schematic drawing of the canal wall down procedure, which includes mastoid tip removal and sacrificing of incus and head of the malleus. The tensor tympani tendon is cut. A fascia graft is placed under the remnant of the tympanic membrane anteriorly covering the middle ear, the facial canal and the labyrinth. Silastic sheeting is used in the middle ear to prevent adhesions. In the presence of stapes superstructures it is tried to attain a pexi of the graft to the head of the stapes. No ossicular reconstruction is done at primary surgery.

functions as a guide for the examiner when monitoring the ears. In this report we selected to present the state of hearing expressed as the mean air-bone gap at 500, 1000 and 2000 Hz. Also, the presence of a closed middle ear was recorded. The retractions or atelectasis did not influence this parameter. The frequency of residual or recurrent cholesteatoma was based on either the operative

Table 1. Postoperative evaluation in ear surgery

	Surgeon's view	Patient's view
Function	A-B-gap S-N-loss	SRT
Anatomy	Closed middle ear Ear canal volume TM mobility	Safe for water
Pathology	Recurrent disease Residual disease	Stability Draining or not

records or the findings at any follow-up visit during the first two postoperative years.

Results

So far, 157 cholesteatoma ears have entered our study. Depending on our health care system in Sweden, all new cholesteatoma ears in the population of 700 000 came into the trial. This represents five new cholesteatoma/100 000 inhabitants per year. At the present time 100 ears have passed the two years' follow-up assessment. Table 2 illustrates the results. In accordance with our one year results the favourable hearing after canal down surgery should be noted.

The difference in frequency of recurrent or residual cholesteatoma is significant within the 95 % confidence limits but may be due to the fact that the canal up ears have been constantly re-explored but only rarely the canal down ears. Future follow-up will tell us whether this difference will persist or not in favour of canal down surgery.

Discussion

In order to have a sufficient number of ears entering our study within a certain time limit, three ENT-departments were involved. This also meant that fourteen surgeons with various skills and experience had to do the surgery. It may be argued that it is an advantage to have a small number of surgeons as it will lead to greater uniformity of treatment reducing the variability and giving more significant results.

On the other hand, the aim of a study should be to obtain results which can be general and hold for surgeons with different experiences. Also, we found it should be important to find out which surgical procedure worked out best in a certain kind of health care system.

Prior to our trial, some surgeons felt one procedure superior to the other, especially in selected cases. This could cause some disturbances in the patient/doctor relationship, as the surgeon felt he was not doing what was best for his patient. Therefore, all surgeons involved in this study had to be clearly motivated to conduct the study and no specific preference was to be given to any of the techniques throughout the

Table 2. Two years follow-up (N=100)

	Canal-Down %	Canal-Up %
1. A-B-gap less than 30 dB	78	68
2. Closed middle ear	80	80
Combined 1 and 2	62	64
Resid. or recurr. cholesteatoma	6	54

trial. The surgeons had to strictly follow the manual and no deviations could be accepted.

In medical trials, for evaluation of drug efficiency, some kind of blindness in recording the results is commonly used. This means that the examiner is unaware of which drug is used in a certain patient, sometimes both the patient and the examiner are unaware of what kind of medication has been used - double-blind evaluation. In surgical trials, this kind of evaluation is very difficult to reach, as the surgical scar or findings in the ear will tell the examiner immediately what has been done. In our study the patient was informed regarding the trial, the findings in surgery etc. but he was not generally informed in detail regarding the specific kind of surgery performed. The follow-up could not be done blindly, as the examiner, when noticing drainage, perforations or canal size, could easily conclude what kind of surgical technique had been used. On the other hand, audiometry including tympanometry was done by a technician with no information whatsoever regarding the kind of surgery performed. Therefore, audiometry may meet the requirement of blindness.

In assessment of the outcome after surgery we have found it advantageous not to have the ears examined by the same person as the surgeon. Most of the data in this report have been collected by the surgeon himself, but hopefully the assessments in the future will be collected by somebody not involved in the surgical procedure. We have also considered some kind of weighing the parameters but decided not to do it at the present time in order to minimize confusion in interpreting the results.

In ear surgery, functional, anatomical and pathological aspects should be considered. As appears in table 1, the outcome may be seen from the surgeon's as well as from the patient's point of view.

The primary purpose of this paper is not to present the outcome of our study, as cholesteatoma surgery needs many years follow-up to evaluate recurrences of the disease as well as stability of function and morphology. It is hoped that this communication will stimulate other surgeons to do clinical trials as we are convinced this is the only way to find out the best surgical techniques and materials used in ear surgery.

This study was performed in cooperation with the Departments of Oto-Rhino-Laryngology in Vänersborg (Tage Hallquist, MD), Uddevalla (Ingemar Månsson, MD, PhD) and Göteborg (Anders Tjellström, MD, PhD).

References:

1. HOLMQUIST J., TJELLSTRÖM A., HALLÉN O. Cholesteatoma surgery in a randomized propective study. Proc. XIIth ORL World Congr. Budapest, Hungary 1981.
2. TJELLSTRÖM A., HOLMQUIST J., HALLÉN O. Canal wall up or down. Cholesteatoma and Mastoid Surgery Proceedings II. International Conference Tel Aviv, Israel, 461-466, 1981.

Computerized multicentre clinical study to evaluate postoperative results in middle ear surgery

C. Deguine

Introduction

Data processing has radically changed the means of memorisation, storage and analysis of medical files. It offers new possibilities of circulating information more widely. The technical imperatives of handling data have introduced a new exactness in the scientific progress.

To take advantage of this progress, in order to evaluate postoperative results in middle ear surgery, it is not only possible but also desirable to extend the studies to a large number of centres to gain a wider and more diversified experience.

We offer here a concrete example thanks to a commercial firm which had initiated a multicentre clinical trial to test a tympanic bioprosthesis. This tympanic xenograft is a product made of the jugular vein of the calf, prepared according to the method of professor Zini, Italy.

Methodology

Forty-two otologists, representing 13 countries accepted to collaborate in this trial which includes 2 steps:

— the otology step: filling in the standard case report form by the surgeon in order to collect all the raw data,

— the computer step: centralization of all the raw data and their analysis.

The preparation of this standard patient case report is a delicate and fundamental task. It represents a compromise between the necessity to take into account a maximum number of parameters and the need to maintain a schematic format to be of practical and objective use. A first case report sheet has been used to initiate the trial and serve as an initial test of feasibility. When the participants reported their first observations, it quickly appeared that certain data which looked initially essential to some of them, were not needed, and various data were of minor importance. In the light of this first experience, we have gathered critics, remarks and suggestions from each participant. A new optimal format was designed to take into account the variety of pathologies and surgical techniques which would lead to valid conclusions.

Case report sheet (CRS)

The standard case report sheet includes 3 parts:

— the preoperative patient evaluation,
— the surgical technique,
— the anatomical and functional results.

The choice of the various data to be recorded in each part has not met with unanimity and will be the subject of several comments. The various sections have been designed and written so as to make sure that an answer will be given in all cases. Indeed, the absence of an answer may mean that the question is of no concern to the surgeon but for the computer technician it means that the question has not been considered, which diminishes the reliability of the reporting.

Preoperative patient evaluation (table 1)
There is no doubt that the general condition of the patient plays a rôle in the quality of the results of chronic otitis surgery. We limited ourselves to mention the possible existence of an associated important pathological disease. Though the condition of the opposite ear is an essential parameter of the surgical indications, it has no influence on the postoperative evolution of the ear operated on. However, several participants having requested it, we have incorporated a corresponding section both on the anatomy and audiometry.

The function of the Eustachian tube has a determing rôle in the evolution of chronic otitis. In the absence of universal and significant tests, we had to limit ourselves to a subjective evaluation based on the clinical experience of each one.

Surgical techniques (table 2)
Though the clinical trial is only concerned with tympanic repair, it is not possible to limit the surgery report to this sole consideration.

Five aspects of the tympanoplasty surgery must be analysed:
— mastoid surgery,
— EAC (bony and epidermal) surgery,
— mucosa surgery,
— ossicular chain surgery,
— drum surgery.

This description of surgery of the ossicular chain is indeed extremely summarized. However, it covers the majority of the techniques currently used. An open section enables the surgeon to report particular or original techniques.

Postoperative evaluation
Of course, the postoperative evaluation is conducted on natomical and audiometric results. The third-month evaluation is sent together with a complete patient observation (table 3).

The next evaluations are reported on separate forms which take into account modifications and incidents that may occur in the long run. The participants are requested to send their evaluation

Table 1

MULTICENTER EVALUATION WITH NEOTYMP XENOIMPLANT — Case Report N°

Hospital :
Adress :
Chief surgeon

Surgeon
1- Chief
2- Experimenced
3- Occasional
4- Training
5- Resident

PATIENT PRE-OP

NAME :	Sex : 1 - M 2 - F	Age	Birthdate (YMD) : .. - .. - ..

GENERAL CONDITION

Noticeable associated affection
....

CONDITION OF THE OPPOSITE EAR

Anatomical
1- Normal
2- Pathol.

Audit.
1- Normal
2- Partial deafn.
3- Total deafn.

OPERATED EAR

Pathology
1- Simple chronic otitis
2- Cholesteatoma
3- Tympanosclerosis predom.
4- Atelectasia predom.
5- Trauma

9- Other ....

Otorrhea
1- No (1 Year)
2- No (3 monthes)
3- Yes

Previous surgery
1- No
2- Mastoïdectomy
3- Radical
4- Modified radical
5- Myringoplasty
6- Not precised

9- Other ....

Eust. Tube Evaluation
1- Patent
2- Intermittent poor
3- Permanently poor
4- Closed

AUDIOGRAM

	125	250	500	1000	2000	4000	8000
B.C.							
A.C.							

after 3 months, 6 months, 1, 2, 3 or 5 years and to send their raw data as soon as available to the centralizing computer office (table 4).

The study of the functional results is made by using the complete audiogram. The computer offers a real advantage for analysing numerical results and to record an infinite number of figures. No information can be lost. All sorts of calculations may be made combining frequences, auditory gains or losses (A.C. or B.C.), depending on the method of evaluation chosen.

Data processing stage

Once centralized, the data are computerized. It will be the responsibility of the computer

Table 2

SURGERY		Date of OP (Y.M.D.) : .. - .. - ..	
Anesthesia 1- Local 2- General (intub.) 3- Local + General 9- Other	EAR CANAL SURGERY Bony canal 1- Intact 2- Sauceriz. 3- Post wall open 9- Other	OSSICULAR CHAIN SURGERY Condition of the chain 1- complete 2- Reconst. on stapes 3- Reconst. on footplate 9- Other	TYMPANIC MEMBRANE SURGERY Perforation (at time of reconstruction) Size: 1- Large 2- Medium 3- Small Site: 1- Tot.Destruc. 2- Central 3- Ant-sup 4- Ant-inf. 5- Post-sup 6- Post-inf. 7- Attic
Incision 1- Transmeatal 2- Endaural 3- Posterior 9 Other.......	Bony canal Reconstruction 1- No 2- Attic wall 3- Post wall 4- Total reconstruction 9- Other	Stapes 1- No explor. 2- Mobile 3- Fixed 9- Other	Material (comparative study) 1- Neotymp 2- Fascia 3- Perichondrium 4- Tymp. homog. 9- Other ....
MASTOID SURGERY 1- No 2- Partial 3- Modified radical 4- Partial oblit. 5- Oblit. Palva 6- Oblit. Sheehy 7- CAT 9- Other	Material 0- No reconstr. 1- Cartilage autog. 2- Cartilage Homog. 3- Bone autog. 4- Bone homog. 5- Ceravital 9- Other	Reconstruction 0- Complete oss.chain 1- One stage 2- Staged procedure 3- No reconstruction	Neotymp 1- Compl. moulded piece 2- Large piece 3- Small piece
MUCOSA SURGERY Condition 1- Normal 2- Inflam. 3- Polypoïd 4- Fibrosis 5- Tympanoscl. 9- Other	Skin : Condition 1- Normal 2- Inflamm. 9- Other	Oss. Chain Material 0- No reconst. 1- Bone autog. 2- Bone homog. 3- Cartil. autog. 4- Cartil. homog. 5- Plastipore 6- Proplast 7- Ceramic (type ....) 9- Other.......	Application 1- Overlay 2- Underlay 9- Other .... Contention Fibrin glue Y / N Sponge Y / N Other ....
Residual Mucosa 1- Normal 2- Ostium 3- Ostium + promontory 4- Hypo + Meso-tymp. 9- Other	Skin : Restoration 1- Preserved 2- Partial ablation 3- Free graft skin 9- Other	Particular case (Diagram)	Packing/duration (days) .... Antibiotics Y / N Post-op ear drops Which one ? Duration (weeks)
		Material in M.E. Silastic Y / N Gelfoam Y / N Fibrin glue Y / N Other	Use of Neotymp 1- Good 2- Average 3- Poor

Table 3

POST-OP EVALUATION ⩽ 3 MONTHS

ANATOMICAL RESULTS

Immediate post-op symptoms ☐

1- None
2- Pain
3- Head aches
4- Dizziness
5- Vomiting
6- Infection
7- Sudden deafness
8- Facial palsy
9- Other ....

Cicatrisation ☐

Nbr of weeks : ....

Neotymp ☐

1- Normal
2- + thin
3- + thick
4- very thick

Possible cause of failure ☐

1- None
2- Infection
3- Allergy
4- Post-op care
5- Mechanical incident
6- Baro-traumat.
7- Bleeding at surgery
8- Eust.tube function
9- Other ....

Otorrhea ☐

1- None
2- Immed. tempor.
3- Immed. persist.
4- Late tempor.
5- Late persist.

Ant.Angle ☐

1- Normal
2- Rounded
3- Oblit.

Residual perforation ☐

1- None
2- Temporary
3- Permanent

Size ☐

1- None
2- Small
3- Medium
4- Large

AUDITORY RESULTS

AUDIOGRAM

	125	250	500	1000	2000	4000	8000
B.C.							
A.C.							

IMPEDANCEMETRY (facultative)

Possible cause of conductive deafness ☐

1- No gap
2- Identified
3- Supposed
4- Unknown

☐

1- Thick graft
2- Columellar problem
3- Poor ventilation
4- Fibrosis
5- Tympanosclérosis
6- Footplate fixation
7- Staged surgery
9- Other ....

Table 4

LONG TERM EVALUATION

If patient out of sight, last examination date (Y.M.D.) : .. - .. - ..

6 Monthes | 1 Year | 2 Years | 3 Years | 5 Years

ANATOMICAL RESULTS

Neotymp
1- Normal
2- + thin
3- + thick
4- very thick

Graft position
1- Normal
2- External migration
3- Atelectasia
4- Ant; retraction
5- Post. retraction
6- Attic. retract.

Ant. Angle
1- Normal
2- Rounded
3- Oblit.

Residual perls
1- None
2- Externe
3- Interne

Residual perforation
1- None
2- Initial
3- Secondary
4- Temporary

Eut. tube evaluation
1- Patent
2- Intermittent poor
3- Permanently poor
4- Closed

Cavity condition
1- Healed
2- Moisty
3- Cholest. retention
9- Other ....

Possible causes of failure
1- External otitis
2- Acute otitis media
3- Allergy
4- Secretory otitis
5- Poor Eust.tube
9- Other ....

AUDITORY RESULTS

AUDIOGRAM

	125	250	500	1000	2000	4000	8000
B.C.							
A.C.							

IMPEDANCEMETRY
(facultative)

Possible causes of deafness
1- No gap
2- Identified
3- Supposed
4- Unknown

1- Thick graft
2- Columellar problem
3- Poor ventilation
4- Fibrosis
5- Tympanosclerosis
6- Footplate fixation
7- Staged surgery
9- Other ....

technician, or better, of the clinician trained in computer and statistical sciences, to evaluate the results and to establish objectively their significance in relation to the raw data and the dispersion of the answers.

The computer used is an IBM-PC with a Lotus 1.2.3. programme. The CRS is the first stage. It is the fruit of the collaboration of a group of otologists using a wide variety of techniques. Most of the sections offer open items and will be completed while daily experience with the format progresses. It will probably be necessary to create a few new sections.

Nevertheless, we believe that this work may be used as a starting point for other clinical studies orientated towards their other subjects. This is the reason why we thought it useful to present it here. Therefore, more extensive and more reliable information would be made available to the otologist within a context of increased objectivity to evaluate the postoperative results and establish the indications of a specific surgical technique.

Data processing in otosclerosis

J.R. Causse, J.B. Causse, J. Bel, P. Michaux, R. Cezard, Ch. Parahy, B. Zoller

Introduction

The application of data processing techniques to patients' files is particularly recommended in the otospongiotic/otosclerotic disease, since the parameters defining history, symptoms, operative technique and follow-up to surgery are relatively simple, easily identifiable, accurate and limited in number. The use of data processing in an otology clinic allows an improved approach to medical and surgical problems, thus increasing the knowledge of the otospongiotic/otosclerotic process and leading to better functional results in affected patients.[1] Moreover, the computer constitutes an ideal means of making research easier and more reliable.

Data processing for otosclerosis in our otology clinic

We started in 1970 on two bases: first, only a significantly wide range of parameters allows accuracy, sharpness, variety and reliability in the information given, their methodical processing thus providing a correct frame of each case; second, data processing in stapes surgery must be based not only on the intra-operative data, but also on the extensive study of collected data showing various aspects of the patients' status, which may affect the functional results, such as preoperative data, history, general status, clinical and audiometric evaluation, vestibular function, etc. This program has grown steadily since 1970 and has been operational since the end of 1972.

Computer

Our first computer in 1972 was an IBM 3, mod. 6, rapidly replaced by an IBM 32, with 16 K bytes main storage, 9 million characters disk storage, input/output through diskettes, display stations with typewriter keyboards and screens, multiple magnetic support combinations, debugging, providing full data protection, printer speed 110 l.p.m.

We are currently planning to change our IBM 32 for a compact IBM 36, with 256 K bytes main storage, 60 million characters disk storage, input/output through diskettes, printer speed 280 l.p.m., 6 display stations including keyboards and color display. This equipment is much more compact and silent (46 dB) and can currently be extended to 1 Mega byte main storage, 800 Mega bytes disk storage, etc. (sch. diag. 1).

Collection of data

A significant amount of material has been gathered from 1959 to the present time (January 1984) based on over 27 700 stapedectomies and over 180 000 otology

Schem. diag. 1 - IMB 36 Compact

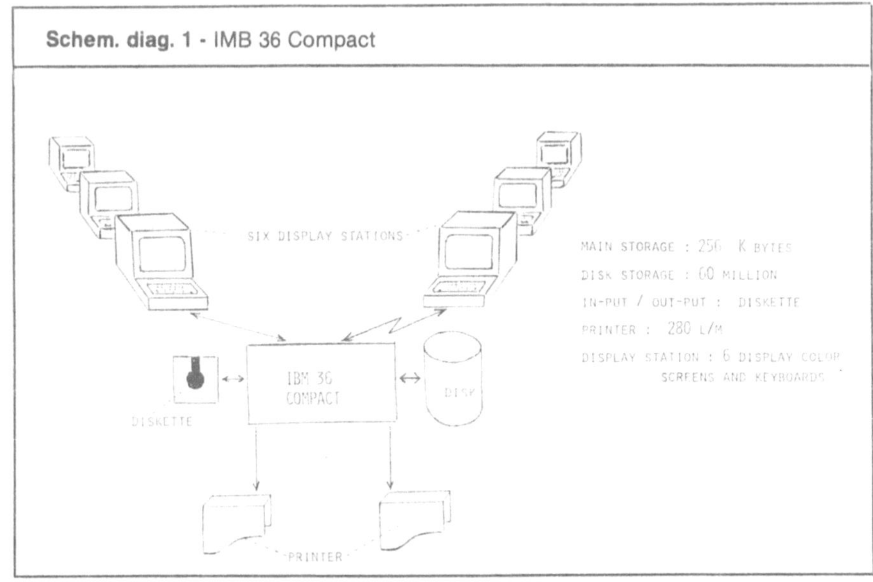

outpatients in our otology clinic. The data collected within this period of twenty-five years going from 1959 to 1984, were studied during the first fifteen years of this period using both conventional and computed data processing methods in order to verify that the statistical results correspond. A wide range of data was selected for the record of each patient, starting from his first consultation, continuing throughout the various medical or surgical stages marking his route to the latest audiometric check-up.

Parameter processing system

We have selected an extremely large number of parameters in the standard-list, but their methodical arrangement allows rapid selection and provides a correct frame of each case. Moreover, the checking off of the selected items for each patient never requires more time than 15' for the first consultation, 8' for subsequent consultations, 3' for the operation, 4' for each post-operative check-up, after brief training. In fact, this procedure is relaxing, because it is methodical due to the standard-list, and rapid, thanks to the preselection of data.

Data processing has been divided into five parts. They are:

— *Parameters of first consultation* (the standard-list consists of 787 coded parameters). History is prepared by assistant nurses and confirmed by the clinician. Clinical data cover the whole ENT area. Audiometric check-up consists of pure tone and speech audiometry, Bekesy audiometry, speech Weber test, impedance measurement, acoustic stapedius reflex elicitation, measurement of loudness recruitment (Metz test), and sometimes if needed, Sisi-test, tone decay test, ECochG and BERA. The classification of audiometric stages is that of Shambaugh, completed in order to make it flexible and more extended. The notation is in real figures. The routine vestibular test battery is made up of torsion swing test and J.B. Causse's vertebro-basilar insufficiency (deprivation) nystagmus test (VBIN test) with ENG tracing recording, which gives useful information in otospongiosis before and after surgery, and when needed, caloric test, optokinetic test and rotatory ENG test. This extensive examination leads to a "possible diagnosis", thus to the treatment, either medical or surgical, in accordance with the selected diagnosis.

— *Parameters of preoperative examination* (148 coded parameters). These are much reduced due to the notation of the current status in comparison with the previous one (unchanged, improved or worse) and of the audiometric and vestibular status in real figures. This chapter ends with "probable diagnosis", "therapeutic decision" and "prognosis".

— *Parameters for operation* (433 coded parameters). After defining the situation of the operation and its type and indicating the surgeon's name, we have analysed each operative step: incision, skin elevation, bony resection, chorda tympani, middle ear, facial nerve, mucoperiosteum, etc., going through to the stapedectomy/stapedotomy itself. The classification of anatomical states of footplate and niche was developed from Shambaugh's original classification with minor modifications. Operative techniques and difficulties encountered are noted, together with possible complementary techniques. The anatomical result is given, as well as the prognosis (good or reserved). The chapter ends with "final diagnosis".

— *Parameters of immediate follow-up* (95 coded parameters). These include local anatomical complications, subjective disturbances, such as increased tinnitus and/or vertigo, and audiometric surveillance by bone conducted audiometry as early as the first postoperative day. Indications for immediate medical therapy must also be checked off.

— *Parameters of postoperative check-ups*,including the functional results (183 coded parameters). We quote the functional results of each operated ear at the end of each postoperative check sheet. Coding is done in real figures, similar to that of preoperative consultations. It is thus easier to follow the progression of hearing and to detect a decline immediately. The functional result itself, obtained from a comparison of the figures, consists of four parts:

- audiometric value, given by pure tone audiometry;
- social value, calculated in accordance with speech audiometry;
- rough value, when the audiometric figures have been recorded without our supervision;
- long-term stability, quoted in dB loss/year on the four conversational frequencies, or better three, by suppressing 4000 Hz in order to eliminate the incidence of presbycusia on the result.

— *Parameters concerning the general status of the patient and anesthesia* (601 coded parameters). This only concerns general anesthesia, but any clinician can code them, if local anesthesia is performed by the surgeon.

— *Research.* This mass of 2247 coded parameters has been extremely helpful to us, for it provides quantity, quality and accuracy of data, which allows extensive research on a multitude of variable factors, not only at the level of clinical statistics concerning the patient and his pathology, but also concerning the otospongiotic disease itself, such as the clinical aspects of the disease, the enzymatic mechanism, its triggering by an immune factor, the mode of NaF action on this mechanism, the genetics of otospongiotic inheritance, etc.

Resulting "flashes"

The result of this data processing is an immediate "flash" of the required data. The information can be given either through a very rapid printing of a "flash" or through multiple color display stations reproducing characters, figures, tables, columns and therefore audiograms (IBM 36), thus improving flexibility, reliability and productivity.

The lack of room prevents us to give some examples of flashes, taken from patients' files, and tables taken from clinical research on patients, as well as the data processing studies published by other authors.

The complete text of this shortened paper, containing all information desired, is available on request.

Comments on resulting information

Files for inpatients and outpatients

Our data processing may seem rather complicated at first sight, but we believe that after brief training, the clinician will see it to be rapid, objective, valid and reliable, moreover full of human feeling with respect to the patients, this last quality being generally considered as absent from data processing methods. In fact only 10 % of the coded parameters have to be selected for any one patient among this mass of data. Moreover, once the operator is trained, the checking off of the selected items does not take more time than dictating or recording the information. A useful method consists of data selection by assistant nurses well-schooled in this procedure, particularly where history and audiometry items are concerned. The framework, always identical for each patient, ensures a basic structure which lightens the physician's job and constitutes an objective tool for the establishment of valid files, reliable and easy to consult.

Statistical data concerning medical and surgical problems

Proper data processing allows the clinician to solve many problems.[1,3]

— *Surgical problems.* At the time we rapidly retrieved information allowing us to compare various types of stapedectomy. We can give an example of an easy and rapid comparison of techniques (table 1).

A recent example of the advantages of this data processing is given by the study made on 6 724 operations performed by J. Bernard Causse between July 1977 and April 1983, in order to compare the respective advantages of the ablation of the complete posterior third of the footplate and those of the 0,8 mm small fenestra located at the posterior third of the footplate, using in both techniques a diamond burr and adding in both cases a large vein graft interposition, as well as an early vigorous postoperative inflation of the middle ear.[4,5,6]

Thanks to the J. Bernard Causse technique, consisting of a 0,8 mm small fenestra located at the posterior third of the footplate, no dead ear occurred during the first postoperative month, and only 14 cases of slight cochlear deterioration were observed in a total of

Table 1. Statistical data - evaluation of long-term success (1960-1975)

15 YEAR STAPEDECTOMY STATISTICAL DATA
EVALUATION OF LONG-TERM SUCCESS OF 16,822 STAPEDECTOMIES PERFORMED
BETWEEN JANUARY 1ST 1960 AND JANUARY 1ST 1975
ACCORDING TO THE TECHNIQUE USED

TYPE OF OPERATION	NUMBER	LONG-TERM SUCCESS (5 TO 15 YEARS)	
		NUMBER	PERCENT.
- STAPEDECTOMIES			
+ VEIN + STAPES REPOSITION (PORTMANN)	859	791	92.08
+ VEIN + POLYTHENE STRUT (SHEA I)	1 050	963	91.71
+ VEIN + STEEL WIRE (KOS + PORTMANN)	13*	12	92.30
+ GELFOAM + STEEL WIRE (SCHUKNECHT-HOUSE)	10*	7	70.00
- TEFLON PISTON (SHEA II)	174	162	93.10
- TEFLON INTERPOSITION (CAUSSE)	14 716	14 444	98.15
TOTAL :	16 822	16 379	97.36
- REVISION-OPERATIONS			
CONDUCTION	173	96	55.50
PERILYMPH FISTULA	7*	6	85.72

* NOT SIGNIFICANT (TOO FEW CASES)

6 724 operations performed by J. Bernard Causse.

Early vigorous inflation has limited postoperative rotatory vertigo to only 14 cases and slight imbalance to only 27 cases in 6 724 operations.

The percentage of decibel improvement of postoperative bone conduction is interesting to consider. Analysis of postoperative bone conduction levels according to frequencies, showed an overall improvement, but it was greater for low frequencies when the technique used was the ablation of the complete posterior third of the footplate (table 2). An unexpected conclusion is that it would seem more interesting to perform a stapedectomy of the posterior third of the footplate on Spanish-speaking patients, in which low frequencies phonemes are predominant. For French-speaking patients, using the 1000 Hz frequency on a large scale, both techniques seem to be of equal interest. As for Scandinavian, Anglo-saxon and German patients, it seems to be better to perform a 0,8 mm stapedotomy in the posterior third of the footplate (sch. diag. 2).

— *Medical problems.* Another example of the usefulness of computed data processing is the management of patients treated with sodium fluoride. The accurate surveillance of NaF therapy is all the more indispensable as NaF has been strongly criticized because of possible toxicity and fluorosis. Computerized surveil-

Table 2. Bone conduction improvement according to the type of operation performed

AVERAGE DECIBEL IMPROVEMENT IN BONE CONDUCTION
ONE YEAR AFTER THE OPERATION
ACCORDING TO THE FREQUENCY AND TO THE TYPE OF OPERATION PERFORMED
STATISTICAL DATA FROM 1977 THROUGH 1983
IN 6,724 STAPEDECTOMIES/STAPEDOTOMIES

	200 Hz	500 Hz	1000 Hz	2000 Hz	4000 Hz
0.8MM SMALL FENESTRA LOCATED AT THE POST. 1/3 OF THE FOOTPLATE	8,487	10,641	12,948	16,350	9,102
ABLATION OF COMPLETE POSTERIOR 1/3 OF THE FOOTPLATE	9,633	11,166	13,166	14,166	2,833

lance has allowed us to demonstrate that NaF is safe and effective.[7]

Research into the otospongiotic disease

The flexibility of the computer and the reliability of its memory make computed data remarkably helpful for research.

— *Research in the genetics of the otospongiotic disease.* [2] Computerized investigations led us to believe that the otospongiotic disease is an autosomal dominant genetic hearing loss with about 40 % penetrance of genes. Data processing on 614 families, comprising 1 465 affected members, has easily shown the rate of inheritance in otospongiosis and allowed us to establish the various percentages of penetrance of genes according to kinship.[2]

— *Research into the enzymatic mechanism.* We have made extensive use of the computer for the study of the enzymatic mechanism in the otospongiotic disease and the mode of NaF action on the enzymatic balance.[8]

Conclusion

There is no doubt that electronic storage and distribution of information is becoming a necessity in modern day medicine. The computer is a flexible tool for displaying data from disk files based on user-specified selection criteria. The physician can search his files, by combining keywords, characters and numbers to review or retrieve information in a form that meets his requirements. All

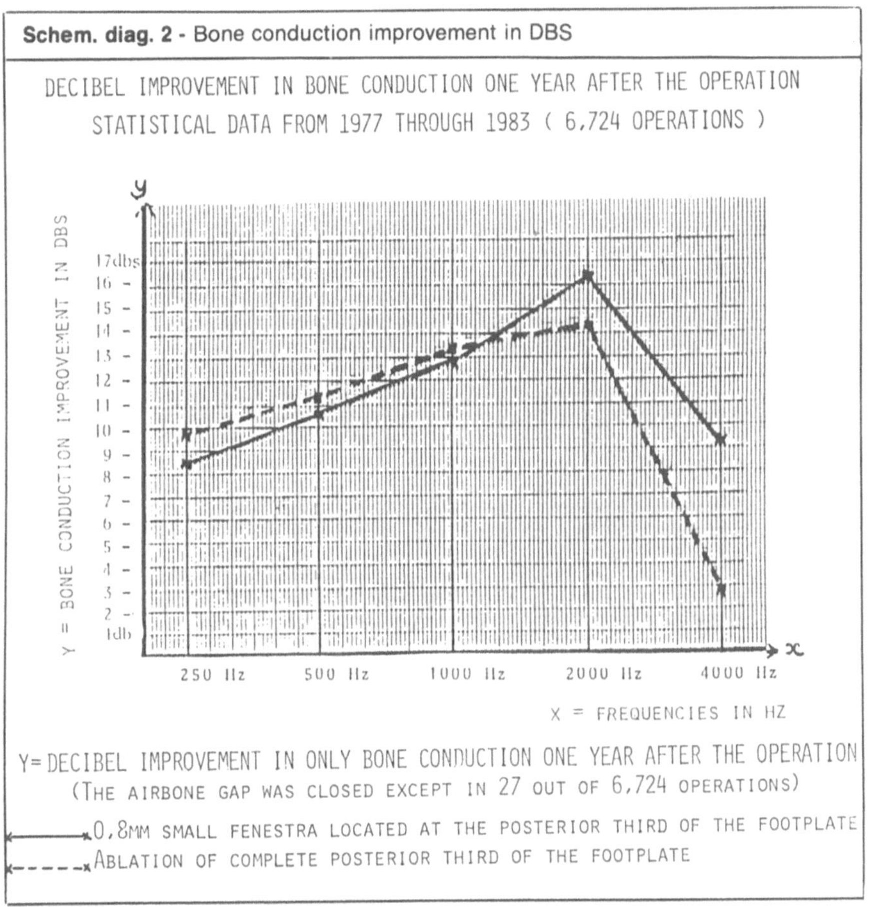

Schem. diag. 2 - Bone conduction improvement in DBS

charts and graphs can be automatically displayed on the computer through color display stations and/or printers. The combination of diskettes with a fix disk allows great flexibility and large possibilities of data storage for a low cost.

The application of data processing to patients' files and to research is particularly easy in otosclerosis. But one must not fall into the trap of utilizing too few data, as this would give a pale caricature of the desired picture instead of a precise frame. The data processing that we present for otosclerosis, is the result of this objective. We do not claim that our procedures are the best, but we would like to stress that the data processing we use, is a living tool, easy to use, flexible in solving day-to-day problems, very effective in the management of patients' files and powerful in the field of research.

References:

1. CAUSSE J.R., CAUSSE J.B. Eighteen-year report on stapedectomy *Clin. Otolaryng.* 5, 49.59, 329-337 and 397-402, 1980 - 6, 67-72, 1981.
2. CAUSSE J.R., CAUSSE J.B. Otospongiosis as a genetic disease. Early detection, medical management and prevention. *Amer. J. Otol*, 5/3, 211-223, 1984.
3. CAUSSE J.R., BEL J., MICHAUX P., CEZARD R., CANUT Y., TAPON J. avec la coll. de M. DESIRE et D. MASSOL: Apport de l'Informatique dans l'Otospongiose - 1ère partie: Systématisation des paramètres d'otospongiose pour ordinateur - *Ann. Otol.* (Paris) 91/1-2, 21-40, 91/3, 133-156, 91/4-5, 217-232, 1974 et 92/7-8, 389-416, 1975 - 2e partie: Statistiques sur 15 ans de stapédectomies - Ann. Otol. (Paris) 93/3, 149-178, 93/6, 393-428 et 93/9, 543-576, 1976.
4. CAUSSE J.B. Etiology and therapy of cochlear drops following stapedectomy. *Amer. J. Otol*, 1, 221-224, 1980.
5. CAUSSE J.B., CAUSSE J.R. The interest of bone conduction audiogram as early as the first postoperative day - XVIII Congr. Pan-americano ORL, Puerto Rico Nov. 1982.
6. CAUSSE J.B., CAUSSE J.R., PARAHY C.: J. Bernard Causse stapedotomy technique and results - 7th Shambaugh-Shea Intern. Workshop on Otology, Chicago, March 1984.
7. CAUSSE J.R., SHAMBAUGH G.E., CAUSSE J.B., BRETLAU P. Enzymology of otospongiosis and NaF therapy. *Amer. J. Otol.* 4, 206-214, 1980.
8. CAUSSE J.R., URIEL J., BERGES J., SHAMBAUGH G.E., BRETLAU P., CAUSSE J.B. The enzymatic mechanism of the otospongiotic disease and NaF action on the enzymatic balance - *Amer. J. Otol.*, 3/4, 297-314, 1982.

Computerized audiological monitoring in normal and pathological subjects

ABSTRACT

R.A. Bertrand

As computers are rapidly becoming integrated in medical practice, they are more frequently used for analysis of screening audiometry of large populations. Their application can be used for evaluation and analysis of screening tests of large populations of school children, adult populations, and especially noise-exposed industrial populations. The screening test gives us not only the degree of hearing loss but also the audiometric pattern for a probable diagnosis and identification of those subjects who should have clinical investigations. The computers allow us to determine the relationship between the noise-induced hearing loss according to the exposure and also the project hearing loss in relation to the environment.

We present our experience in the surveillance of large groups of noise-exposed subjects, describing the methodology used to acquire the hearing levels, the computer analysis of these results and the various interpretations and studies that can be obtained. Finally, the rôle of the otolaryngologist will be explained in relation to the results obtained.

Computerized postoperative evaluation of otological surgery

ABSTRACT

J.J. Shea

A simple yet effective prepunched IBM card is described by which otologic data can be collected and analyzed.

The card is divided into four parts:
- patient history,
- preoperative hearing,
- operative findings and procedure,
- postoperative hearing.

The information at operation is punched into the prepunched card with a ball point pen after operation by the surgeon and later by the audiologist. The cards are read by a card reader and analyzed in any way desired.

The number of operations which close the A-B gap to within 10 dB and those made worse can be easily determined.

I have used this system for the last 28 years to collect data from 32 000 otologic operations.

A "Politzer Society" survey

ABSTRACT

L. Feenstra

In April 1980 questionnaires were mailed to thirty members of the Politzer Society from thirteen different countries. Seventeen of them responded, presenting seventeen opinions. Two categories of answers were met. The one consists of the "peripheral hospital" approach i.e. collecting only the data relevant for the case in question or relevant to the answers of the (research) questions posed.

The other one consists of the "University" approach, i.e. a variety of collecting all data one can think of to feed punch cards or computers.

The first group likes to keep the data collecting workable and not too cumbersome, the second group hunts for all data for the sake of completeness.

Both groups point to the many conflicting prejudices or opinions about the state of art and to the unlikelihood of solving the question to everybody's satisfaction.

SCIENTIFIC EXHIBITION

Patho-anatomical findings - A routine procedure

M. De Cock, J.F.E. Marquet

Material and methods

Using the techniques of allograft requires a total eradication of all pathological tissue. This routine eradication during surgery of any tissue suspected of containing pathology, has provided us with a large number of specimens, since drums, tympanic membrane remnants - including the fibrous annulus - and each diseased ossicle are systematically removed. More than 1 100 slides have been prepared and analysed.

After their removal, all materials are preserved in 4 % formaldehyde buffered to a PH of 5,7. Each specimen is stained for histopathological examination. The hematoxylin flochsin safran and Masson's trichrome staining methods are routinely done. On some specimens the ultrastructure of the eardrum has been studied by E.M. These different techniques have been applied not only on original material, but also on implanted allografts.

In order to compare patho-anatomical findings to their original site, three photographs are taken systematically: a preoperative otoscopic view and pictures of both the medial and lateral side of the removed specimen. Complete notes concerning the case history and surgical reports added to this material, are the basis for further analysis and studies of the pathological anatomy of the middle ear.

Histological evaluation

The tympanic membrane

As a rule, we may assert that the pathological picture of the tympanic membrane in chronic ear pathology must be considered as a representation of the whole middle ear cleft pathology. A perforation only - regardless of its size - is a sign of an underlying pathology. Its dimensions - e.g. small, medium, large, subtotal or total - may never be handled as a criterion with regard to the pathology. Consequently, we advocate a total myringectomy in the great majority of cases.

— *Normal situation*

Performing the total myringectomy in most cases gives the opportunity to examine also the normal condition. The three layers of the pars tensa (epidermis, lamina propria, mucosa) as well as the inner circular and outer radiate lamina have been described a century ago (Politzer in 1869, Gerlach in 1869). In electron microscopic studies, Lim (1968-1970) has observed the ultra-structural details of the tympanic membrane. The pars flaccida - first described by Shrapnell (1832) - consists of epidermis, lamina propria and mucous layers. The pars flaccida, contrary to popular conception, is thicker than the pars tensa (Lim, 1970).

— *Implanted allografts*

Implanted allografts also present three layers. There is no difference between the structure of the pars tensa and that of the pars flaccida. The ultra-structure of the epidermal layer of these grafts presents, after three years of implantation, similar findings to that of a normal eardrum (figure 1). Under the epidermis one can see a connective tissue layer with outer radiar and inner circular fiber arrangement in the pars tensa. Whether this is newly formed tissue or a remainder of the allograft is difficult to say. However, it seemed to be old grafting material which had not been completely resorbed after more than three years (figure 2). The medial side of these tympanic allografts consists of one layer of flattened cells with microvilli. At this moment some complex discussions are going on about the "immunological rejection" phenomenon in using allografts. Although, no immunological studies were performed on this subject, postoperative photomicrographs and histological studies, as well as the long-term anatomical data, confirm that formaldehyde-fixed donor collagen possesses mild antigenicity. The host response is minimal, and not relevant to the clinical success of the tympanoplasty.

— *Pathological findings*

An essential patho-anatomical topic concerning the tympanic membrane, lies in the study of the mucocutaneous junction at the edges of perforations and of the pathology studied in relation to each of its constituent tissues, namely in the skin or squamous epithelial layer, the mesochymatous layer and its collagenic fibers and the mucosal layer.

The limit of the mucocutaneous junction. A great variability has been found regarding the size and

Fig. 1. E.M. view of an allograft. Epidermal layer: detail of stratum corneum and stratum granulosum as described by Lim (1968)

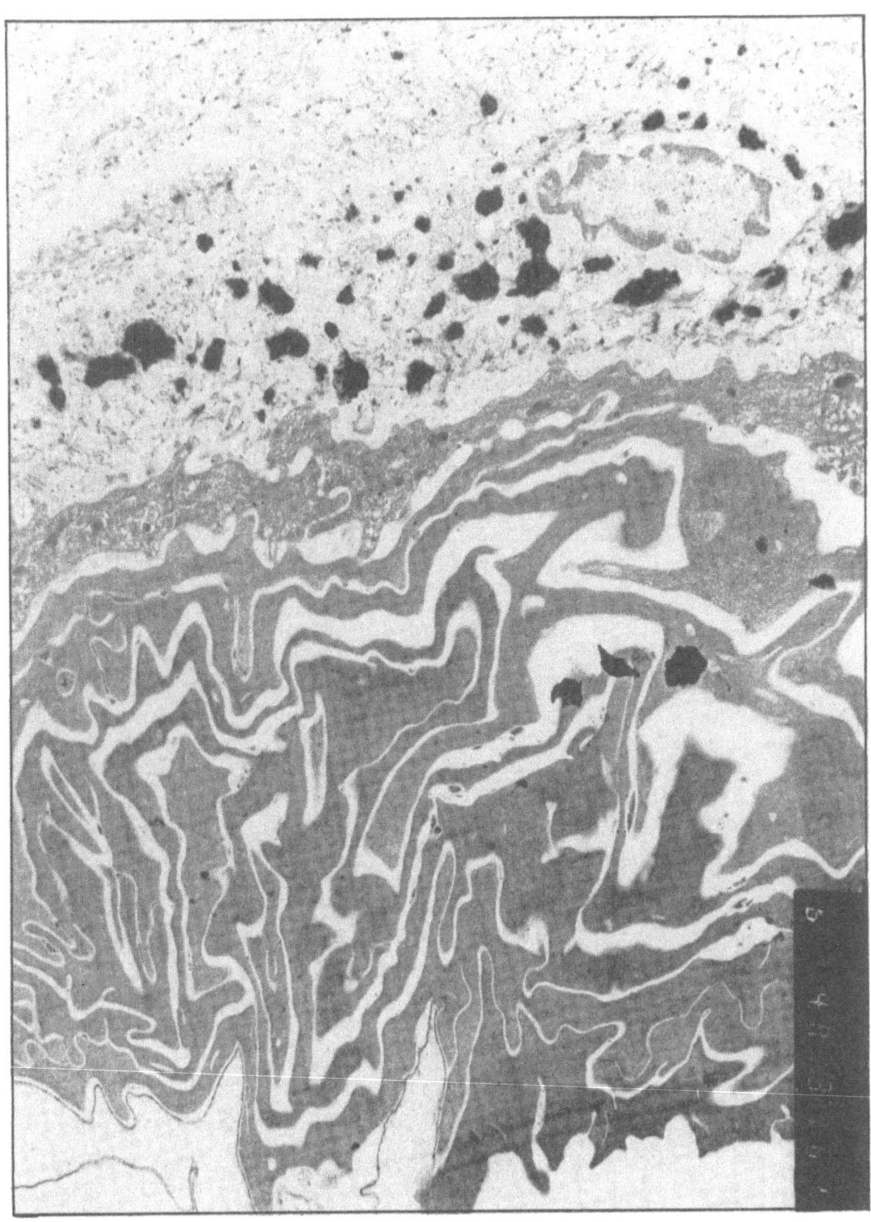

Fig. 2. Allogenous tympanic membrane, 3 years after transplantation: presence of an epithelial layer - lamina propria of the host collagen fibers and fibrocytes - mucosal layer with microvilli

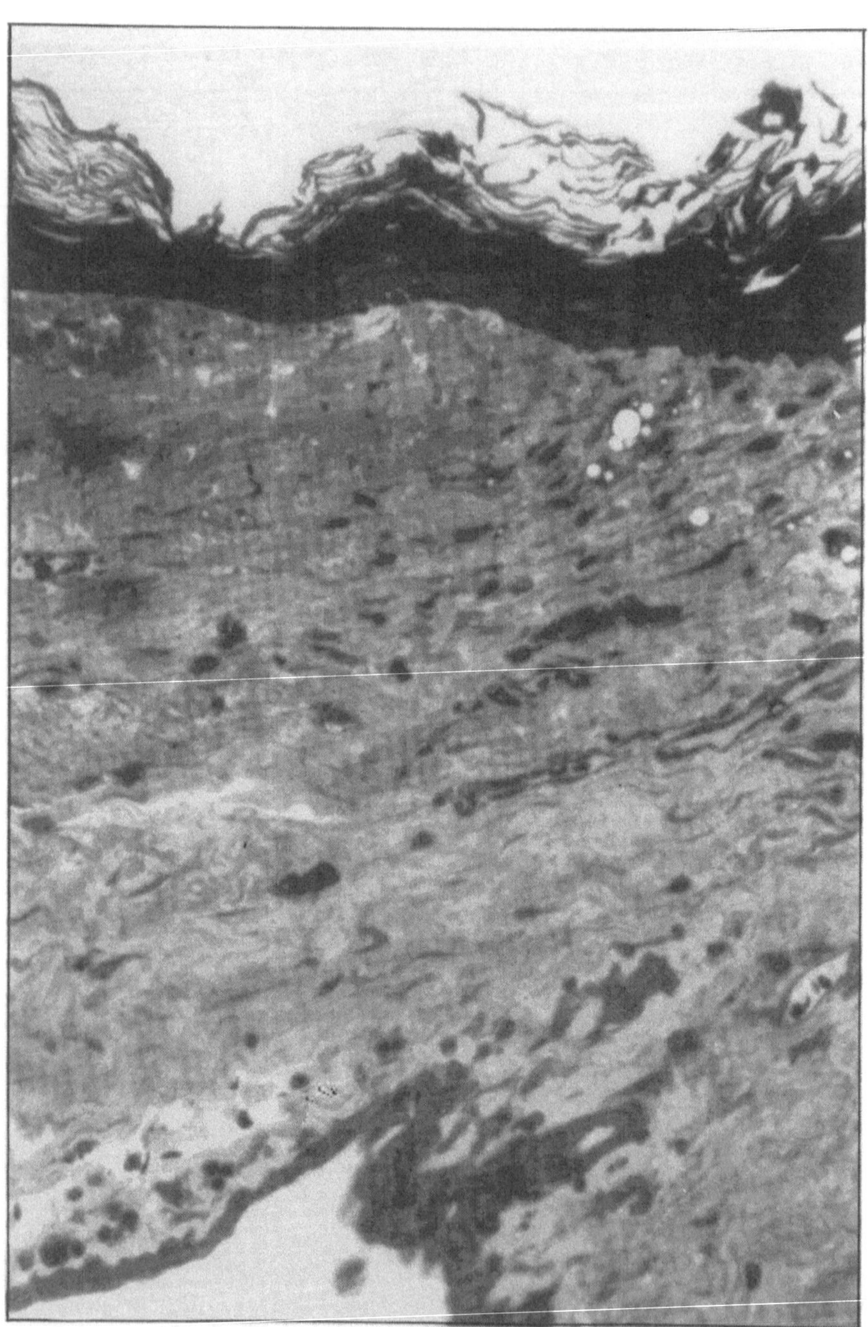

the location of the mucocutaneous junction. Wet and fibrous or tympanosclerotic drum remnants are often covered laterally by mucosal epithelium with granulation tissue and polyps being the evidence of inflammation. The edges of a dry perforation do not give any guarantee about the site of this junction. While immigration of squamous epithelium towards the attic recess or even on the promontorium is a well-known phenomenon, the covering of the medial side of the tympanic membrane by epidermis is otoscopically rather unexpected, but does appear in many cases (figure 3).

The squamous epithelial layer. There are two aspects of the problem:

- the invasive property of squamous epithelium, and
- its reference with underlying tissue.

In a large number of cases, ingrowth of meatal skin into the fibrous annulus has been observed. This shows the risk of a later development of iatrogenic pearls attempting to remove the epidermis from its area, and consequently the need to remove it totally. . A similar ingrowth of epidermis in hyalinized or tympanosclerotic drum remnants has also been discovered. A healing process of the tympanic membrane may enclose squamous epithelium behind the drum, resulting in a non-infective cystic cholesteatoma. In previous tympanoplasty, especially when fascia has been used, papillar ingrowth of basal epidermic layer is often observed. On the contrary, a denser and structured underlying tissue web such as the tympanic membrane allograft, favors a correct but not hypertrophic skin overgrowth. Ossicles or bony structures overgrown by

Fig. 3. Edge of perforation

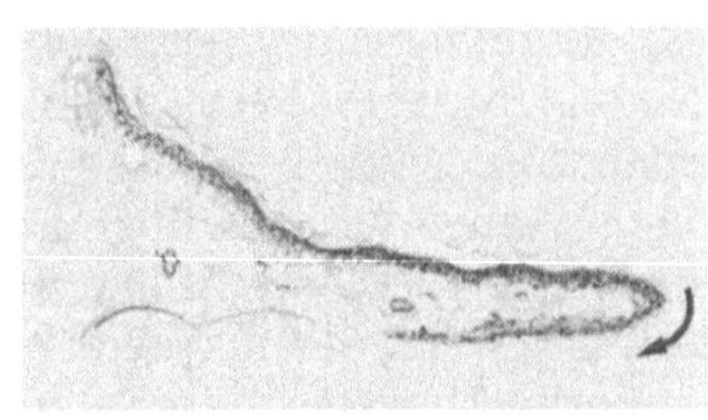

A: Ingrowth of stratified epithelium

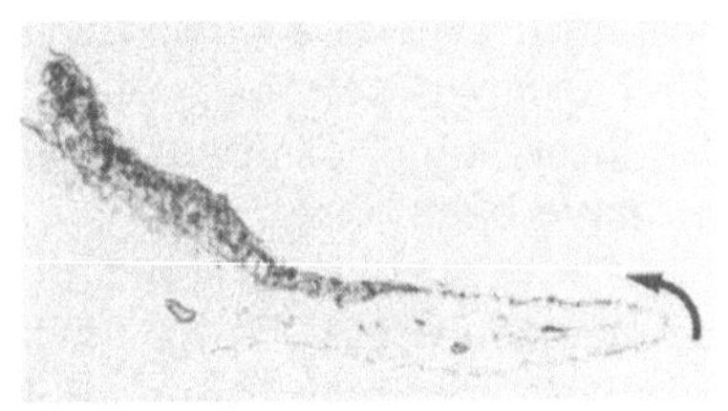

B: Mucosal overgrowth

squamous epithelium, as, for instance, after a perforation of the pars flaccida or after retraction pockets, are compatible with normal dermis. With increased thickening of the underlying granulomatous tissue, the thickness of the basal lining always increases and osteitic lesions are more frequently present.

The fibrous layer. Lysis of the collagenic web is found after inflammatory reactions, generally of infectious origin. Regrowth and subsequently spontaneous closure of the perforation mainly occurs following an identical pattern, called the "Snake Head" (figure 4). If not, a permanent perforation remains. Intermediary stages are also observed:

- a replacement membrane being only constituted by a very thin intermediate layer of collagenous fibrous tissue, in between a thin layer of epidermis and mucous membrane;
- a fibroblastic invasion of the submucosal layer followed by thickening and fusion of the collagenous web. In this type a hyalinization appears with deposits of scattered intracellular and extracellular calcium and phosphate crystal forms, the so-called tympanosclerosis plaques. In a later stage, ossification figures have been observed.

The mucosal layer. Being part of the whole mucosal lining of the middle ear cleft, identical pathoanatomical pictures have been noticed in the mucosal layer, as well as elsewhere in the middle ear cleft. During non-specific inflammatory processes ciliated columnar cells and globlet cells increase, and gland-like structures appear. The middle ear mucosa reacts by hyperplastic and metaplastic transformation. In the submucosa inflammatory cells appear, vascular dilatation and edema occur, new capillaries develop and a profileration of fibroblasts and collagen fibers are observed. This leads to the formation of granulation tissue with hystocytes, lymphocytes, plasma cells and other mononuclears. Polyps and cystic formations have been discerned. Specific inflammatory processes, like tuberculosis and even carcinomatic tissue, have been met.

Ossicles

Osteitis, the most common lesion noticed in removed ossicles, is often ignored and disregarded, when using conservative surgical techniques. Osteitic lesions might be found isolated, after an acute or subacute otitis, or associated, as, for example, embedded in infectious granuloma, or combined with cholesteatoma matrix or even embedded in tympanosclerosis. Histologically, granulation tissue is nearly always seen in association with bone destruction, together with an increased blood flow in the capillary proliferations and a marked histiocytosis. However, sterile lysis of ossicles, caused by mechanical agents - such as prosthesis - does exist. Osteogenic lesions are less

Fig. 4. Tympanic perforation: differentiation and immigration of the epithelial cells during the healing process. "Snake Head" appearance

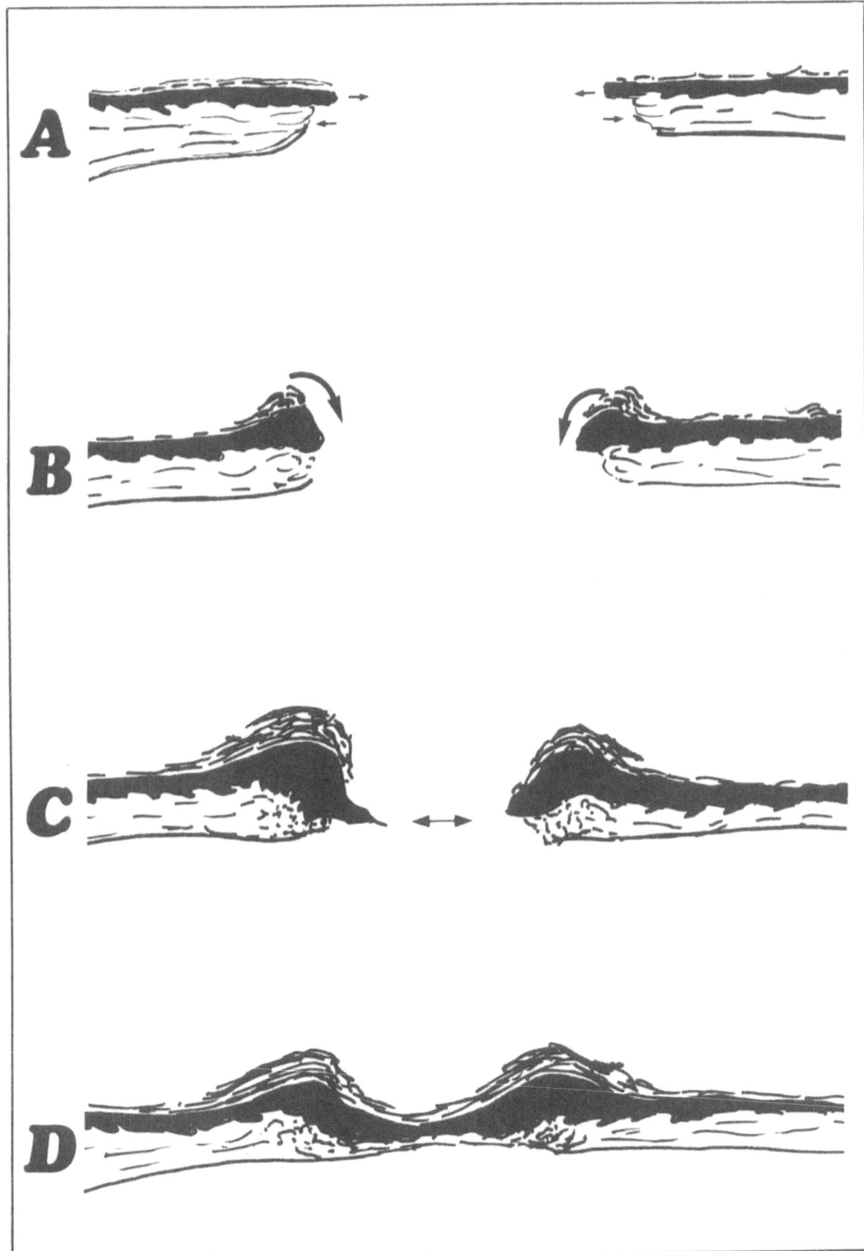

commonly found on removed ossicles, because they mostly involve the bony wall of the middle ear or the otic capsule itself. Nevertheless, they are observed in tympanosclerosis, in implanted ossicles, and even as ossified fibbrosis in a polyethylene strut.

The pathological findings of arthrosis and arthritis of the ossicular joints are totally ignored. Another paper will be devoted to this type of pathology.

Conclusion

The surgical techniques developed as a consequence of the use of allografts, have proved to be of great value in obtaining the main goals pursued in chronic ear surgery, namely eradication of the pathology, anatomical restoration of the middle ear and functional improvement. Using allograft techniques demands a total eradication of all suspected pathological tissue. As a consequence, this made our attitude towards pathology more radical.

Removal of the pathology is obtained by a TOTAL myringectomy, including the annulus remnants and, when necessary, remnants of ossicles and mucosal pathology. In cases of cholesteatoma, this technique allows an entire removal of the matrix "en bloc" together with the embedded ossicles and tympanic remnants.

Another consequence and advantage is the large collection of specimens providing us with the opportunity of a routine histological examination. Systemic patho-anatomical examination of each collected specimen has been of particular value, for each slide has been studied, bearing in mind the case history, the surgical reports and the pre-, per- and postoperative iconography. A systematic method of study is essential.

Literature:

1. BOEDTS D. The tympanic epithelium in normal and pathological conditions. *Acta Oto-Rhino-Laryngol.* Belg. 32, 295-420, 1978.
2. LIM D.J. Human tympanic membrane: an ultrastructural observation. *Acta Otolaryngol.* 176-186, 1970.
3. MARQUET J. Cholesteatoma or keratoma. A pathological approach. *Acta Oto-Rhino-Laryngol.* Belg. 84, 5-11, 1980.
4. MARQUET J. The patho-anatomical findings as indication of homografts. *Proc. XIIth World Congress*, Budapest, 1981.

Labyrinthine fistula and pre- and postoperative bone conduction

F. Debruyne

The influence of a labyrinthine fistula on the pre- and postoperative cochlear function was studied by comparing bone conduction (BC) thresholds in 2 samples of patients before and after cholesteatoma surgery.
Group I consisted of 40 patients

(40 ears) with a fistula of the lateral semicircular canal (the endosteum was intact in 33 cases; in 7 cases a small perilymph flow was seen; in 2 cases there was also a fistula of the superior canal).

For group II, 40 ears were selected, with an extensive cholesteatoma, but without erosion of the bony semicircular canals.

Figure 1 shows that the mean *preoperative* BC thresholds were slightly higher in the ears with fistula than in the ears without these findings; at 4000 Hz the difference was statistically significant: 8,65 dB ($p<0{,}01$).

In group I, the cholesteatoma epithelium was completely removed from the fistula, just before the reconstructive phase of the intervention; the bony defect was covered with fascia.

Postoperative BC thresholds were measured two months after surgery. The averaged differences between the pre- and postoperative thresholds were found to be similar in both groups (see below).

Fig. 1. Mean preoperative bone conduction thresholds with the standard deviations

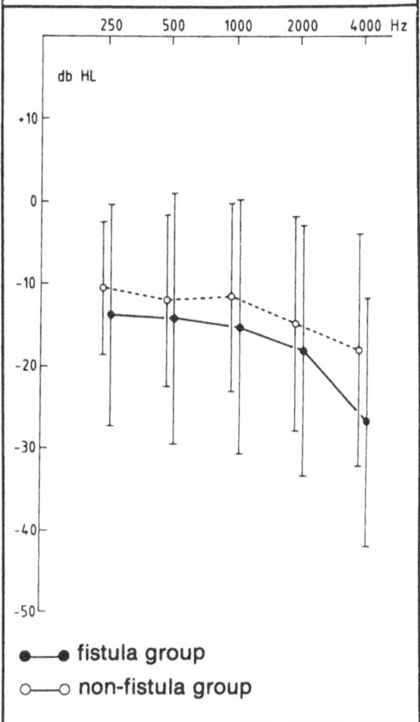

Conclusion

It can be concluded from this statistical study that:

— cochlear function, especially at high frequencies, is more likely to be disturbed in patients with a labyrinthine fistula;

— matrix removal from a limited labyrinthine fistula can be done without risk of additional cochlear damage.

	250	500	1000	2000	4000	Hz
Fistula group	-0,58	-0,58	-0,29	-0,44	-1,76	dB
Non-fistula group	-0,51	+0,89	-0,51	-0,64	-1,67	dB

Photography of the ear

ABSTRACT
M.N. Daouk

Photographic documentation of the ear has a great educational value. The classical transmicroscopic photography of the ear has its inadequacies and this is why the endoscopic photography of the ear is becoming widely accepted.

The use of some of the fiberoptic endoscopic equipment that is available commercially on the market along with standard photographic equipment has made this technique possible. The whole tympanic membrane could be included in one frame. The equipment is already available in the office of many otolaryngologists. It can also be gas-sterilized and used in the operating room. The technique is simple and does not require a lot of knowledge of photography.

One poster shows the technique. Two other posters show a wide range of ear pathology photographs, using the endoscopic photography of the ear.

Anatomy of the retrotympanum

M.C.H. Gersdorff, J.-P. Maisin

Before considering the surgical techniques for removal of any diseased tissue from the retrotympanic mucosa of a cholesteatoma lodged within it, it is helpful to recall its specific embryology and anatomy.

Embryology
The posterior tympanum, or retrotympanum, is derived from the second branchial arch. Lodged between the otic capsule and the tympanic ring, initially the retrotympanum is virtual. Its individualization and development are linked with two phenomena. On the one hand, the outward rotation of the annulus tympanicus away from the otic capsule individualizes the posterior region. On the other hand, expansion of the endothelial pouches, particularly the saccus posticus,

leads to reabsorption of the second arch mesenchyma, making from it the latero-hyoid part, and ensuring the development of the retrotympanum. In this "valley", the ossification of Reichert's cartilage will, in the neonatal period, result in the formation of Proctor's styloid complex composed of three eminences or protuberances: Politzer's styloid eminence, the pyramidal and chordal eminences (figures 1a, 1b, 1c).

Fig. 1a. The styloid complex: three eminences

English	Latin	French
Pyramidal eminence (pyramid)	eminentia pyramidalis	Eminence pyramidale (pyramide)
Styloid eminence	eminentia styloïdea	Eminence styloïde
Chordal eminence	eminentia chordae	Eminence cordale

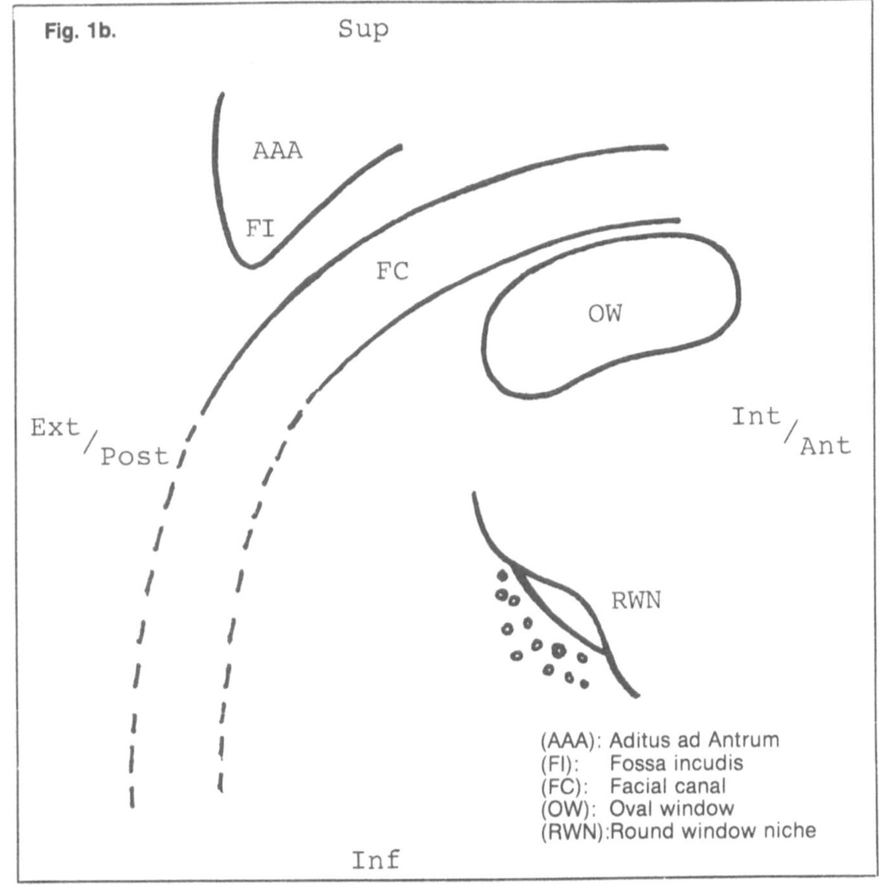

Fig. 1b.

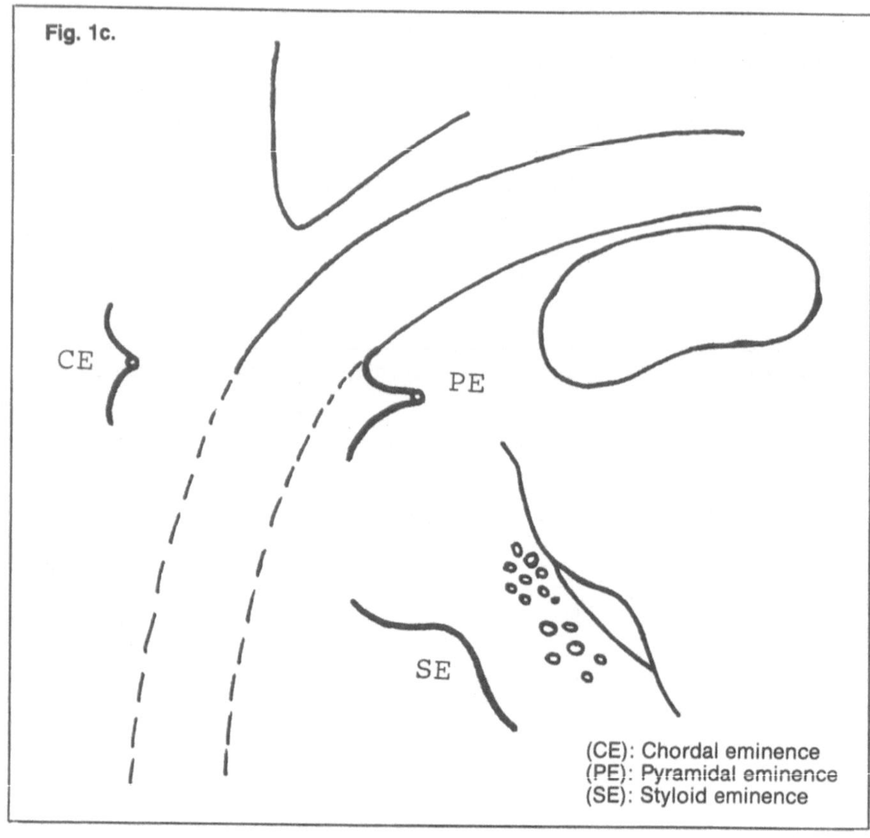

During the same period, in the way in which a mountain range is created, the bony bridges develop between these eminences and the neighbouring structures, outlining the valleys known as sinuses. While these structures are being formed, the anatomy of the region becomes more complex with the development of the facial canal. Lying over the outer face of the otic capsule and initially bare, the facial nerve, that of the second arch, is progressively sheathed by a bony canal, thus becoming an integral part of the retrotympanum.

These developments are described in detail by Proctor[1] and Guerrier.[2]

Anatomy

In the adult, systematic anatomical study of the posterior wall begins with the projections or eminences. In the middle lies the one most evident at surgery, the pyramidal; below is the styloid eminence, while above and towards the back lies the chordal (figures 2a, 2b). Arising from these eminences, with between them the promontory and the posterior lip of the round window niche, lie — more or less clearly evident — numerous ridges, bridges or crests: outwards and transversally, the chordal ridge; downwards and longitudinally, the pyramidal ridge; inwards and transversally, the ponticulus and lastly, below and frontwards, the subiculum (figure 2b). Above, obliquely, the region is bounded by the facial nerve canal.

It should be noted that Andrea[3] reports a doubling of the ponticulus, the posterior tympanic ridge, being united in 22 % with the ponticulus according to Guerrier.[2] These ridges or bridges with

Fig. 2a. Bony ridges (bridges) of the retrotympanum

English	Latin	French
Chordal ridge	Crista chordae	Crête cordale
Ponticulus	Ponticulus (promontorii)	Ponticulus
Posterior tympanic ridge	Crista tympanica posterior	Crête tympanique postérieure (Andréa)
Pyramidal ridge	Crista pyramidalis	Crête pyramidale
Subiculum	Subiculum (promontorii)	Subiculum

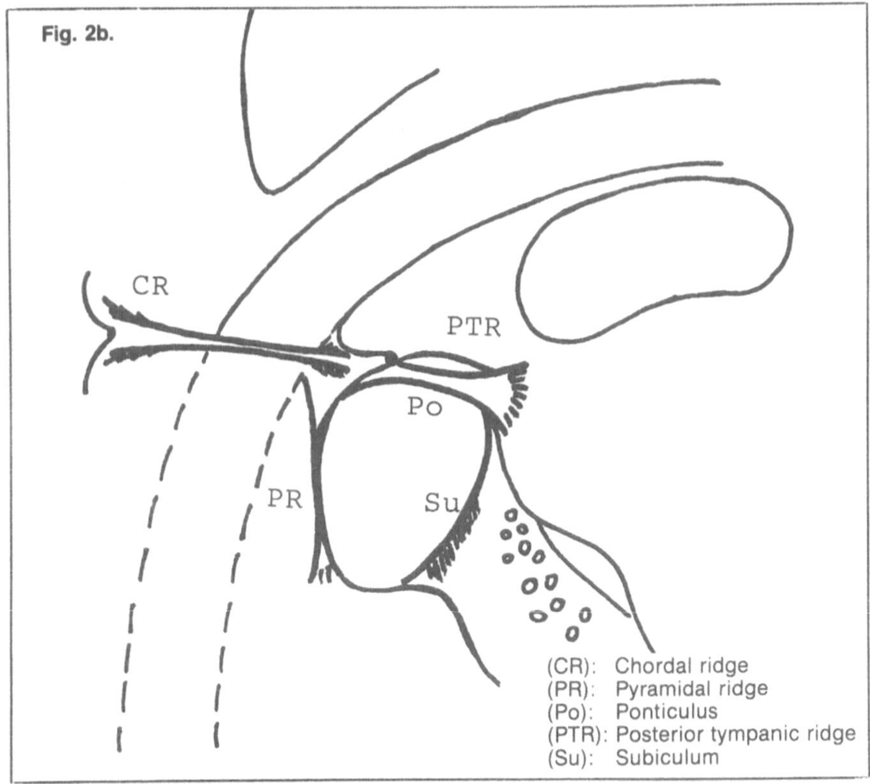

the facial canal demarcate the retrotympanic sinuses:

— *two supra-pyramidal or external sinuses*: the supero-external, facial sinus (or facial recess), and the infero-external, lateral tympanic sinus;

— *two infra-pyramidal or internal sinuses*: the supero-internal, posterior tympanic sinus and the infero-internal, sinus tympani (figures 3a, 3b).

The facial sinus, known to surgeons as the facial recess, is Schwalbe's posterior and superior sinus, also called by Sappey "fossette supra-pyramidale". It is situated between the facial canal and the chordal ridge. It is, in reality, a series of cellular structures grouped around a single clearly individualized cell. Its average depth is 2,5 mm, for 1 to 2 mm in width and 0,5 to 1 mm in height.[2] This sinus may be in direct contact with the facial canal.

Proctor's *lateral tympanic sinus* of Schwalbe's posterior and inferior sinus, called by Grivot "fossette pré-pyramidal", is situated between the chordal and the pyramidal ridges, outside of the pyramid and above the hypotympanum. Its major axis varies from 1,5 to 2,5 mm. Its depth is 2,5 mm.[2]

The *posterior tympanic sinus*, defined by Proctor, is separated

Fig. 3a. Sinuses of the retrotympanum

		English	Latin	French
External or Supra-pyramidal sinuses	Sup.	Facial sinus (facial recess)	Sinus posterior et superior (Schwalbe)	Sinus tympanique post. et sup. (récessus facial) (fossette supra- ou sus-pyramidale de Sappey)
	Inf.	Lateral tympanic sinus (Proctor)	Sinus posterior et inferior (Schwalbe)	Sinus tympanique post. et inf. (fossette pré-pyramidale de Grivot)
Internal or Infra-pyramidal sinuses	Sup.	Posterior tympanic sinus (Proctor)	Sinus tympani posterior	Sinus tympanique post. (de Proctor)
	Inf.	Sinus tympani	Sinus tympani (inferior)	Sinus tympanique (fossette infra- ou sous-pyramidale d'Huguier)

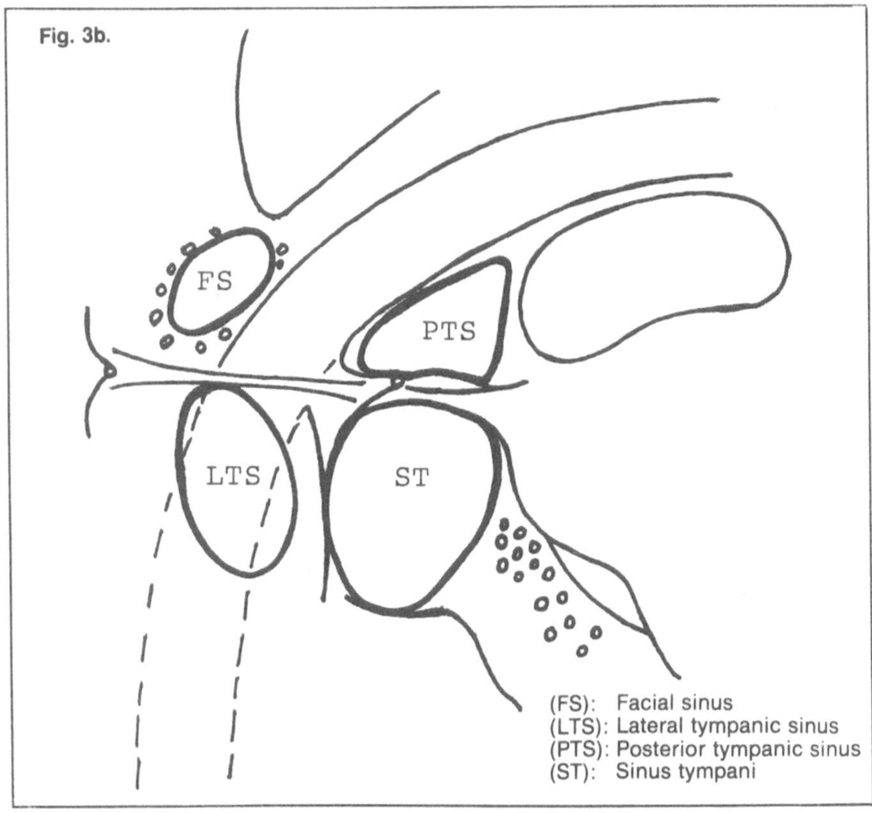

from the tympanic sinus by the ponticulus, being situated between the latter and the facial canal.

The *sinus tympani* is generally oval in shape, bounded by the ponticulus, pyramidal ridge and subiculum. Its major axis measures between 2,5 and 3,5 mm, its minor axis between 1 and 2 mm and its depth is from 2 to 3,5 mm. More detailed description of this anatomy has been given by Proctor [4,1] and Guerrier.[2]

From the *surgical point of view*, one may thus consider there are:

— *External or supra-pyramidal sinuses*, which are the facial sinus or supero-external sinus, and the lateral tympanic sinus or infero-external sinus, separated by the chordal ridge.

— *Internal or infra-pyramidal sinuses*, which are the posterior tympanic or supero-internal sinus, and the sinus tympani or infero-internal sinus, separated by the ponticulus.

The *anatomical variations* of the retrotympanum concerning the surgeon are essentially those of the *facial nerve canal*. Firstly, the congenital bony dehiscences in the facial canal: these vary from 0,5 to 3 mm and are very frequent (55 % according to Baxter[5], 57 % according to Dietzel[6]). They essentially concern the tympanic segment (91 % as against 9 % for the mastoid segment).

At tympanic level, dehiscences are often adjacent to the oval window (83 %), with protrusion in 26 % of cases. Concerning the mastoid segment, dehiscences are seen mainly towards the facial sinus (79 %) against 21 % towards the tympanic sinus or the retrofacial cells. A protrusion of the nerve is found in 12 %.[7]

Apart from dehiscences and protrusions it must be borne in mind that there may be anatomical variations in the course of the facial canal. From the surgical point of view, it is therefore necessary:
— to bear in mind the possibility of dehiscences, protrusions or abnormalities along the course of the facial nerve in the retrotympanum;
— to identify the upper facial canal (tympanic segment) before arriving at the retrotympanum and the mastoid segment of the canal, if necessary having reference to the classic landmarks: cochleariform process, lateral semicircular canal, promontory, round window niche,... particularly in exeresis of cholesteatoma;
— to take into account any abnormality, even minor, of the external or middle ear, these being possibly associated with an abnormality of the facial canal or the facial nerve itself;
— to consider as subject to caution any soft tubular structure in this region, even outside of the classic course of the facial nerve.

References:

1. PROCTOR B. Surgical anatomy of the posterior tympanum. *Acta Oto-Rhino-Laryngol.* Belg. 25, 911-928, 1971.
2. GUERRIER Y. Anatomie chirurgicale des parois de la caisse du tympan. Monographies Chouvin-Blache, vol. 6, 1977.
3. ANDREA M. Regiao posterior da caissa da tympano. Etude anatomo-chirurgicale. Thèse. Lisbonne, 1975.
4. PROCTOR B. The development of the middle ear spaces and their surgical significance. *J. Laryngol. Otol.*, 78, 631-646, 1964.
5. BANTER A. Dehiscence of the fallopian canal. *J. Laryngol. Otol.*, 85, 587-594, 1971.
6. DIETZEL K. Über die Dehiszenzen des Facialiskanals. *Z. Laryngol-Rhinol-Otol.*, 40, 366-376, 1961.
7. PROCTOR B., NAGER G. The facial canal: normal anatomy, variations and anomalies. *Ann. Otol. Rhinol. Laryngol.*, suppl. 97, 91, 33-61, 1982.

Posterior tympanotomy

ABSTRACT

B. Ars

The purpose of our work is to analyse the rôle played by the tympanic part of the temporal bone. We have used two types of methods: a classical one: morphology, with embryological and anatomical study, and another more modern method: biophysics.

The first part concerns the results of the morphological observations; the illustrations and a brief commentary of the figures give the main point which may be drawn from them. The second part is devoted to anatomy: we take the tympanic part as the reference point in our anatomo-surgical systematization of the tympanic cavity. Thanks to this systematization, the individual morphological variants observed in anatomo-surgical systematization of the tympanic cavity. Thanks to manner. On the basis of this systematization we propose some advice on clinical and surgical aspects. The demonstration of the physical importance of this tympanic part supports the results of this study.

Our biophysical study demonstrates clearly the fundamental rôle played by the tympanic frame in sound transmission.

The various theoretical and experimental arguments have led us to advocate a surgical technique of approach to the tympanic cavity: the posterior tympanotomy is more suitable for a better functional result.

Clinical, peroperative and histopathological data base

E. Koekelkoren, F. Abes, L. Moeneclaey, S. Peeters, J.F.E. Marquet

Introduction
The micro-electronic revolution of the last decade has brought the computer and its software into our society as a common tool. Also in medicine, the computer is far integrated, not only in information and communication systems, but also in diagnostic and therapeutic investigations. In our department, we apply the possibilities of the microprocessor by setting up a program of data base: data collecting, data proceeding and statistics. The aim of this program consists of gathering and preserving data, so that this information can be used at any time and for all purposes, e.g. in studies, tests or investigations about a special topic.

Method
Considering the impossibility of predicting the future interests of investigators on one hand, and the fact that the data may not be influenced by our actual interests on the other hand, the program must be established so as to conform with the following criteria:

— the listing has to be comprehensive, without being too extensive,
— the program must achieve a uniform way of collecting, preserving and proceeding data,
— the system ought to be permutable with other existing and future programs,
— practical feasibility.

In giving our program a concrete form, we decided to make three divisions:
— the preoperative findings: clinical data;
— the peroperative findings: mostly done by means of the operation microscope;
— the postoperative findings: the histopathological data.

In each division we evaluate several points on the following subjects: tympanic membrane, tympanic cavity, mucosa, ossicles and joints.

Results: Listing for clinical and preoperative evaluation

Table 1.

```
Name :......................

Nr. Patient :              [ ][ ][ ][ ][ ]

Surgical case :            [ ][ ][ ][ ][ ][ ][ ]

Male    L:1   R:2          [ ]
Female  L:3   R:4

Birth year :               [ ][ ]

Pre-operative statement of hearing loss :
        0   no hearing loss
        1   mild degree
        2   moderate degree
        3   severe degree

Operation formula :                              Color code:
[ ][ ][ ][ ][ ][ ][ ][ ][ ][ ][ ][ ][ ][ ][ ]    Y  yellow
|  T  | + |  M  | + |  I  | + |  S  | + |  W  |CC|   B  blue
                                                 O  orange
                                                 R  red

Origin of the biopt tissue :
        1   tympanic membrane
        2   covering tissue
        3   ossicles
        4   mucosa
        5   tumor
        6   varia

Cholesteatoma present :      [ ]

Alfachymotrypsin used :      [ ]
```

Table 2.

TYMPANIC MEMBRANE

Tissue type : 0 original
1 autograft
2 allograft
3 mixed type

Involved by cholesteatoma : ☐

Tympanic membrane otoscopic statement :

0 mobile
1 immobile

0 dry
1 wet

0 thick
1 thin

0 without granulation
1 with granulation

0 without polyposis
1 with polyposis

0 keratinizing
1 non-keratinizing

0 no perforation
1 perforation (P)

0 without retractionpocket
1 with retractionpocket (R)

0 without tympanosclerosis
1 with tympanosclerosis (T)

superior
1 2
3 4
7
5 6
inferior

Muco-cutanous junction :

0 ill defined
1 well defined lateral to the lamina propria
2 well defined medial to the lamina propria
3 well defined lat. and med. to the lam. propria
4 well defined at the edge of the perforation

Collagen :

0 no interruption
1 interruption of collagen (IC)

Table 3.

TYMPANIC CAVITY

Per-operative statement, fibrous tissue :

0 not present
1 present

0 not infected
1 infected

MUCOSA

Per-operative statement, mucosa :

	Tympanum	Atticum	Mastoid
Normal	☐	☐	☐
Smooth	☐	☐	☐
Granular	☐	☐	☐
Polypoid	☐	☐	☐
Scarred	☐	☐	☐

Per-operative statement, inflammatory submucosal changes :

	Tympanum	Atticum	Mastoid
Congestion Edema	☐	☐	☐
Glue ear	☐	☐	☐
Cholesterol granuloma	☐	☐	☐
Tympano-sclerosis	☐	☐	☐
Involved by cholesteatoma	☐	☐	☐

Table 4.

OSSICLES

Tissue type :

	Malleus	Incus	Stapes
0 original	0	0	0
1 autograft	1	1	1
2 allograft	2	2	2
3 prothesis	3	3	3

Per-operative statement :

	Malleus	Incus	Stapes
0 no involv.	0	0	0
1 involved	1	1	1

Ossicular chain :

0 intact

1 not intact

Involved by cholesteatoma :

☐ Malleus ☐ Incus ☐ Stapes

JOINTS

Per-operative statement :

	I.M.joint	I.S.joint	Annular lig.
Abnormal mobility	☐	☐	☐
Ankylosis	☐	☐	☐
Luxation	☐	☐	☐
Tympanosclerotic changes	☐	☐	☐
Squamous epithelial infiltration	☐	☐	☐

COMMENTS OR REMARKS

This part of the program contains four subdivisions:
— identification and general information (table 1). By means of a uniform way of numbering, permuting with other programs is very easy. A simple operation formula, namely the tympanic-ossicular formula - introduced by us several years ago[1] - summarizes the postoperative state. This formula is very easily surveyed and suitable for computer use;
— evaluation of the tympanic membrane (table 2). Here we introduced a tympanic diagram which is very useful in registration of the localization of a pathological finding by using an abbreviation;
— evaluation of the tympanic cavity and the mucosa (table 3). To localize the pathological findings, the middle ear is divided into three areas: tympanum, atticum and mastoid;
— evaluation of the ossicles and the joints (table 4).

To be complete, there is, beside the statements of the listing, also a statement for comments and remarks about special notes on the case.

Listing for histopathological evaluation

Table 5.

```
Name :.........................

Computer case : [ ][ ][ ][ ][ ]

Nr. biopt :     [ ][ ][ ][ ][ ][ ]

Film    :1  Slides :2
Picture :3  T.V.   :4   [ ]

Staining : standard with silver staining [ ]

Immunofluorescence : [ ]

Origin of biopt :                studied
     1   tympanic membrane         [ ]
     2   mucosa                    [ ]
     3   ossicles                  [ ]
```

Table 6.

TYMPANIC MEMBRANE

Anatomo-pathological statement, epidermal epithelium :

- ☐ non-keratinizing
- ☐ papillary formation ☐ irregulary ingrowth
- ☐ perforation

Muco-cutanous junction :

0 ill defined
1 well defined lateral to lam. prop.
2 well defined medial to lam. prop.
3 well defined lat.and med.to lam.prop.
4 well defined at the edge of theperfo.

Anatomo-pathological statement, lamina propria :

- ☐ collagen absent
- ☐ collagen interrupted
- ☐ disorderly arranged collagen fibers
- ☐ tympanosclerotic changes
  - ☐ hyalinisation
  - ☐ calcification
  - ☐ osteocytes
  - ☐ ossification

Anatomo-pathological statement, presence of :

- ☐ retractionpocket
- ☐ cholesteatoma
  - ☐ papillary ingrowth
  - ☐ inflammatory changes of surrounding stroma
  - ☐ granulation tissue in surrounding stroma

Anatomo-pathological statement, mucosal layer :

0 simple squamous epithelium
1 cuboidal epithelial changes
2 columnar epithelial changes
3 squamous epithelial changes

Mucosal glandular hypertrofy ☐

Table 7.

MUCOSA

Origin of biopt : 1 tympanum
2 atticum
3 mastoid

Anatomo-pathological statement, epithelium :

Tympanum	Atticum	Mastoid	
☐	☐	☐	simple squamous epith.
☐	☐	☐	pseudo-stratified ciliated epith.
☐	☐	☐	cuboidal epith. changes
☐	☐	☐	columnar epith. changes
☐	☐	☐	squamous epith. changes
☐	☐	☐	keratinizing

Anatomo-pathological statement, presence of :

Tympanum	Atticum	Mastoid	
☐	☐	☐	goblet cells
☐	☐	☐	increased number
☐	☐	☐	tubular glands
☐	☐	☐	glandular hypertrofy
☐	☐	☐	glandular hyperplasy

Anatomo-pathological statement, acute inflamm. changes :

Tympanum	Atticum	Mastoid	
☐	☐	☐	congestion and edema
☐	☐	☐	leucocytes infiltration
☐	☐	☐	round cell infiltration

Anatomo-pathological statement, chronic inflamm. changes :

Tympanum	Atticum	Mastoid	
☐	☐	☐	fibrosis
☐	☐	☐	cholesterol granuloma

Anatomo-pathological statement :

Tympanum	Atticum	Mastoid	
☐	☐	☐	tympanosclerotic changes
☐	☐	☐	hyalinisation
☐	☐	☐	calcification
☐	☐	☐	osteocytes
☐	☐	☐	ossification

Table 8.

OSSICLES

Origin of biopt : 1 malleus
2 incus
3 stapes

Anatomo-pathological statement, epithelium :

Malleus	Incus	Stapes	
☐	☐	☐	simple squamous mucosal epith.
☐	☐	☐	pseudo-stratified ciliated epith.
☐	☐	☐	cuboidal epith. changes
☐	☐	☐	columnar epith. changes
☐	☐	☐	squamous epith. changes
☐	☐	☐	keratinizing
☐	☐	☐	glandular formation
☐	☐	☐	increased number of goblet cells

Anatomo-pathological statement :

Malleus	Incus	Stapes	
☐	☐	☐	vascular congestion
☐	☐	☐	vascular and peri-vascular inflamm. cell infiltration

Anatomo-pathological statement, bone structure :

Malleus	Incus	Stapes	
☐	☐	☐	osteocytes live
☐	☐	☐	bone absorption
☐	☐	☐	with granuloma
☐	☐	☐	in presence of osteoclasts
☐	☐	☐	new bone formation
☐	☐	☐	peri-vascular areas involved
☐	☐	☐	cortical areas involved
☐	☐	☐	peri-vascular and cortical areas involved
☐	☐	☐	new bone formation with tetracyclines

Table 9.

JOINTS

Origin of the biopt : 1 incudo-malleolar joint (I.M.J.)
2 incudo-stapedial joint (I.S.J.)
3 annular ligament (A.L.)

Anatomo-pathological statement :

I.M.J.	I.S.J.	A.L.	
☐	☐	☐	absence of the joint
☐	☐	☐	abnormal joint
☐	☐	☐	abnormal joint cartilage
☐	☐	☐	abnormal joint lumen
☐	☐	☐	abnormal joint synovium
☐	☐	☐	abnormal joint ligaments

Anatomo-pathological statement, inflammatory changes :

I.M.J.	I.S.J.	A.L.	
☐	☐	☐	peri-articular inflamm. changes
☐	☐	☐	synovial inflamm. changes
☐	☐	☐	presence of squamous keratinizing epithelium
☐	☐	☐	excluding the joint
☐	☐	☐	including the joint

Anatomo-pathological statement :

I.M.J.	I.S.J.	A.L.	
☐	☐	☐	tympanosclerosis
☐	☐	☐	hyalinisation
☐	☐	☐	calcification
☐	☐	☐	osteocytes
☐	☐	☐	ossification

All biopsies taken during surgery are elaborated into histological slides at the laboratory of our department. During the anatomo-pathological study of the specimens the listing for histopathological evaluation (tables 5, 6, 7, 8, 9) is followed and completed. This listing contains the same subdivisions and subjects as those of the clinical and peroperative evaluation (cf. supra).

In this way the computer program can be used in several directions:
— in the vertical direction: delivering data about clinical, peroperative and finally histopathological findings;
— in the horizontal direction; delivering data about the tympanic membrane, the tympanic cavity, mucosa and the other subsequent subjects.

Conclusion

In our department we postulated that the most important criterion to meet is "the practical feasibility": since the value and the result of a program depend on its continuity, it is a prerequisite that the performance of this program is simple and easily surveyed. Therefore, completing the listing may only take a short time and may not be strenuous. The used codes have to be simple and clear, so that each co-operator, regardless of his experience, can use the program in daily practice without becoming stressed.

The main difference between the first and the second part of the program exists in the performance. In relation to the first part, namely the listing for clinical and peroperative evaluation, there are three different ways of answering provided:
— by circling the appropriate answer;
— by marking one or more right answers;
— by using a code.

In the second part, more properly, the listing for histopathological evaluation, only the possibility of circling or marking is left. The underlying idea is that no answer on any topic corresponds to the negation of the stated topic, this in contra-distinction with the first part. In this way, completing the lists becomes very easy and can be done in a minimum of time, still without losing data. So when we look up a particular case, the computer gives only the filled in answers in the listing for clinical and peroperative evaluation, while it will show an answer to each statement of the listing for histopathological evaluation, namely the asked answer itself or its opposite.

Discussion

By presenting here our method of collecting, proceeding and preserving data of clinical, peroperative and histopathological evaluation, we are not claiming that this is "the only and best way" to handle the problem. We just want to demonstrate "one possible way" of data processing, by storing interesting information, for present and future usefulness.

As far as the problem of a computerized data system is concerned, one point must be seen very clearly: the pitch of this matter is the conflict between being comprehensive and detailed without getting too extensive on one hand, and the practical feasibility without becoming too generalized, on the other hand.

Reference:

1. MARQUET J., GRAFF A., Postoperative evaluation of middle ear surgery. *Audiology*, 21, 20-32, 1982.

Pre- and postoperative radiological evaluation in middle ear surgery

ABSTRACT

E.V. Claus, F.E. Offeciers, M. Lorré, P. Van de Heyning, J. Claes, J.F.E. Marquet

The multidirectional polytomography allows a three-dimensional reconstruction of the anatomical and pathological structures of the temporal bone.

This conventional technique is still of great value as long as most of the radiological departments do not dispose of a CAT-scan or NMR.

Apart from a clear didactic value, the multidirectional polytomography is helpful in diagnosis, preoperatively for the clarification of surgical landmarks as well as for postoperative evaluation.

Some typical pre- and postoperative cases are shown of cholesteatoma and reconstructive middle ear surgery by means of tympano-ossicular allografts, of traumatic lesions of the middle ear, and of congenital atresia of the external auditory canal and middle ear. Some unusual postoperative images are also shown.

Pre- and postoperative evaluation of tubal dysfunction by means of endoscopy

K. Yamashita

Introduction

According to a survey of our own cases, postoperative middle ear complications, including ear effusion, retraction, perforation, recurrent cholesteatoma and others, were found more frequently in cases with middle ear cholesteatoma than in those with chronic otitis media. In these cases, tubal dysfunction seems to be one of the most important causes of the complications. Endoscopic observation of the Eustachian tube revealed interesting and important information about the site and the mechanism producing tubal dysfunction from the visual aspect.

Method

Endoscopy of the Eustachian tube was performed using the flexible fiberscope with and without an instrumentation channel by the procedure which was introduced by the author.[1] A relatively free approach allowed a detailed examination of the tubal orifice. And the tubal lumen of the cartilaginous portion was examined using the flexible fiberscope with a channel for air insufflation permitting insertion of the scope. The sound of air flow into the middle ear cavity was constantly monitored by an auscultation tube or recorded by a microphone placed against the ear canal of the side being examined. The visual findings of the tube were recorded by photography or videotape.

Results and Conclusions

In cases with epitympanic cholesteatoma or middle ear atelectasis, middle ear effusion, epitympanic retraction pocket, and/or atelectasis occurred more frequently after tympanoplasty (65 % of 57 cases) than in those with chronic otitis media (18 % of 102 cases).

By endoscopic observation of the structure and movement of the Eustachian tube, the following findings have been observed and considered as important factors altering the surgical results:

— adenoid enlargement and tubal tonsils on the tubal torus obstructed the tubal orifice even in cases of the adolescent or adult in spite of good passage of tubal lumen (figures 1,2). In such cases, Nd-YAG laser surgery under endoscopy was one kind of effective treatment before tympanoplasty;

— in some cases with high-arched palate and hypoplastic velum, abnormal stricture or obstruction of the tubal orifice was observed (figures 2,3). In these cases, it was difficult to

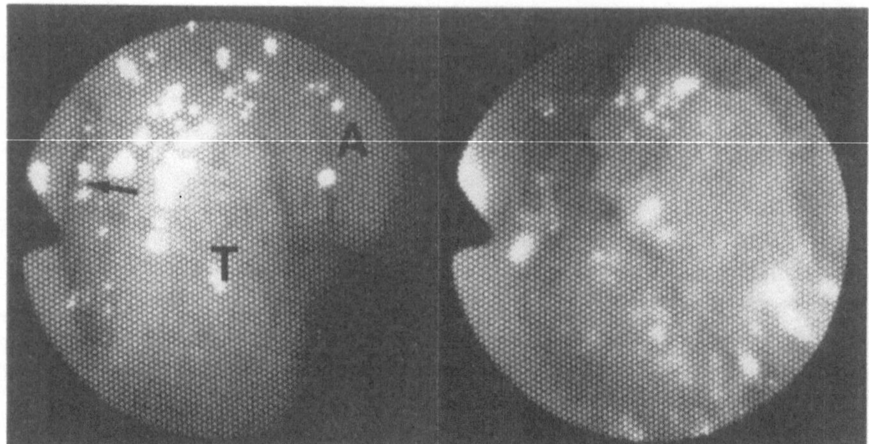

Fig. 1. Left: Severely obstructed tubal orifice (arrow) by hypertrophied tubal tonsil on the torus (T) and enlarged adenoid (A). Right: Marked hypertrophy of tubal tonsil inside the orifice, pneumatic endoscopic findings, right side, 38-year old male with cholesteatoma and middle ear effusion

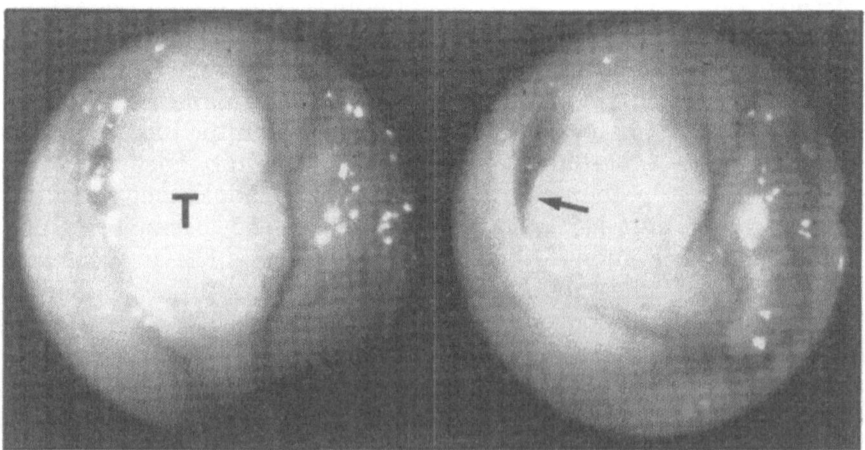

Fig. 2. Hypertrophied tubal tonsil (T) on a hypoplastic torus. Left: At rest. Right: On swallowing action, the tubal orifice (arrow) is obstructed by the torus, right side, 13-year old boy with cholesteatoma and middle ear effusion

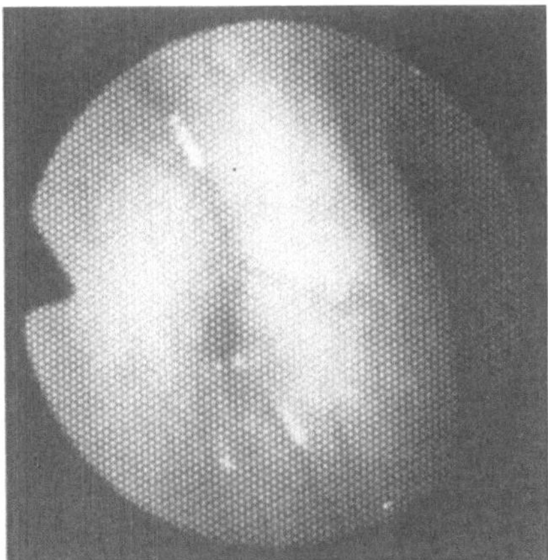

Fig. 3. Abnormal stricture of the tubal orifice in a case with high-arched palate and micrognathia, right side, 29-year old female with cholesteatoma and middle ear atelectasis

obtain a good result after tympanoplasty;
— severe middle ear complications are found in about 25 % of the cases with cleft palate. In such cases, the pharyngeal orifice is blocked by the eminence formed by the levator muscle during the swallowing action because of the wrong direction of the muscle (figure 4), or the hypoplastic torus and tube itself which may cause both opening and closing failure in combination (figure 5). These points should be considered in order to improve palatoplasty.

When tympanoplasty is performed in cases with chronic otitis media or middle ear cholesteatoma, it is extremely important to perform examinations to obtain an accurate picture of the condition of the Eustachian tube pre- and also postoperatively.[2] In the conventional tubal inflation test using catheter, stenosis around the tubal orifice can be overlooked and contradictory results can be obtained such as poor tubal function despite good pas-

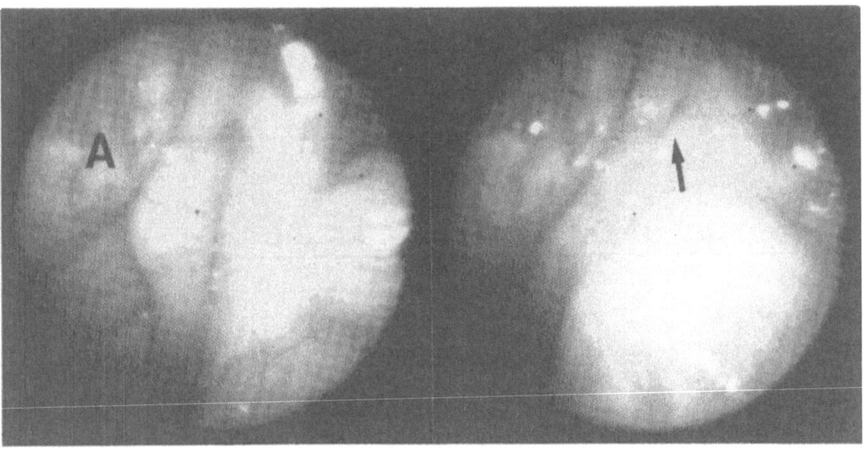

Fig. 4. Block of the tubal orifice (arrow) on swallowing action (right) due to abnormal direction of the levator muscle in a case with cleft palate (postoperative) and cholesteatoma, left side, 12-year old boy. A: Hypertrophied adenoid

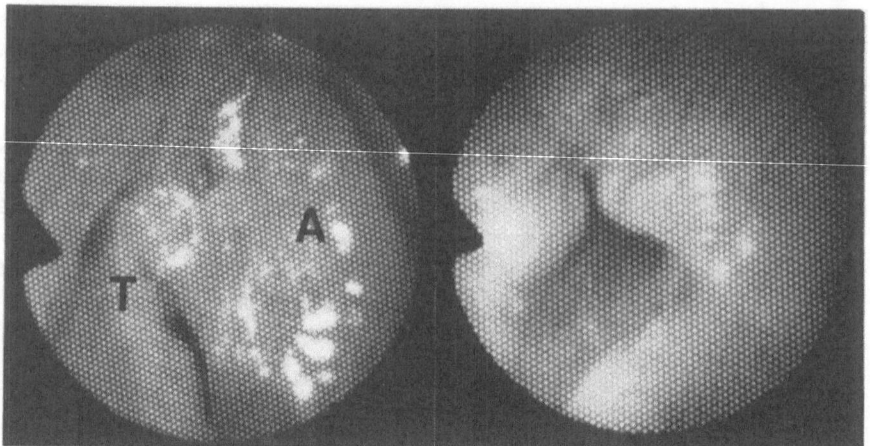

Fig. 5. Left: Hypoplastic tubal torus (T) and adenoid enlargement (A). Right: Intraluminal view showing floppy tube, right side, 12-year old girl with cleft palate (postoperative) and cholesteatoma

sage of air through the catheter, because the tip of the catheter is inserted directly into the cartilaginous portion.

As shown here, tubal endoscopy may reveal interesting and important findings relating to tubal function. Thus, this procedure may play an important rôle as a pre- and postoperative examination tool for tympanoplasty.

References:

1. YAMASHITA K. Pneumatic endoscopy of the Eustachian tube. *Endoscopy,* 15: 257-259, 1983.
2. ZÖLLNER F. Anatomie, Physiologie, Pathologie und Klinik der Ohrtrompete und ihre diagnostisch therapeutischen Beziehungen zu allen Nachbarschaftserkrankungen. Springer, Berlin, 1942.

Endoscopy of the Eustachian tube

ABSTRACT

K. Yamashita

The author introduced a systematic procedure of endoscopy of the Eustachian tube using the flexible fiberscope with and without an instrumentation channel. A relatively free approach allows a detailed examination of the tubal orifice. And the tubal lumen of the cartilaginous portion is examined using the fiberscope with a channel for air insufflation permitting insertion of the scope. The sound of air-flow into the middle ear cavity is constantly monitored by an auscultation tube placed against the ear canal of the side being examined. This method can be a useful and complementary clinical examination procedure for evaluating tubal dysfunction.

Bacteriological examination of middle ear secretions

P. Van Cauwenberge, M. Rysselaere, G. Declercq

Introduction

The controversial reports concerning the bacteriology of secretory otitis media (SOM) are mainly due to the fact that, even when bacteria are present in the middle ear effusions, their number is scant, contrary to what happens in chronic and acute suppurative otitis media, where a rich flora with heavy growth of bacteria is usually present.[1] This means that there is a need for highly sensitive bacteriological techniques and for a standardization of the methods used. In this present report we will describe our techniques which are used in a standardized way and which guarantee the detection and identification of bacteria with quantitative as well as qualitative information. The value of this standardized bacteriological method, in which the direct microscopic examination plays a very important rôle, is demonstrated by analyzing the results obtained in 87 consecutive children with secretory otitis media (SOM).

Standardized methods

Sampling

When dealing with an intact eardrum, the external ear canal is sterilized with a 70° alcohol solution, during 90 seconds. Then, the alcohol solution is carefully aspirated from the external ear canal and eardrum until the surface is completely dry. Tympanostomy is performed and the middle ear effusions are aspirated with a sterile canula.[2] We use the Juhn Tym Tap and, in order to avoid aspiration of a possibly remaining alcohol solution on the external surface of the eardrum, we introduce the tip of the siliconized canula in the tympanostomy opening. The effusions are collected in a sterile plastic collector which is immediately closed and transported to the microbiology laboratory. In the laboratory, different smears are made for direct microscopic examination; inoculation for aerobic and anaerobic culture is performed without any delay. In our material there is only a time lapse of maximum 5 minutes between sampling on the one hand, and smearing and inoculation on the other hand. If the tympanic membrane is perforated and otorrhoea is present, the secretions from the external ear canal should be aspirated before introducing the sterile canula into the perforation to collect a specimen for bacteriological examination.

Direct microscopic examination

Direct microscopic examination of the middle ear gives us valuable information about the concentration of bacteria present in the secretions - and their morphological properties - and also about the rôle of inflammatory cells present in the secretions, and even about the function and morphology of these cells. The presence of intracellular bacteria not only gives us indications about the pathogenicity of these bacteria but also about the phagocytic function of macrophages, histiocytes and other cells present. With fluorescence acridine orange staining we can, in addition, distinguish dead from living bacteria.[3]

— *Gram stain.* The smear is air-dried and heat-fixed. Cristal-violet solution is applied during one minute and then washed with tap water. Then, lugol iodine solution is applied for one minute and also washed with tap water. The smear is decolourized with 95% ethylalcohol and again washed with tap water. Then, counterstaining is performed with fuchsine solution during 30 seconds, after which the preparation is washed with tap water and blot-dried.[4]

— *Giemsa stain.* The smear is air-dried and fixed in absolute methanol during 5 minutes. Then, the freshly prepared Giemsa solution is applied for 20 minutes (1 drop Giemsa into 10 drops of a phosphate buffered solution). After 20 minutes the smear is washed with tap water and air-dried.[5]

— *Acridine orange stain.* To study the viability of the bacteria present, no fixation is used in this method. One drop of the specimen is mixed with 1 drop of acridine orange solution (0.003 % in Hanks buffered saline solution). A coverglass is put on the smear and the preparation is immediately observed under a Leitz fluorescent microscope.[6] Dead organisms have a red or orange colour, living organisms give a green fluorescence.[3]

Aerobic and anaerobic culture

The specimen is inoculated as soon as possible on:

— an enriched medium preferably warmed in the incubator; incubation is performed at 37 % in a CO_2 enriched atmosphere (anaerobic jar + gas generating kit CO_2 system),

— anaerobic culture (anaerobic jar + gas generating kit anaerobic system),

— liquid medium (brain heart infusion broth).

For anaerobic culture, we use an anaerobic blood agar base (Gibco) to which 50 ml/l defibrinated sheep blood is added. For aerobic culture we use chocolate agar + chemical enrichment (Vitox oxoid).

Bacteriological results in SOM

To examine the value of our standardized bacteriological method and the information provided by the different techniques used, we examined the effusions obtained from 87 consecutive cases of SOM, of at least 3 months duration. The specimens were taken from children between 2 and 7 years of age.

Direct microscopic examination
Gram stain (87 ears) showed bacteria present in 40 cases (44 %). Acridine orange stain (87 ears) showed fluorescent (living) bacteria in 37 (42 %) and non-fluorescent bacteria in 23 (24%). Fluorescent and non-fluorescent bacteria were often found together in the same specimen. The Giemsa stain (74 ears) showed bacteria in 23 cases (31 %).

Aerobic culture (87 ears) was positive in 30 cases (34 %), while the anaerobic culture (87 ears) only grew anaerobes in 4 specimens (4 %). Haemophilus influenzae was the most frequently found aerobic bacteria (table 1), but also Branhamella catarrhalis, micrococci and Streptococcus pneumoniae were found in 5 to 10 % of the cases. We noted a very low incidence of Staphylococcus epidermidis and a complete absence of Staphylococcus aureus and Streptococcus pyogenes.

Comparison of different methods (table 2).
In 53 cases (60 %), we found a complete correlation between the Gram stain and the acridine orange stain. The Gram stain gave more information in 11 cases (13 %) while the acridine orange stain was superior in 23 cases (27 %).

Table 1. Bacteria [yeasts] found in culture*

Haemophilus influenzae	13
Branhamella catarrhalis	7
Micrococci (a.o. luteus)	6
Streptococcus pneumoniae	5
Diphteroids	3
Corynebacterium belphanti	2
Staphylococcus epidermidis	1
Propionibacterium acnes	3
Peptostreptococcus	1
[Candida Guillermondi	1]

* 87 ears with SOM of at least 3 months duration; children aged 2-7 years.

Table 2. Comparison of the different methods*	
Gram stain vs. acridine orange stain	
Complete correlation:	53 (60 %)
More information in Gram stain:	11 (13 %)
More information in acridine orange stain:	23 (27 %)
Total	87 (100 %)
Gram stain vs. aerobic and anaerobic cultures	
Positive culture of bacteria seen in stain: (or negative culture with negative stain)	56 (64 %)
Negative culture of bacteria seen in stain:	20 (23 %)
Positive culture of bacteria, not seen in stain:	11 (13 %)
Total	87 (100 %)
Acridine orange stain vs aerobic & anaerobic cultures	
Positive culture of bacteria, seen as fluorescent-green in stain (or negative culture with negative stain):	54 (62 %)
Negative culture of bacteria, seen as red or orange (= dead) bacteria in stain:	8 (9 %)
Positive culture of bacteria, seen as red or orange in stain:	2 (2 %)
Negative culture of bacteria, seen as fluorescent-green in stain:	16 (19 %)
Positive culture of bacteria, not seen in stain:	7 (8 %)
Total	87 (100 %)

* 87 ears with SOM of at least 3 months duration: children aged 2-7 years.

With regard to the relationship between direct microscopic examination and the cultures, we found a positive culture of the bacteria which were seen in the Gram stain (or negative culture with negative stain) in 56 cases (64 %); in 20 cases (23 %) the bacteria seen in the stain could not be cultured, while in 11 cases (13 %) bacteria could be cultured which were not identified in the Gram stain. This means that, based on the Gram stain and culture, we can conclude that in 13 % bacteria that were indeed present (shown by positive culture) were not identified by Gram stain, while in 23 % the bacteria which were really present (seen in direct microscopic examination) could not be cultured, which means that the culture techniques were not sensitive enough or that the bacteria were dead.

Comparison of the results obtained by acridine orange stain and culture gave a positive culture of bacteria seen as fluorescent-green in the staining (living bacteria) or a negative culture with a negative stain in 54 cases (62 %). In addition, bacteria seen as red or orange (dead) in the acridine orange stain did not grow on aerobic and anaerobic culture media in 8 cases (9 %). In 7 cases (8 %) bacteria cultured could not be seen in the acridine orange stain, while in 16 cases (19 %) fluorescent-green bacteria from the acridine orange stain could not be cultured which means that the culture technique was not sensitive enough in these cases; in only 2 cases (2 %) bacteria seen as red or orange in the stain were grown in culture.

Discussion

An important facet of the bacteriology of middle ear effusions is that the quantity of bacteria (if present) is very low.[7] This means that our bacteriological techniques should be as sensitive as possible and that the use of different bacteriological techniques - especially in the direct microscopic examination - can give us more information than if only one technique (for example the Gram stain) is used. In this way, the fluorescent acridine orange staining is a very valuable method which often gives us additional information. It is also possible to distinguish dead from living bacteria with this method. The Giemsa staining, on the other hand, gives better information about the inflammatory cells present in the effusions (not discussed in this paper). Aerobic culturing is discussed in our paper and it confirmed the important rôle of Haemophilus influenzae and the involvement of Branhamella catarrhalis and Streptococcus pneumoniae.[1,7] The anaerobic cultures were only positive in 4 %.

Conclusions

There is a need for standardization of sensitive bacteriological techniques in the bacteriological examination of middle ear effusions or secretions. Direct microscopic examination, making use of 3 different staining methods - Gram, acridine orange and Giemsa - provides very interesting and complementary information. Acridine orange staining is a recent method for direct microscopic examination and completes the information obtained by the Gram and Giemsa staining. With our methods we could demonstrate bacteria present in the middle ear effusions in 42 to 44% by direct microscopic examination, in 34 % with aerobic and in 4 % with anaerobic cultures.

References:

1. VAN CAUWENBERGE P. Otitis media with effusion. Microbiological aspects. *Acta Otorhinolaryng. Belg.* 36, 196-213, 1982.
2. JUHN S.K., MEYERHOFF W.L., PAPARELLA M.M. Clinical application of middle ear effusion analyses. *Laryngoscope* 91, 1012-1015, 1981.
3. BERNSTEIN J.M. Personal communication.
4. BARON J.B., CABAU N. Nouvelles techniques de laboratoire en ophtalmologie. G. Doin & Cie, Paris, 1957, p. 49.
5. LENNETTE E.H. Manual of clinical microbiology. *Am. Soc. Microbiol.* 1980, p. 1015.
6. KRONVALL G., MYHRE E. Differential staining of bacteria in clinical specimens using acridine orange buffered at low Ph. *Acta Pathol.microbiol. Scand.* Sec. B: Microbiol. 85, 249-254, 1977.
7. LIU Y.S., LIM D.J., LANG R.W. et al. Chronic middle ear effusions: immunochemical and bacteriological investigations. *Arch. Otolaryngol.* 101, 278-286, 1975.

Venous hypotensive anaesthetic technique for middle ear surgery - "Protected sleep"

J. Delaruelle, R. Prévinaire, M. Dehaen, B. Bael, P. Spiritus, J.F.E. Marquet

Patho-physiology of the cardio-vascular system in relation to bleeding and oozing during surgery

When hypotensive anaesthetic techniques are discussed in the literature, the authors nearly always mean arterial hypotension. However, arterial hypotension, even at low levels, as a complement to classic curarisation - artificial ventilation anaesthesia does not always result in a sufficient bloodless surgical field, as can be seen especially in microsurgery of the ear, septorhinoplasty or other types of head and neck surgery.

Forces determining exchange		Blood - and - Tissue
	Forces within capillary	Opposite forces within tissues
	HYDROSTATIC PRESSURE exerted by:	**HYDROSTATIC PRESSURE** of tissue
At ARTERIOLAR end of capillary	**B P** - 30 mmHg	10 mmHg **TP**
	is opposed by	
	OSMOTIC PULL	
	exerted by	
	PLASMA PROTEINS	
	(since they cannot pass through the membrane in significant amounts)	**OSMOTIC PULL**
	OP = 25 mmHg	15 mmHg
	EFFECTIVE DRIVING FORCE	
	= 10 mmHg	
	BP (30 - 10) - **O.P.** (25-15)	
	O.P. = 30 mmHg **B.P.** = 10 mmHg	15 mmHg OP 10 mmHg TP
At VENULAR end of capillary	**EFFECIVE PULLING FORCE**	
	= 15 mm Hg	
	O.P. (30 - 15) - **B.P.** (10 - 10)	

Hyperventilation and hyperoxygenation would seem obligatory to combat possible dangerous effects of induced arterial hypotension. This certainly results in a higher arterial and venous pO_2 but does not answer the real question: what about the oxygen availability and utilization at the tissular and cellular level? We cannot discuss here in detail every aspect of this very complex problem.

To clarify and to explain a "reconsidered" anaesthetic approach which the authors present in this paper, we just want to recall some basic physiological data.

We would like to do this by means of a few successive diagrams without much explanation, because we think the diagrams to be sufficiently clear.

Anaesthetic techniques - Hyperventilation with respirator

This technique will result among other things in: pO_2 rise, pCO_2 fall, vasoconstriction, venous pressure rise, immediate postoperative hypoxia during the rebuilding up of the depleted CO_2 stores of the body, more difficult

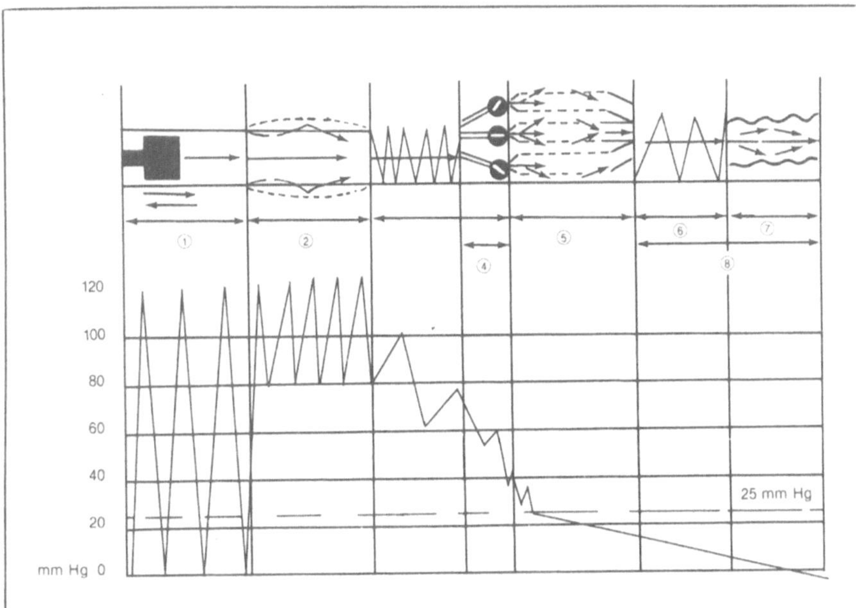

Diagram of the successive vessel areas, linked in series, and of the fall in pressure levels in these areas

1 Pump
2 Elastic arteries
3 Precapillary resistance arterioles
4 Sphincter vessels
5 Capillary exchange vessels
6 Postcapillary resistance vessels
7 Capacity vessels
8 Venous side

oxygen dissociation from hemoglobine.

Normoventilation with respirator
The so-called "normal" parameters which are taken into consideration in assessing normoventilation are unappropriated in our opinion.

One should not compare anaesthetic parameters with the physiological parameters of a normal person during his daily activity (which is done almost everywhere), but rather with normal "sleep"-parameters, at night, during a period of so-called deep sleep (relative hypoventilation, pCO_2 rise, lower metabolic rate, lower blood pressure, relative hypothermia, etc.). Even with normoventilation, artificial ventilation always presents a different pattern of expansion of the respiratory system and brings about a non-physiological cardiac venous return (during expiratory phase instead of during inspiration).

Moderate hypoventilation with spontaneous respiration
Such a technique is only possible when there is no intrinsic surgical need for complete muscular relaxation and curarisation, as for example in head and neck surgery. In such a state parameters should be more or less comparable with deep sleep parameters. Thanks to vasodilation, low venous and arterial pressure, we can obtain an almost normal gradient in capillary blood flow with less dangerous consequences of arterial hypotension. Microsurgical bleeding will be minimal. There are two important difficulties in order to obtain such a spontaneous respiration anaesthetic state:

— Choice of a pharmacodynamic mixture with only mild depression of spontaneous respiration, but still permitting adequate anaesthesia and analgesia. Concomitant minimal disturbance of tissular perfusion and cellular oxygenation.

— Absence of any impediment or valvular resistance to expiration. If this is not achieved, the gradually building up of intrapulmonary pressure will result in venous pressure rise, hindrance to capillary blood flow gradient, bleeding and oozing.

Evaluation of different pharmacodynamic drugs and mixtures
The personality and the background of each particular anaesthetist will undoubtedly play a predominant rôle in the choice of drugs and mixtures in performing such an anaesthetic technique. The drugs - if they fulfil the necessary conditions - are perhaps not so important. Many combinations are possible. The concept "spontaneous respiration - sleep parameters - venous hypotension" is much more important. In this way, we may hope to fulfil the criteria imposed by middle ear microsurgery: minimal bleeding, no

oozing, no middle ear pressure changes.

Anaesthetic procedure

Example
Middle ear surgery, retroauricular approach, man, 52 yrs, 86 kg. Preoperative examinations are normal but for a mild chronic restrictive lung function test (smoker).

Premedication
2 to 1½ hours preoperatively:
per os: 20 mg diazepam
1 hour to 45 min preoperatively:
I.M.: morphine HCl 15 mg
N-allylnormorphine 10 mg
promazine HCl 100 mg
atropine 0,5 mg

Induction
— Installation of an intravenous line in a sufficiently large vein with a not too large indwelling catheter ("floating-catheter" principle). We use a 500 ml, 10 % sorbitol solution.
— Diazepam 40 to 60 mg I.V.
The spontaneous respiration is maintained thanks to the diazepam administrated in the premedication.
— Intravenous diazepam is painful and very irritating for the endovein. Immediate rinsing of the vein with 20 to 30 ml sorbitol is of the utmost importance (three-way stoplock).
— Introduction of not too big an oral airway.
— Inhalation by mask (to and fro or Mapleson-D anaesthetic circuit) of O_2:5 to 61 with halothane (0,5 - 1 %) and ethrane (1 - 1,5 %).
— Surgical preparation of the patient.
— Morphine HCl 10 mg I.V.
The spontaneous respiration is still maintained thanks to the N-allylnormophine in the premedication.
— Laryngoscopy, introduction of a nasal stomach tube.
— Local anaesthetic spray of the larynx and the trachea with 10 % Xylocaïne solution. If there are still bucking or coughing reflexes, a further I.V. 10 mg diazepam and/or 100 to 150 mg thiopentone.
— Anaesthetic mask with O_2, halothane and ethrane for another 5 to 8 min.
— Gentle intubation (without relaxant) tube no. 7 or 8 maximum. Almost no coughing reflex and absence of bucking expresses sufficiently deep anaesthesia.
— Analgesia and anaesthesia for surgery.
If necessary, 10 to 20 mg I.V. diazepam or 100 to 150 mg thiopentone.

Maintenance
— It is standard procedure in our anaesthetic service to maintain spontaneous respiration throughout for head and neck surgery, controlling the degree of anaesthesia and hypotension mostly by playing with the two inhalational agents.
— We use a modified Mapleson-D-circuit without any respiratory valve. The expiratory valve is replaced by a light-weight Y piece, with one part connected to an

expiratory corrugated tube of 30 to 50 cm, open to the air.
— In its lumen, at about 20 to 30 cm from the Y piece, a much smaller suction catheter is secured. A controlled suction of about 15 cm H_2O in this catheter is maintained and this simple scavenging device is connected to a central vacuum system (see figure).

Apart from preventing pollution of the operation room this system also decreases the amount of rebreathing.
— Routine monitoring comprises: ECG, heartrate (HR), bloodpressure (BP), respiratory wave form and rate (RR) by thoracic impedancimetry, capnography in the patient's part of the Y piece and temperature, in the rectum of naso-pharynx (T).
— These parameters are continually controlled and regularly written down on a chart as a manually performed "trend-recording".
— Respiration is sufficiently deep and calm and there is no bronchial hypersecretion.
— Peripheral circulation is adequate as judged from both the

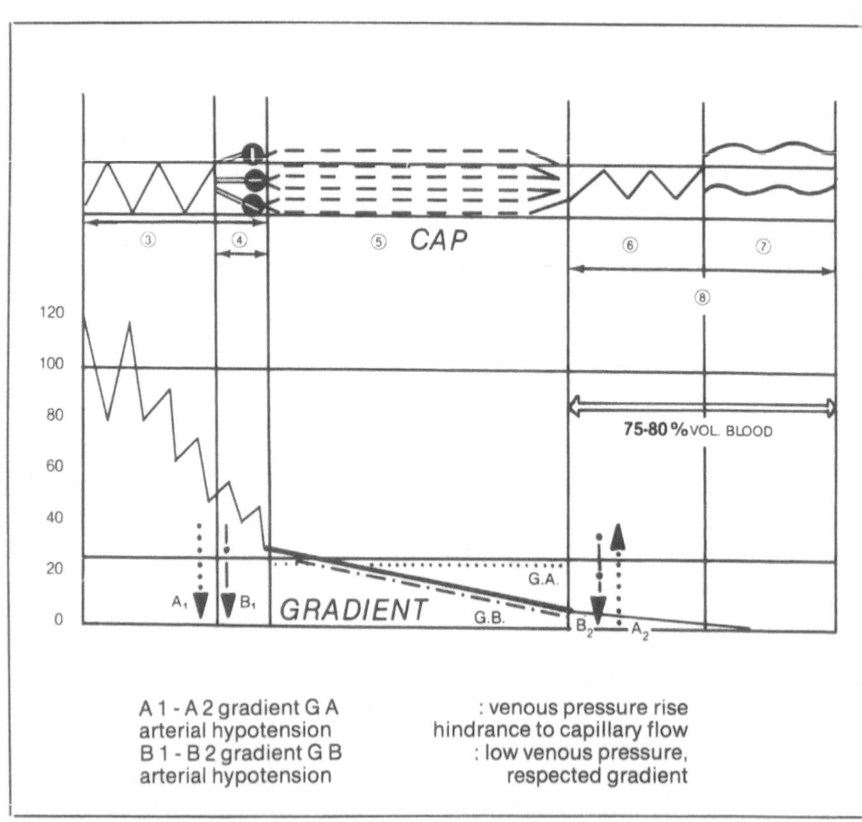

A 1 - A 2 gradient G A : venous pressure rise
arterial hypotension hindrance to capillary flow
B 1 - B 2 gradient G B : low venous pressure,
arterial hypotension respected gradient

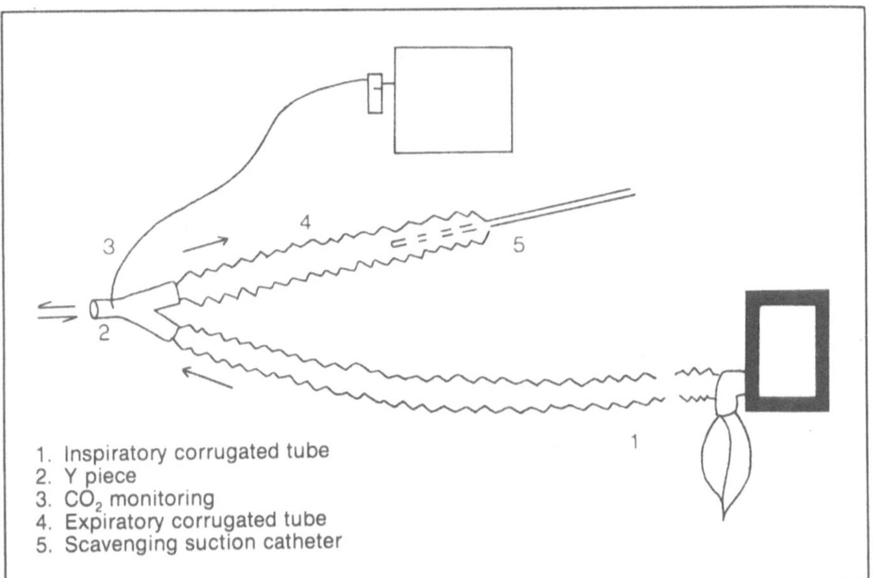

extremities and the microscopic operation field.

— Upon reposition or homograft of the tympanic membrane, the latter does not balloon (no N_2O).

Hypotension

Basic venous hypotension is obtained and slight anti-Trendelenburg further decreases the pressure in the operative field. Due to vasodilation, a relative arterial hypotension is seen. If the systolic pressure remains higher than 100 mmHg or if the heart rate stays higher than 90/ min, we use labetalol (Trandate) in incremental doses of 2 to 4 mg.

Coagulation disorders

If the preoperative laboratory tests show a critical or insufficient amount of fibrinogen, it will often be necessary to administer I.V. incremental doses of fibrinogen. If after several hours of microsurgery, a local fibrinolysis becomes manifest, we use I.V. 50 to 60 units of Botropase, a snake venom.

Termination

— Very gradual returning of parameters to preoperative levels, gradual awakening, residual analgesia.

— Gentle extubation, (aspiration manœuvres of secretion are rarely necessary), and placement of an oral airway.

— Installation of the patient in bed in lateral stabilized position, alternating sides each hour in the recovery ward until consciousness is restored.

An experimental study of homografts of the tympanic membrane with malleus

H. Moriyama, K. Aoki, Y. Honda

The present experiments in cats (96) were performed to explore the process of survival and the taking of transplanted homografts of the tympanic membrane, which were preserved in 4 % and 0,5 % formalin solutions (pH 7.0), and reactions of middle ear mucosa of the recipient. The present study also includes gross and histopathological examinations of the eardrum, observation of fibers of the lamina propria of the transplanted tympanic membrane by means of polarizing microscopy and that of vascularization in the transplanted tympanic membrane and malleus by intravascular India ink injection.

Five weeks after transplantation, the membrane was still very turbid on the whole and showed hyperplasia in the epithelial layer; the middle ear cavity showed edematous changes and the presence of effusion, with a lumen which suggested a delated blood vessel or lymphoduct; the middle ear mucosa showed an increase in the connective tissues accompanied by vascularization and cellular infiltration, indicating strong inflammatory reactions. The Gelfoam packed in the middle ear cavity remained. After eight weeks, the membrane still showed hyperplasia and turbidity, but the hyperplasia in the epidermal layer was reduced. In the middle ear mucosa, no foreign body giant cells were found and the general disappearance of inflammatory changes was seen, although partial cellular infiltration, chiefly by lymphocytes, and an increase in vessel-rich connective tissues were seen. In the malleus, partial vascularization was recognized. After twelve weeks, the membrane became thinner in its peripheral part, but epidermal hyperplasia was still seen in the region near the malleus. In the middle ear mucosa, the inflammatory changes had disappeared for the most part, though cellular infiltration and a picture of Gelfoam intake were partially seen. After 24 weeks (figure 1), the tympanic membrane presented an almost normal picture, and thin epidermal and mucosal layers were seen sandwiching the collagen fibers. The edematous connective tissues had been absorbed, and the middle ear mucosa had become thin and was covered with ciliated epithelium.

When we compared the reactions of the middle ear mucosa after autogenous fascia graft and those after homograft, cellular infiltration, chiefly by lymphocytes, was seen in both graft cases, foreign body giant cells were not found in

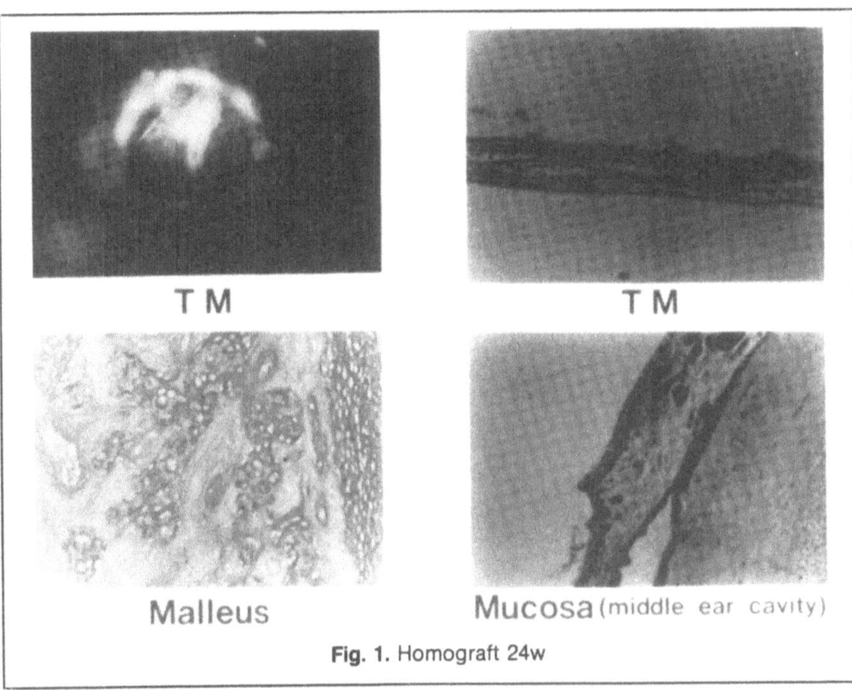

Fig. 1. Homograft 24w

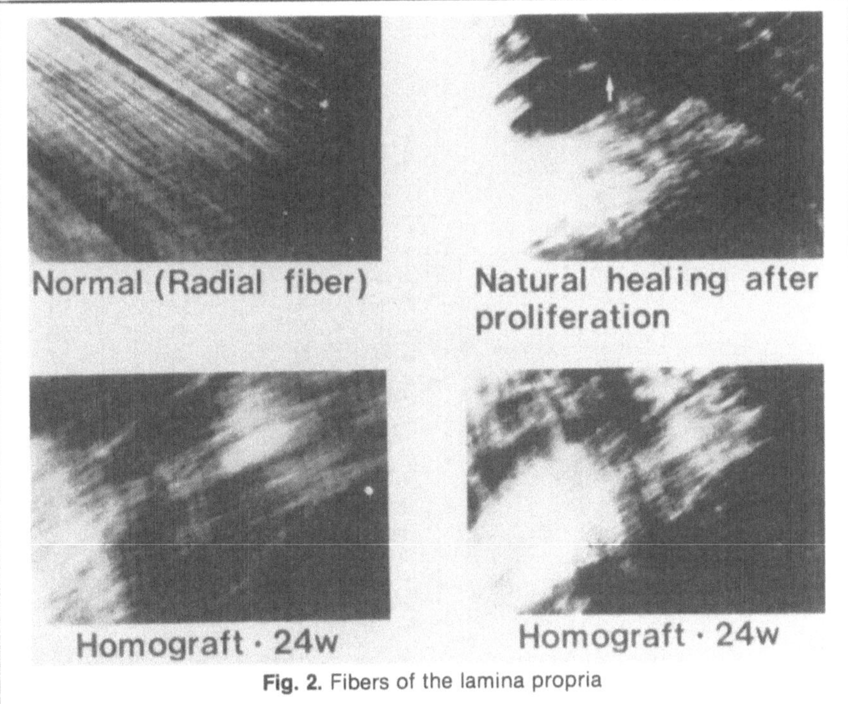

Fig. 2. Fibers of the lamina propria

either of them and similar inflammatory changes were seen in both. Thus, the changes in the middle ear mucosa were thought to occur not because of rejection but because of non-specific stimuli such as Gelfoam. Such changes disappeared gradually, but in some cases the fibrous structures (granulation) were seen in the middle ear cavity.

In the normal membranes, the circular fibers were dense in the peripheral region and became sparse in the central part; in the central part, radial fibers were dominant. In the spontaneously reproduced membranes, the arrangement of the fibers was generally disordered although arrangements were seen in some parts. The homograft tympanic membranes, on the other hand, had slightly loose indistinct fibers, but their arrangement was not disordered, suggesting that the grafted fibers remained (figure 2).

In the grafted membranes, the

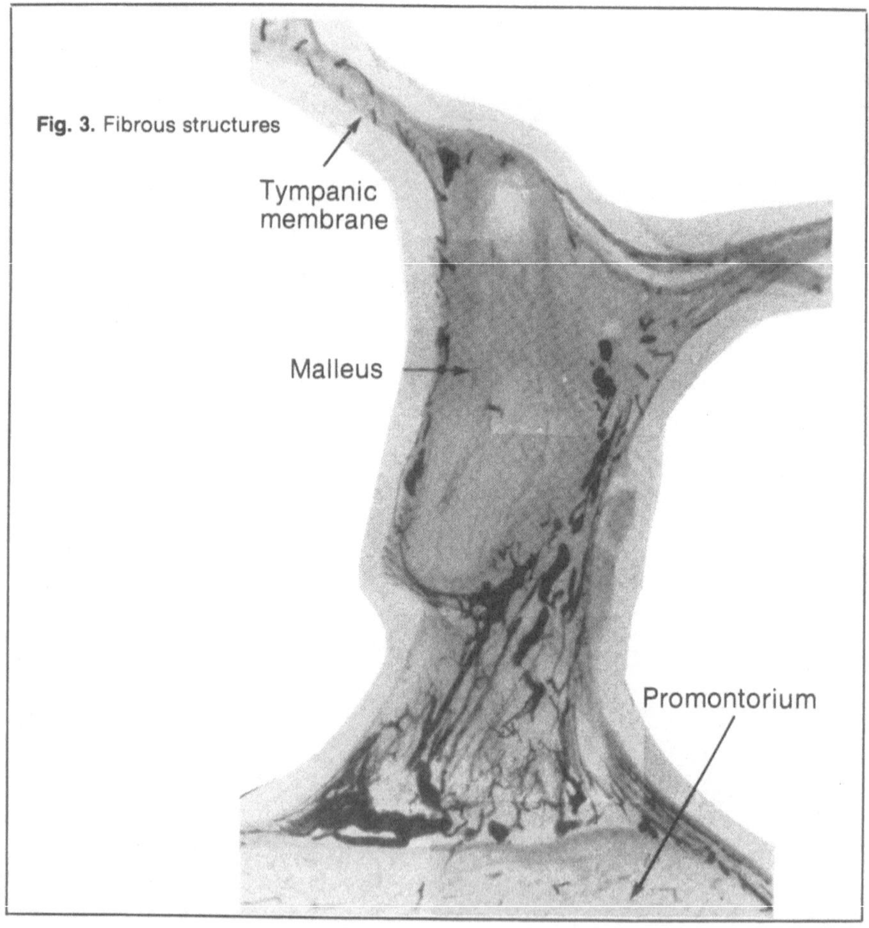

Fig. 3. Fibrous structures

branches which go down the manubrium mallei were not found; instead, there were blood vessels which entered the membrane from the outside and anastomosed with each other at various sites to nourish the membrane. Irrespective of whether the malleus is a normal or grafted one, it is nourished by the vasoganglion in the epidermal or mucosal layer of the membrane. But when vessel-rich, fibrous structures are found in the middle ear cavity, the malleus seems to be nourished in a slightly different way. Such fibrous structures are rich in blood vessels, and a number of vessels, large in diameter, are recognized (figure 3). In these cases, we assume that the tympanic membrane and malleus are nourished chiefly through these fibrous structures.

The above results suggest that the tympanic membrane homograft actually means grafting of the collagen fibers of the intermediate layer, and that this technique is superior to the grafting of other materials like the fascia in that the former makes a thinner membrane than the latter without lateral healing. On the other hand, perforation in the membrane takes place in some cases of tympanic membrane homograft, and we had the impression that postsurgical infection, even if slight, could considerably affect the grafted membrane.

Clinical significance of the tympanic isthmus related to the development of cholesteatoma

I. Miyajima, Y. Honda

Introduction

The term tympanic isthmus, which is a narrow pathway between the mesotympanum and the epitympanic space, was originally proposed by Proctor[1,2,3] (figure 1), whose observations was repeated by Aimi[4,5] and others,[6,7] each of whom agreed on its significance.

The purpose of this study is to examine the anatomy of the tympanic isthmus in a large number of fresh temporal bones and to investigate pathological changes resulting from various middle ear diseases, especially the pars flaccida type cholesteatoma (attic retraction cholesteatoma) and the pars tensa type cholesteatoma

Fig. 1. Diagram to show the right attic view from above

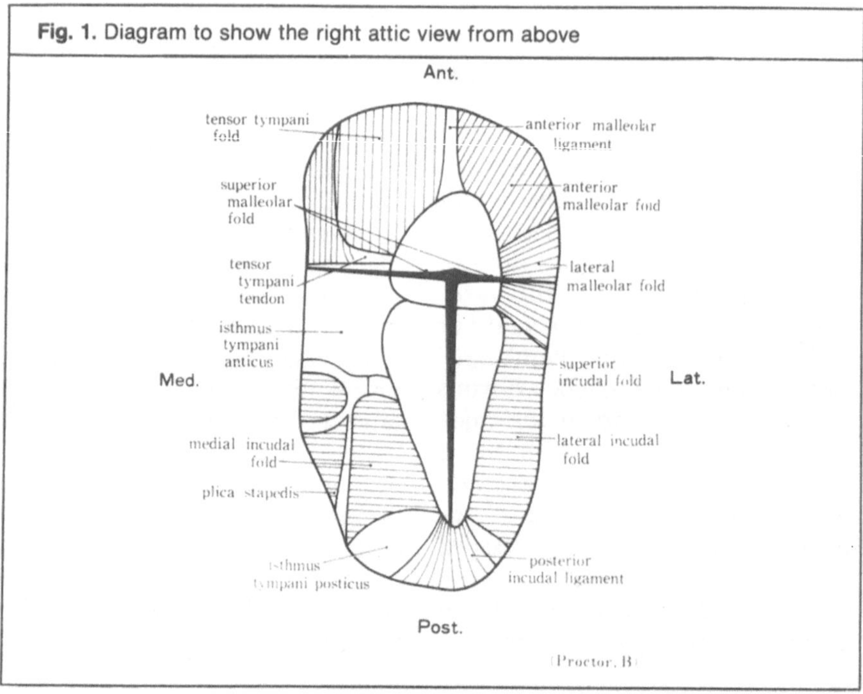

which arises from the postero-superior quadrant (PSQ) of the tense portion of the tympanic membrane.

Materials and method

The anatomy of the tympanic isthmus and its specific anatomical structures were investigated in 170 fresh temporal bone specimens under the operating microscope. Temporal bones[8] were obtained from autopsies for investigation during the period from 1978 to 1983. Almost all of the 170 specimens were fresh ones and the others had been fixed with a 10 % formalin solution.

The method of dissection which we used was the anatomical atticotomy in which the tegmen tympani of the temporal bone was removed and the entire epitympanum was exposed, followed by observation of the attic from above.

In addition to the anatomical investigation as described above, our study has been supplemented with the analysis of large numbers of surgical findings in cholesteatoma.

Results

A total of 170 temporal bone specimens were examined under the operating microscope. Five of these were shown to have middle ear diseases. Three of the specimens came from female patients and the other 2 from male patients. Their age ranged from 43 to 76, with an average age of 61 years. The following items were noted: glue ear with obstructed isthmus (1 specimen); attic retraction cholesteatoma with narrowed isthmuses (2 specimens); chronic otitis media with occlusion of the isthmus by the retracted pars tensa itself (1 specimen) and the PSQ retraction cholesteatoma with obstruction of the isthmus by the retracted PSQ itself (1 specimen).

Pneumatization of the mastoid was inhibited in all of the pathological specimens.

As a representative specimen, the glue ear with obstructed tympanic isthmus is introduced here in figures 2, 3, 4. Otoscopic examination revealed the retraction of the pars flaccida of the tympanic membrane. In short, the attico-antral space was isolated from the tubo-tympanic space by the obstructed tympanic isthmus induced by chronic stimulation of the glue from above, resulting in retraction of the pars flaccida of the tympanic membrane, leaving the mesotympanum intact.

These pathological findings in the isolated epitympanum have been confirmed by the surgical findings in cholesteatoma, especially the pars flaccida type.

Discussion

From the results of cadaver temporal bone dissection and the analysis of surgical findings in cholesteatoma, we have concluded that there are two types of

Fig. 2. Attico-antral space filled with glue (arrow). Malleus head can be found (right ear)

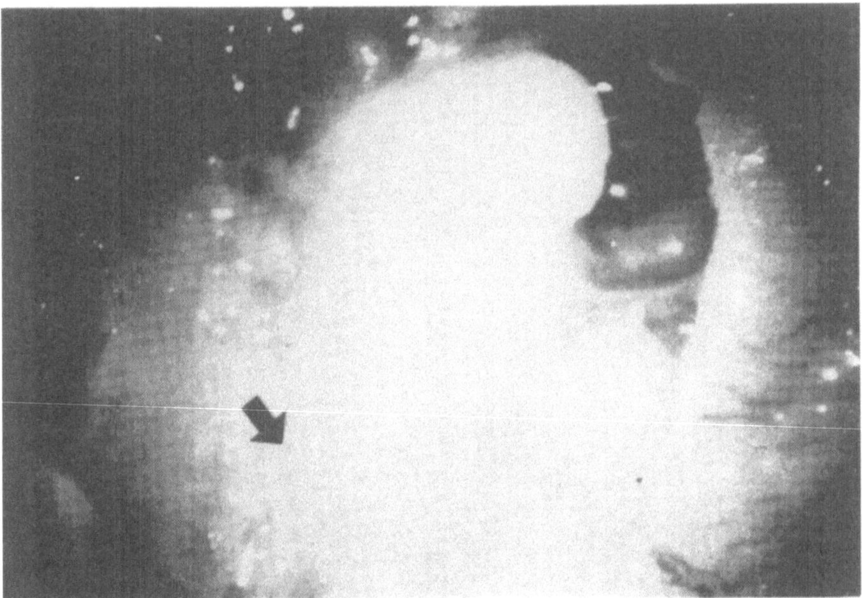

Fig. 3. Same specimen as in fig. 2. After removal of the glue, the tympanic isthmus is found to have been obstructed (arrow)

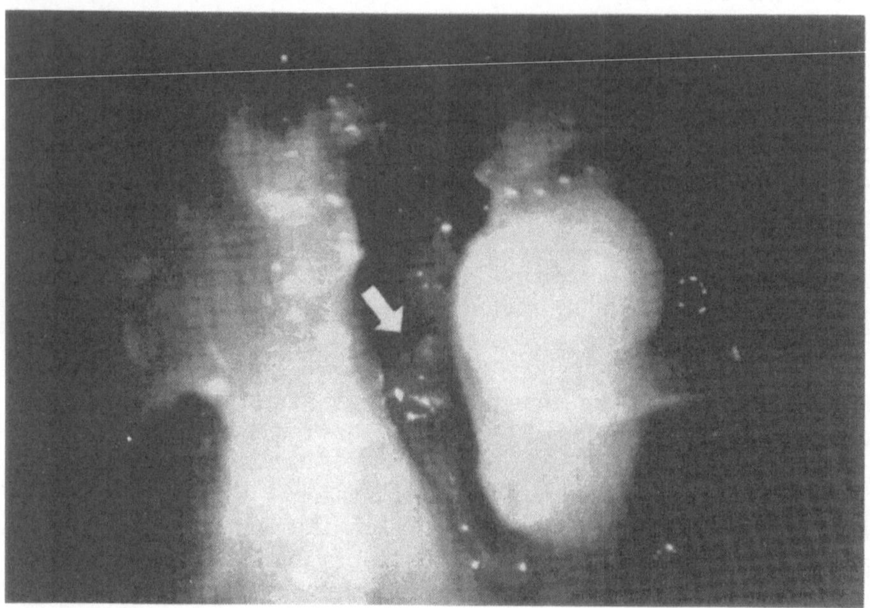

Fig. 4. Observation of the mesotympanum through the control hole (arrow) revealed to be normal. Same specimen as in figures 2,3

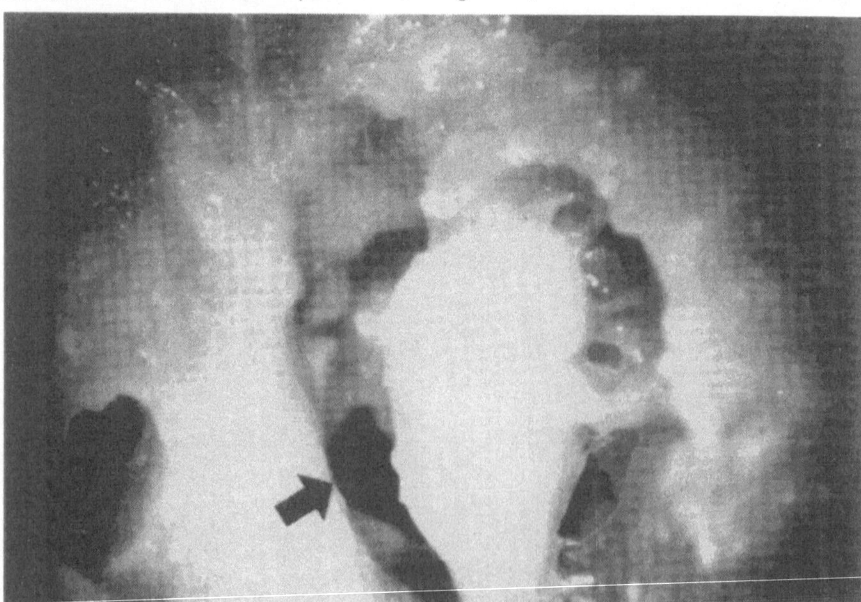

acquired cholesteatoma: one type is the pars flaccida type (attic retraction type), the other is the pars tensa type (PSQ retraction cholesteatoma[9]).

Concerning the pars flaccida type cholesteatoma, the poorly pneumatized mastoid caused by persistent otitis media with effusion in infancy results in the trapped glue in the attico-antral space (Mawson)[10] even if tubal function has been restored later on. Consequently, the tympanic isthmus, which is a physiological narrow space between the epitympanum and mesotympanum, located before and behind the stapes, is closed membranically due to the chronic stimulation from above.

If the pars flaccida of the tympanic membrane is continuously stimulated from behind by the pathological state in the attico-antral space, the long-term slight inflammation will gradually induce the development of division and differentiation of the cutaneous epithelial cells of the pars flaccida, that is, the pars flaccida type cholesteatoma. As a result, the hypertrophic pars flaccida where keratinized desquamated epithelium is found, will become a retraction pocket due to the intratympanic negative pressure in the epitympanum.

It is observed that the development of cholesteatoma has been stopped in the midst of the process when the tympanic isthmus is not completely obstructed or the pneumatization of the mastoid is comparatively good, that is, the epitympanum and antrum are well aerated.

However, the cholesteatoma derived from the pars tensa, namely the pars tensa type cholesteatoma, originates also from otitis media with effusion with severe dysfunction of the Eustachian tube. In this situation, the tympanic isthmus has been gradually obstructed by the back surface of the retracted or adhered tympanic membrane itself from below, followed by the development of retraction cholesteatoma into the epitympanum (figures 5, 6). However, the progression of the retraction is sometimes halted by the growth of granulation or connective tissue in the vicinity of the tympanic isthmus. In addition, when the perforation occurred at the tense portion of the eardrum, the development of the retraction cholesteatoma has been prevented in almost all cases.

Conclusions

Acquired cholesteatoma has been divided into two types. One is the pars flaccida type (attic retraction cholesteatoma) and the other is the pars tensa type (PSQ retraction cholesteatoma).

Furthermore, the pattern of the blockage of the tympanic isthmus has also been divided into two types. One is the membraneous occlusion without retracted pars

Fig. 5. Diagram showing the development of the pars flaccida type cholesteatoma (attic retraction cholesteatoma)

Attic Retraction Cholesteatoma

Isthmus block

(HONDA)

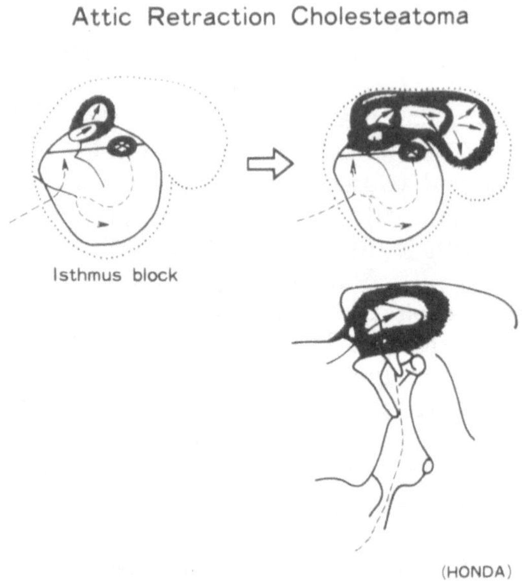

Fig. 6. Diagram showing the development of the pars tensa type cholesteatoma (PSQ retraction cholesteatoma)

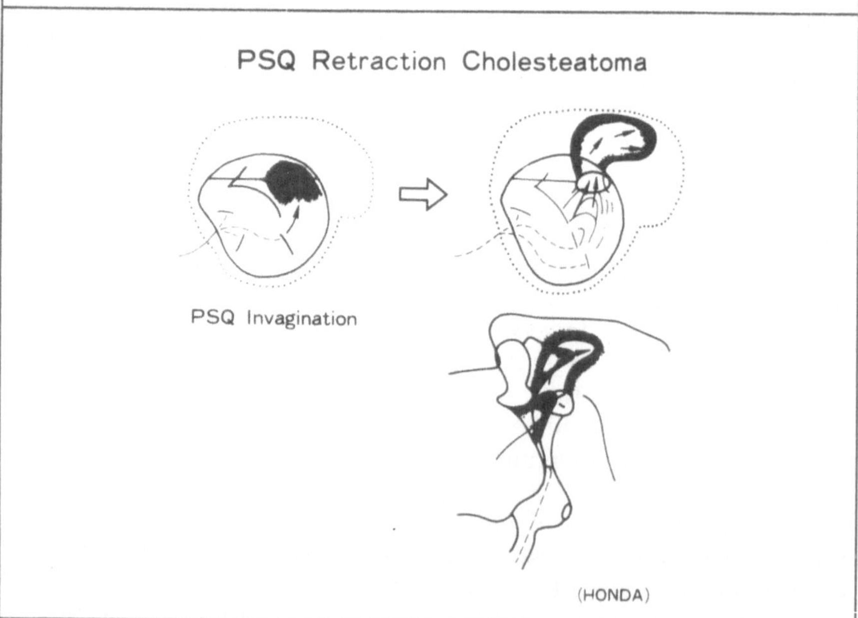

tensa. This occlusion is considered to have been induced by chronic pathological stimulation in the attico-mastoid space. The other is the occlusion by the back surface of the retracted tympanic membrane itself from below. Naturally, a combination of the two patterns should be possible.

While the former type of isthmus blockage is considered to be related to the development of the pars flaccida type cholesteatoma, the latter is related to the development of the pars tensa type.

The common factors of the two types of cholesteatoma, except for the isthmus blockage, are considered to be the poorly pneumatized mastoids and tubal dysfunction especially in the pars tensa type.

The development of acquired cholesteatoma is closely related to the persistent serous otitis media, especially the glue ear.

References:

1. PROCTOR B. The development of the middle ear spaces and their surgical significance. *J. Laryngol.* 78: 631-635, 1964.
2. PROCTOR B. Surgical anatomy of the posterior tympanum. *Ann. Otol.* 78: 1026-1030, 1969.
3. PROCTOR B. Attic-aditus block and the tympanic diaphragm. *Ann. Otol* 80: 371-375, 1971.
4. AIMI K. The clinical significance of epitympanic mucosal folds. *Arch. Otolaryng.* 94: 499-505, 1971.
5. AIMI K. The tympanic isthmus: Its anatomy and clinical significance. *Laryngoscope* LXXXVIII, No. 7. 1067-1081, 1978.
6. WULLSTEIN S.R. Histopathological alterations of the mucosal folds in chronic otitis media. *Acta Otolaryng.* 81: 197-203, 1976.
7. MIYAJIMA I. Clinico-Anatomical study of the tympanic mucosal folds. *Otorhinolaryngology,* Tokyo. 24 Suppl. 3: 1-42, 1981.
8. SCHUKNECHT H.F. Pathology of the ear. 2-3, Harvard University Press. 1974.
9. BHIDE A. Etiology of the retraction pocket in the postero-superior quadrant of the eardrum. *Arch. Otolaryng.* 103: 707-710, 1977.
10. MAWSON S.R. Diseases of the ear. 3rd edition 284-285, Arnold, 1974.

Experimental cholesteatoma
Part 1 - Closed method of the tympanic orifice

S. Sano, Y. Honda

Many cases of middle ear cholesteatoma are of the attic type cholesteatoma. The pathogenesis of this condition has been discussed among many researchers. This paper reports a pathological condition established in animals which is similar to human attic type cholesteatoma.

Method

In normal rabbits anesthetized intravenously, an incision was made below the auricle to expose the bulla of the middle ear. The bulla was opened by a drill under a surgical microscope. From the opened window, the tympanic orifice of the Eustachian tube was confirmed, and a muscular segment was filled in. After confirming that the tympanic membrane was not injured during surgery, the skin was sutured. The animals were kept for a certain period thereafter (3 days to 16 weeks). A total of 122 ears were submitted to this experiment; each was observed under a light microscope after sacrifice of the animal.

Results

Serial sections including the auditory canal, tympanic membrane, and the middle ear cavity were prepared from each specimen. All experimental ears were divided into the following three groups according to the pathological condition:

Group A: The middle ear cavity was filled with pus, showing severe infection. Whole perforation occurred in the tympanic membrane, and inflammatory products were also present in the auditory canal, causing hypertrophy of the epithelium of the auditory canal. However, there was no case of cholesteatoma formed by the migration of the epithelium into the middle ear cavity. Of the 122 ears, 67 were assigned to this group (illustration 1a).

Group B: Exudate occupied most of the middle ear cavity, and bleeding and pus were occasionally noticed. Inflammation in the middle ear cavity was milder than in group A, although the degree varied according to the case. The inflammation was limited to the inside of the middle ear cavity. There was no tympanic perforation, and the pars tensa and the pars flaccida were observed. No inflammatory products were present in the auditory canal. Hypertrophy of the epithelium of the auditory canal was slight. Of the 122 ears, 46 were assigned to this group (illustration 1b).

Group C: Lesions in the middle ear cavity were almost the same as in group B. Most middle ear cavities were filled with exudate. No changes were found in the pars tensa, whereas nine ears showed interesting findings in the pars flaccida. Illustration 2a shows an ear four weeks after surgery. The epithelium of the pars flaccida showed hypertrophy and the pars flaccida formed a retraction pocket. These findings were considered to represent the early stage of the formation of pars flaccida cholesteatoma (P F chole). Capillary formation was marked under the epithelium. The mucosal layer on the back side of the migrating epithelium went on without discontinuance. Exudate was found in the middle ear cavity.

Illustration 2b, like 2a, shows an ear four weeks after surgery. Debris was found in the retraction pocket. No papillary formation of the epithelium was observed, while the pars flaccida was migrating to the attic. There were no changes in the pars tensa.

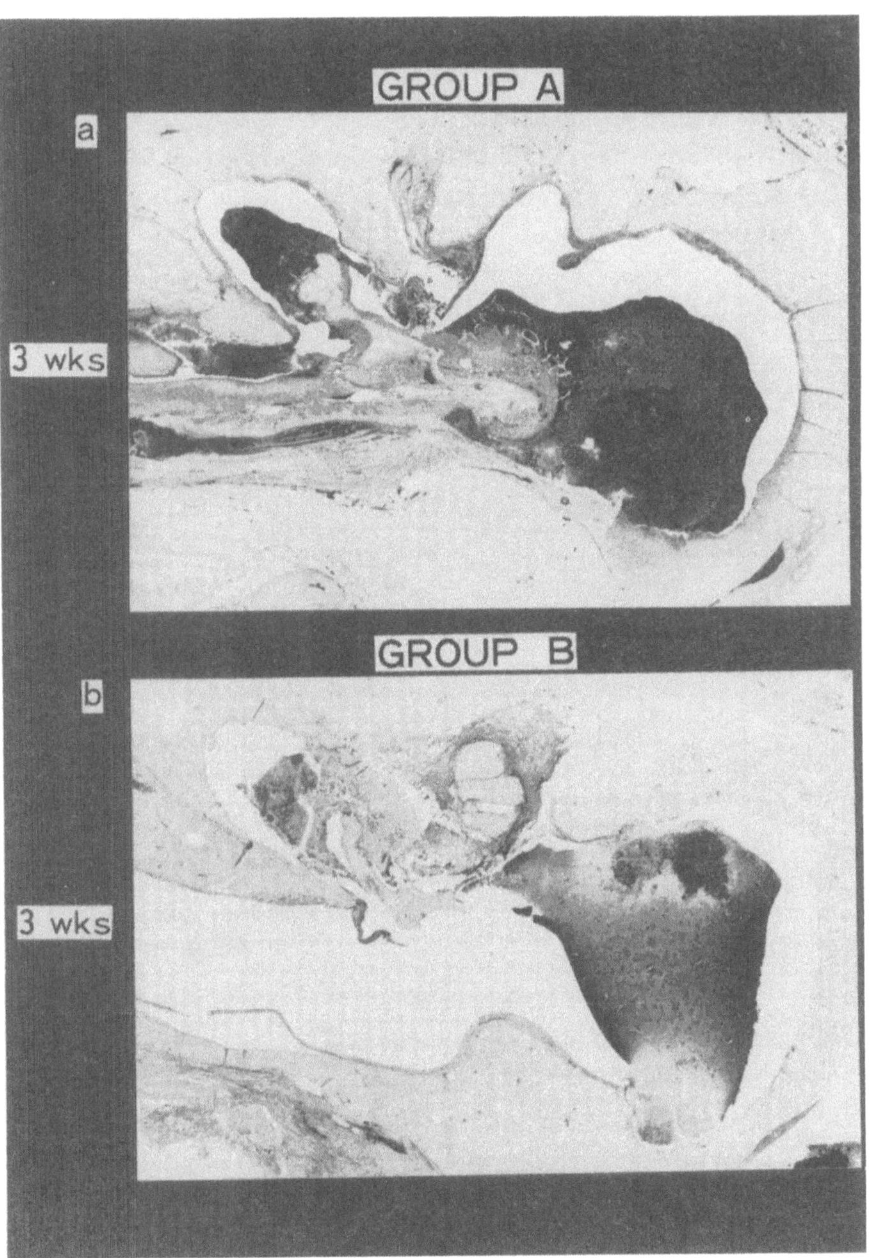

Illustration 1.

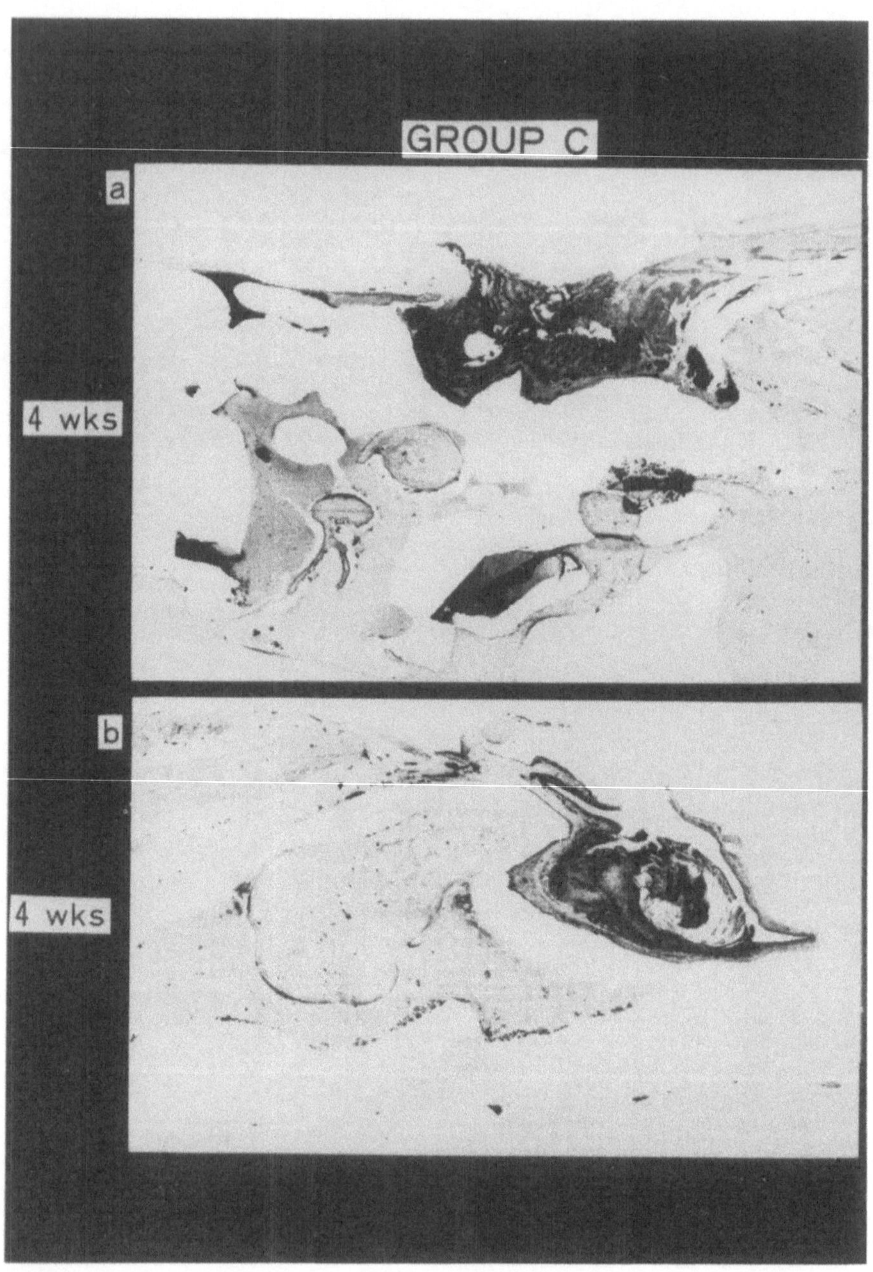

Illustration 2.

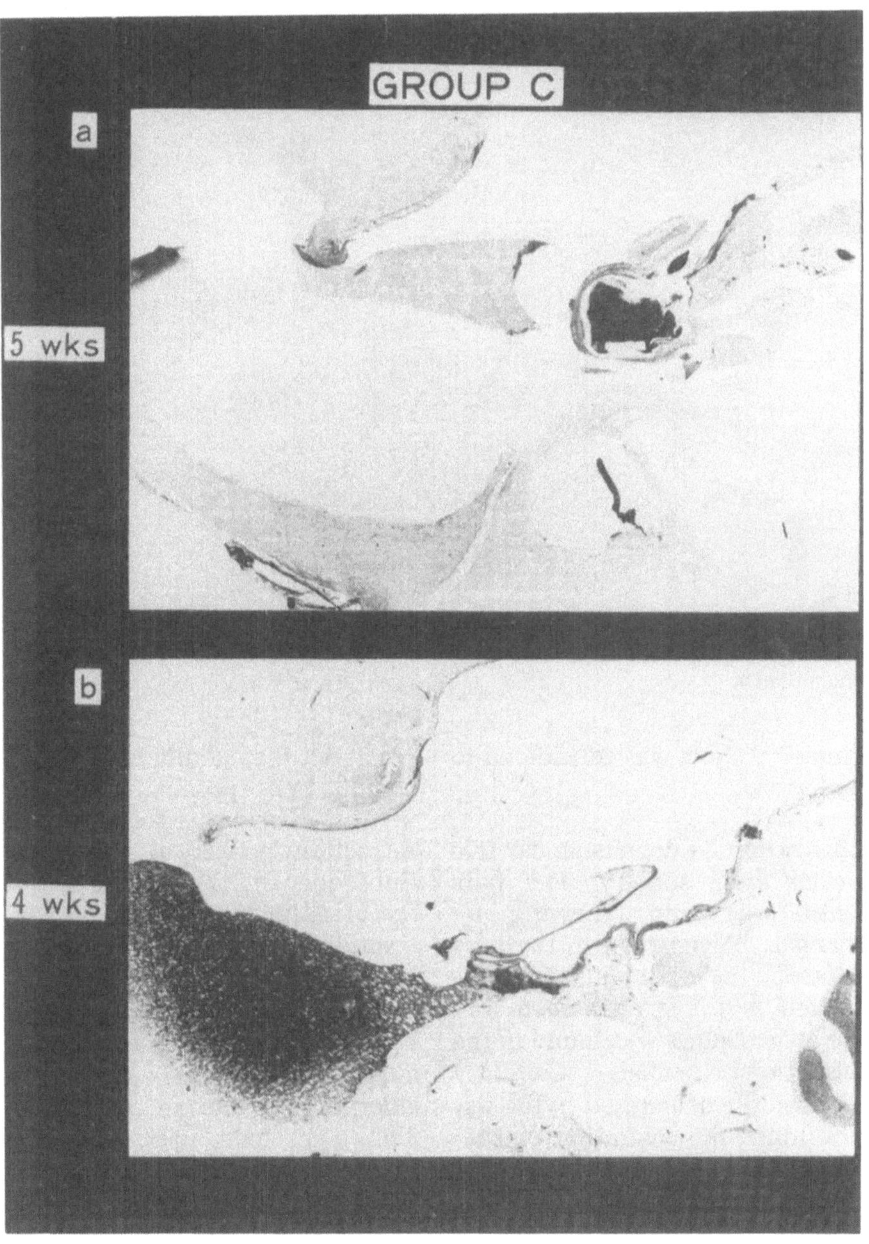

Illustration 3.

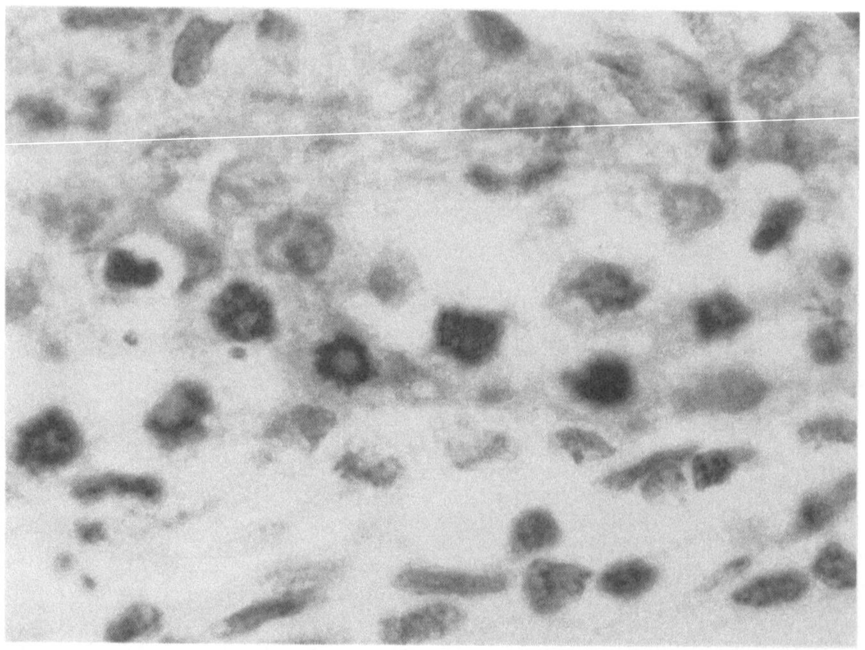

Illustration 4.

Thus P F chole was considered to be formed.

Illustration 3a depicts an ear five weeks after surgery. The pars tensa was thin, showing no changes. In contrast, in the pars flaccida, the epithelium was retracted and migrated deep into the attic. Debris was found in the retraction pocket. Capillary formation was marked in the tissue under the migrating epithelium. Thus, the formation of P F chole was confirmed.

Illustration 3b is of an ear four weeks after surgery. The pars flaccida in this case was retracted and migrated into the middle ear cavity deeper than in the above cases. The migrating epithelium reaches the Fallopian canal, stapes and promontrium. No keratin debris was found in the retraction pocket of this case. Subsequently, the mitotic activity of epithelial cells in the retraction pocket was investigated in P F chole produced experimentally. Colchicine (1 μg/g of body weight) was injected subcutaneously at 11.00 a.m. in consideration of diurnal rhythm. At 3.00 p.m., four hours after the injection, the animals were sacrificed. Pyknotic cells in the epithelial cells of the severely infected pars flaccida (group A) showed regressive changes, and no mitotic cells were observed. The migrating epithelium of the auditory canal in group C had the highest mitotic activity (illustration 4), differing significantly from the corresponding activity of the pars flaccida in the control group and group A.

Comment

Friedmann and Fernandez et al. reported that they produced experimental cholesteatoma. Their reports ascribed the mechanism of the formation of cholesteatoma to epithelial pearls and papillary formation of basal cells in the deep epithelium of the auditory canal followed by perforative purulent otitis media. In our experiments, retraction of the pars flaccida occurred when no tympanic perforation occurred and simultaneously when mild inflammation persisted in the middle ear cavity. When the middle ear was under such conditions, although there were no marked changes in the pars tensa, marked mitosis occurred in the epithelial cells from the pars flaccida to the auditory canal, resulting in retraction of the pars flaccida. The retracted epithelium showed further mitosis and developed into cholesteatoma. In the pars flaccida at this time, the epithelium, subepithelial tissue and the mucosa were retracted all together into the middle ear cavity. There was no growth of granulation tissue in the middle ear cavity. Unlike Rüedi's experiments, our experiments showed no passage of the basal cells of the epithelium through subepithelial tissue and granulation tissue in the middle ear cavity to form a cholesteatoma.

Experimental cholesteatoma

Part 2 - Consequence of intratympanic pressure to the pars flaccida

N. Mizorogi, Y. Honda

Two different types of experiments are introduced here.

Obstruction of the pharyngeal orifice of the Eustachian tube

The procedure was carried out for the purpose of confirming whether or not the retraction phenomenon on the pars flaccida as mentioned in Part 1, was observed.

Experimental methods: eighty-eight rabbit ears were used. The pharyngeal orifice of the Eustachian tube was electrically coagulated through the oral cavity. The animals were sacrificed between one and six months after the treatment, and specimens were prepared.

Results: during the first two weeks with obstruction (figure 1),

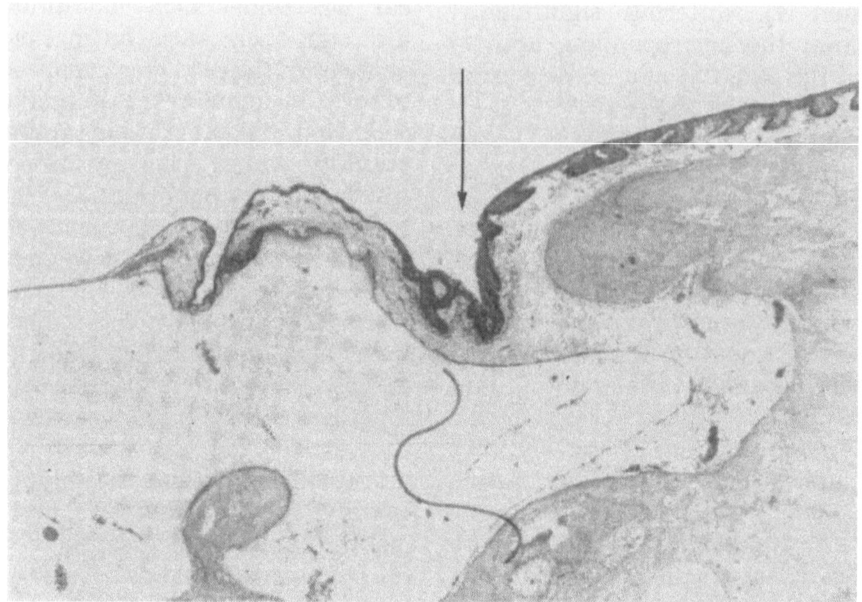

Fig. 1. Retraction of the pars flaccida observed at 2 weeks after obstruction of the pharyngeal orifice of the Eustachian tube

there was retention of exudate in the typanum, without tympanic perforation. After more than a month, the tympanic membrane was perforated because of inflammation. Of the 88 ears, tympanic perforation occurred in 27, which were, therefore, not followed up. Of the 61 ears without perforation, seven showed marked changes in the pars flaccida, 15, slight thickening of both the pars flaccida and the pars tensa and 39, no marked changes.

The changes in the pars flaccida in the seven cases included proliferation of the epidermal layer and the connective tissue layer which occurred despite the absence of any marked changes in the pars tensa. Four out of seven ears showed retraction of the pars flaccida. After six months, a marked, localized retraction of the pars flaccida, containing a large amount of debris composed of exfoliated epithelial cells, was observed in some cases. This finding may be designated as retraction cholesteatoma (figure 2).

Discussion: obstruction of the pharyngeal orifice provoked marked changes in the pars flaccida, as did obstruction of the tympanic orifice in Part 1. After obstruction of the pharyngeal orifice, the tympanum was subjected to negative pressure, followed by retention of an exudate. Simultaneously, cell proliferation was initiated in the epidermal

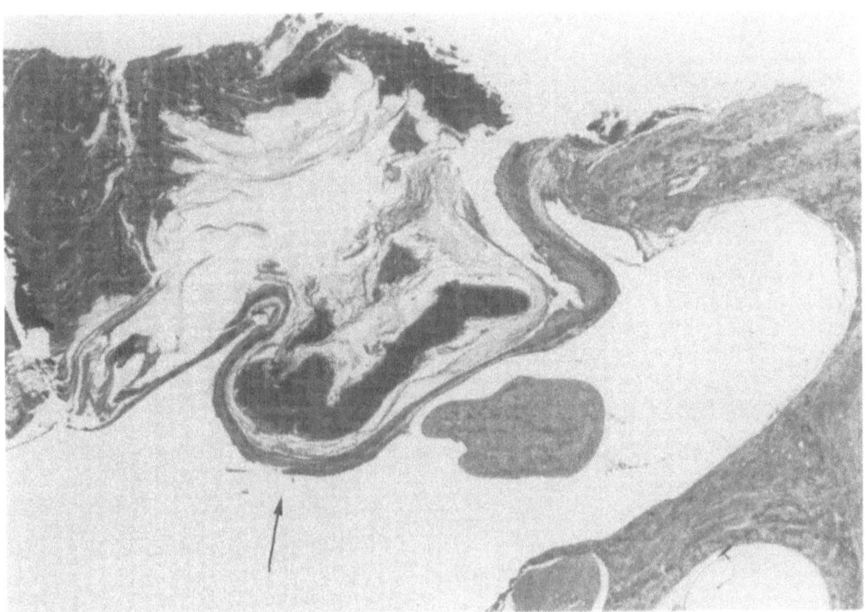

Fig. 2. Retraction cholesteatoma observed at 6 months after obstruction of the pharyngeal orifice of the Eustachian tube. Accumulation of debris can be seen in the external auditory meatus

and intermediate layers of the pars flaccida, whereas the pars tensa infrequently experienced marked changes. This phenomenon is attributable to the stimulation by the pooled fluid and the negative pressure and is identical, in principle, with the responses of the tympanic membrane which appear when the tympanic orifice is obstructed. However, if the tympanic membrane becomes perforated, these changes are no longer present.

Stimulation of the tympanic membrane from the outside

In our present experiment, stimulations as mild as inducing no tympanic perforation were given from the outside (figure 3).

Methods: rabbits were used for this experiment. Gelfoam containing 2 % benzpyrene dissolved in olive oil was uniformly spread on the external surface of the tympanic membrane. The external auditory meatus was obstructed by suturing the skin layer at the orifice. Two to eight weeks after this treatment, the animals were sacrificed for preparation of specimens.

Results: the total number of ears studied was 105, of which tympanic perforation was observed in 10. Of the remaining 95 ears, 25 showed retraction of the pars flaccida into the tympanic cavity, whereas 38 showed bulging into the external auditory meatus. In the remaining 32 ears,

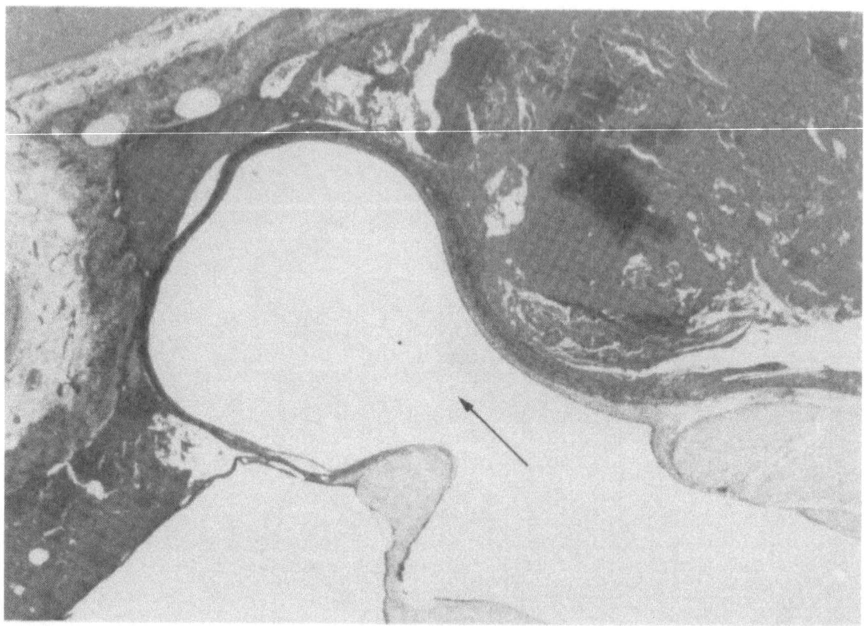

Fig. 3. Extrusion of the pars flaccida observed in stimulation of the tympanic membrane from the outside. Stimulants can be seen in the external auditory meatus, color in the middle ear cavity is white

the pars flaccida was thickened at a normal site.

Conclusions: in these experiments, ears with no tympanic perforation presented three different morphologies of the pars flaccida:

— retraction into the tympanic cavity,

— bulging into the external auditory meatus and

— thickening at a normal site.

Therefore, when the pressure of the tympanic cavity is equal to that in the cavity of the external auditory meatus, the pars flaccida thickens at a normal site, whereas when the tympanic cavity is in negative pressure, the pars flaccida retracts into the middle ear cavity. On the other hand, when the external meatus is in negative pressure, the pars flaccida protrudes into the external auditory meatus.

The result of these experiments show that the retraction of the pars flaccida is influenced by negative pressure in the middle ear cavity.

An experimental study of the effect of middle ear infection upon the pneumatization of the mastoid

K. Aoki, S. Esaki, Y. Honda

Introduction

It is generally believed that a cause-and-effect relationship exists between chronic otitis media and suppressed growth of the pneumatized cellulae in the temporal bone. However, we are not yet certain whether otitis media occurs and becomes chronic in the case of suppressed growth of the cellulae or whether otitis media induces suppressed growth of the cellulae. The congenital inheritance theory[1,2,3] and the acquired inflammation theory[4] are still controversial. Therefore, in the present experiment we used the temporal bones of pigs, in which the growth of the cellulae was very good and the individual difference was not significant. An experiment was performed to study the morbid state of the middle ear, especially in the infant, as well as its effect on the growth of cellulae.

Materials, methods and results

We studied the effect of middle ear infection in three ways - tympanic membrane perforation test, Eustachian tube stenosis test and middle ear paraffin infusion test - in the early stage of life upon the development of pneumatization of the mastoid, using 24 pigs. In 5 pigs of one group in which paraffin was infused into the left middle ear by perforating the tympanic membrane through the external auditory meatus, a marked suppression of the growth of cellulae was observed.

In the normal group, the thickness of the bone cortex was as thin as 1 to 2 mm at any stage after birth. As pigs have very well-developed cellulae in continuity in the lower tympanum and almost reach adulthood 6 months after birth, their use in experiments on the growth of cellulae is beneficial. In the case of normal growth, pigs already have cellulae 2 days after birth, and the process of development of cellulae is as follows: osteoids are first formed in the bone metabolic layers underneath the periosteum over the surface of the mastoid processes and then the mastoid processes themselves gradually enlarge, while the cellulae develop to the trabecular bone in the bone metabolic layers underneath the epithelium at the extreme tip of the bone cortex adjacent to the epithelium of the pneumatized cavities. This process continues until about 6 months after birth (figure 1).

In the treated group, observation

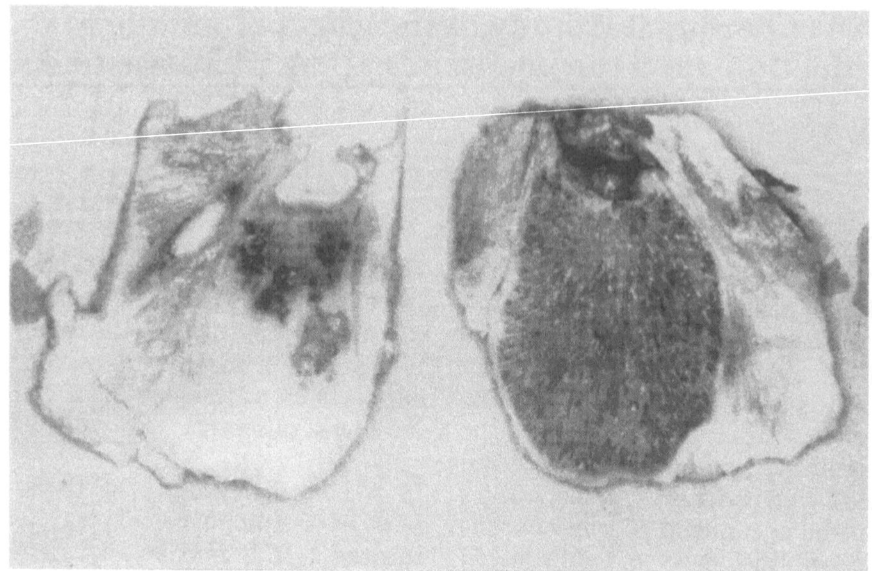

Fig. 1. Thickness of the bone cortex: a: treated; b: normal.

of the process of development of cellulae revealed strong suppression of growth in all cases. Histologically, the marked changes were the continuity of the middle ear inflammatory changes and this inflammatory stimulus strongly affected the bone metabolic layers beneath the epithelium of the pneumatized cavities and the periosteum, reducing vascularization, osteoblasts, and osteoclasts and suppressing bone metabolism. This suppression of the bone metabolic layers underneath the epithelium of the pneumatized cavities was strong so that the subsequent formation of cellulae was not observed and the pneumatized cavities remained small. From these findings, it was naturally considered that the inflammatory stimulus given to the cavity of the middle ear was stronger and longer in respect to bone metabolism beneath the epithelium of pneumatized cavities in the inside than to the metabolic layers beneath the periosteum on the outside. Therefore, there was a difference in growth between the mastoid processes and the pneumatized cavities (formation of the cellulae) when an inflammatory stimulus was given so that the process of formation of the trabecular bone, or pneumatization, was intensely suppressed, and the hypertrophied cortex was formed. In comparison with the normal group, the thickness of the bone cortex was more than tenfold (figure 1).

Discussion

Whether suppression of the growth of cellulae is due to congenital inheritance or to acquired changes due to inflammation, is a very important clinical question in regard to therapy and prophylaxis for otitis media in view of the strong correlation between a morbid state of chronic otitis media and the suppression of the growth of cellulae. This experiment was undertaken to elucidate these relationships. We do not deny the congenital inheritance theory, but the fact that suppression of the growth of cellulae was closely related to the persistent state of otitic inflammation in the early stages of growth favors the acquired inflammation theory. When overall consideration is given to these findings, as well as the fact that, in cases of suppression of pneumatization of the temporal bone in adults, abnormalities in the tympanic membranes were often observed, together with the previous history of the subjects showing otitis media in infancy, the acquired inflammation theory in regard to the suppression of pneumatization appears to be more plausible.

References:

1. DIAMANT M. Otitis and pneumatization of the mastoid bone. *Acta Otolaryng.* Suppl. 41, 1, 1940.
2. DIAMANT M. The "pathological size" of the mastoid air cell system. *Acta Otolaryng.* 60, 1, 1954.
3. GOTO T. et al. Repneumatization after antrotomy. *J. Otolaryngol. Jpn.* 49, 609, 1946.
4. WITTMAACH K. Schleimhautkonstitution und Pheumatisation. *Arch. Ohren Heilk,* 132, 261, 1930.

Cholesteatomatous invasion of the middle ear: classical points of entrance and their pathways

J. Claes, J.F.E. Marquet

Introduction

The mucosal folds of the middle ear cleft are generally considered to play a major rôle in middle ear ventilation, the formation of effusions, cholesterol granulomata and cholesteatomata.[1,2] Together with these folds however, many of the other normal structures of the middle ear also have great influence on the development of the pathology. Besides the folds, the ossicles, the muscle tendons and the compartments of the middle ear, some of the ossicular ligaments also have great importance in this matter.

Four types of pathogenesis of cholesteatoma are classically described,[3] we consider migration and invagination of epithelium as the most frequently encountered and therefore most important mechanism.[4] Papillary ingrowth of epithelium[5] might also be an important mechanism when weakness of the fibrous middle layer of the drum is present.

The malleal ligaments (figure 1).
A clear distinction must be made between the anterior and posterior malleal ligaments and the striae tympanicae, with which they are often confused.[6]

○ The anterior malleal ligament is a very strong and short structure that binds the anterior tympanic spine to the base of the anterior malleal process. This ligament lies clearly medially and superiorly to the stria tympanica anterior, which belongs to the tympanic membrane. It must also be distinguished from the anterior malleal process, which is connected by fibrous structures to the anterior petro-tympanic fissure and which forms an articulation allowing slight three-dimensional movement of the malleus.

○ The posterior malleal ligament connects the base of the lateral process of the malleus to the pretympanic spine; it lies clearly medially and superiorly to the stria tympanica posterior.

○ The lateral malleal ligament, together with the lateral malleal fold, forms the roof of Prussack's space.

○ The superior malleal ligament has a purely static function and is of no importance in the pathogenesis of cholesteatomata.

Fig. 1. The malleus with AML, PML, STA and STP, view from anterior, superior and medial.

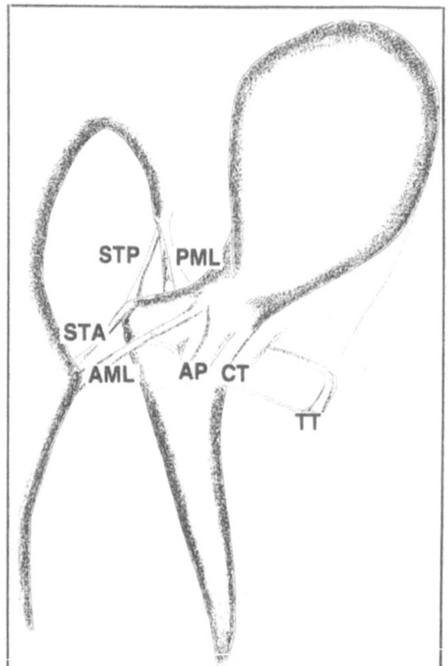

The mucosal folds of the middle ear
As described by Proctor, these folds occur in constant anatomical postions.[1] Some of them have

Abbrevations used in the illustrations
AML: Anterior Malleal Ligament
PML: Posterior Malleal Ligament
STA: Stria Tympanica Anterior
STP: Stria Tympanica Posterior
AP: Anterior (Malleal) Process
CT: Chorda Tympani
TT: Tensor Tympani tendon and muscle
TTF: Tensor Tympani Fold
LIF: Lateral Incudal Fold
MIF: Medial Incudal Fold
IF: Interossicular Fold
PMF: Posterior Malleal Fold
ATI: Anterior Tympanic Isthmus
PTI: Posterior Tympanic Isthmus

particular importance in the development of cholesteatoma.

○ The lateral incudal fold is a very strong barrier preventing cholesteatomatous invasion of the posterior attic laterally to the incus.

○ The tensor tympani fold, on the contrary, does not always form and also shows very often defects. This fold, therefore, is no barrier to cholesteatomatous invasion, which - as described later in this paper - will easily occur from the anterior attic into the anterior mesotympanum and protympanum.

○ The medial incudal fold and the interossicular fold have their importance in the formation of anterior and posterior tympanic isthmus.

○ The lateral malleal fold forms the roof of Prussack's space, its absence or weakness might play a major rôle in the central pathway of cholesteatomatous invasion, described later.

○ The superior malleal and incudal folds and the stapedial folds have much less importance.

Anterior and posterior tympanic isthmus (figure 2). Ossicles and mucosal folds separate the attic from the tympanum in such a way that only three connections exist. A first connection is inconstant and formed by the defects or absence of the tensor fold, thus opening the anterior attic to the anterior tympanum. The anterior tympanic isthmus is the second and con-

Fig. 2. Anterior and posterior tympanic isthmus. View of the ossicles from superior.

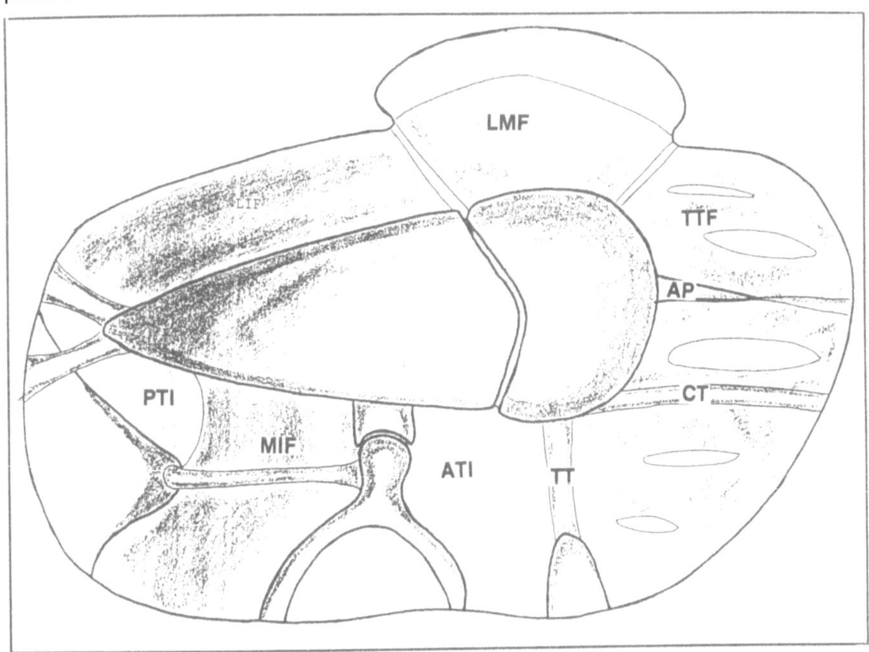

stant opening bounded anteriorly by the tensor tympani tendon, posteriorly by the stapes and long crus of the incus and laterally by the interossicular mucosal fold. The posterior tympanic isthmus is the third, also very constant, opening bounded anteriorly by the medial incudal fold, posteriorly by the facial recess and pyramidal recess, medially by the stapes and its tendon and laterally by the medial face of the short process of the incus.

Points of entrance and pathways
Several authors have published their vision on the development of cholesteatoma in relation to middle ear anatomy[7,8] especially in relation to the postero-superior quadrant.[9,10] Clinical observations have led us to consider three classical pathways of cholesteatomatous invasion of the middle ear:

— strong central retraction of the flaccid part of the drum leads to a moulding of the malleous head and cholesteatoma invades the anterior and posterior attic immediately. This form of cholesteatoma is often seen in the older patient[11] (figure 3).

Two more common pathways observed have their points of entrance through defects in the lamina propria of the flaccid drum part. These defects may be acquired postinfectious lesions caused by lysis of the collagen middle layer of the drum.[12] J. Marquet and D. Boedts however

Fig. 3. Central retraction of the flaccid drum part, view from lateral.

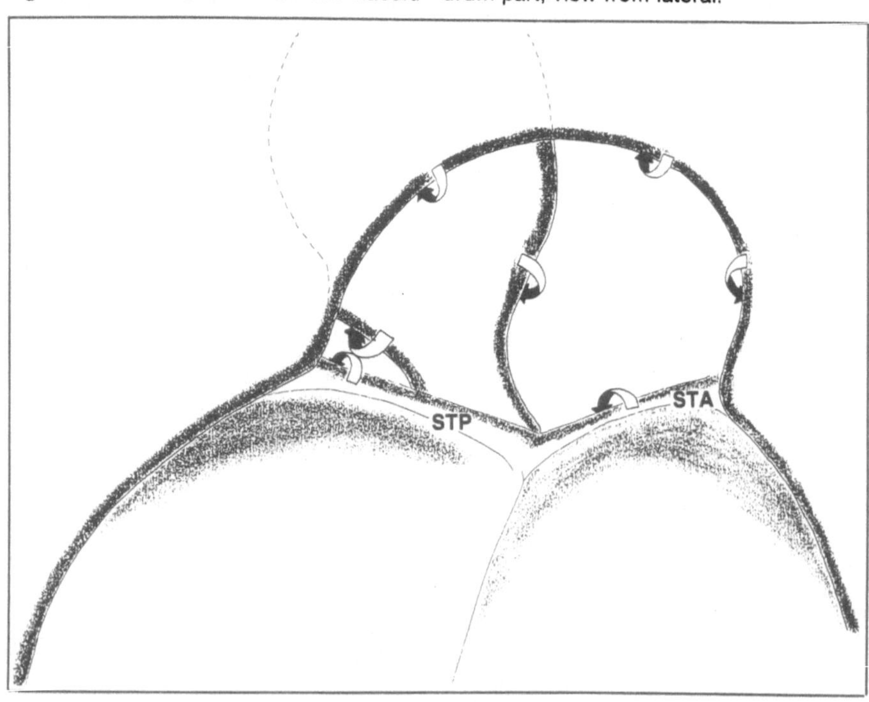

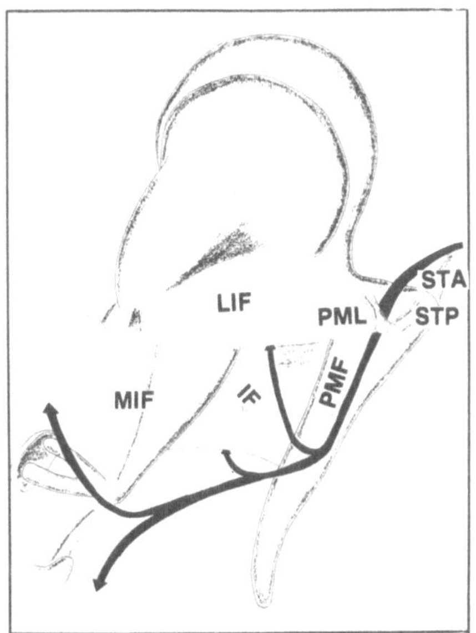

Fig. 4. Posterior pathway of invasion. View of the ossicles from lateral, posterior and superior.

described fibrous middle layer defects in the flaccid drum part of 3,5 % of normal temporal bone dissection specimens, thus suggesting a congenital origin;[13,4]

— through posterior defects the invasion proceeds over the stria membrana tympani and inferiorly to the posterior malleal ligament and laterally to the posterior malleal fold into the posterior space of Von Troeltsch. The lateral incudal fold forms a strong and intact mucosal barrier to the cholesteatoma and directs the expansion to the tympanum and into the tympanic sinus. The long process of the incus is surrounded anteriorly and posteriorly and invasion of the attic occurs upwards through the anterior and posterior tympanic isthmus (figure 4);

— through anterior defects the invasion proceeds superiorly to the anterior malleal ligament and cholesteatoma invades the entire anterior attic. The dehiscences or absence of the tensor fold permits the cholesteatoma to invade the tympanum medially and laterally to the anterior malleal process and chorda tympani and through the anterior tympanic isthmus. This pathway is often observed in younger children and often corresponds to a very small entrance point (figure 5).

The two latter pathways have been demonstrated in a film re-

Fig. 5. Anterior pathway of invasion. View of the malleus from lateral, anterior and superior.

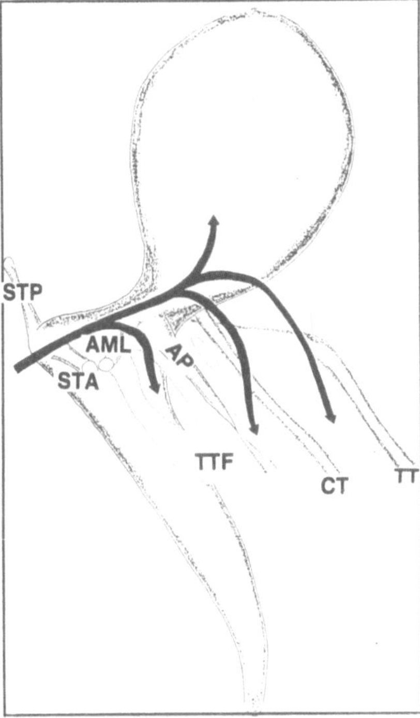

corded during surgery of middle ear cholesteatoma (figure 6). Recognizing these pathways will help us to estimate the extent of disease during micro-otoscopic examination of the patient. Most of all it will help us during surgery when our first task is total eradiction of pathology. The best way to accomplish this is, in our opinion, by dissecting and pushing back the cholesteatoma through exactly these same pathways in the opposite direction.[4] Whenever this is not possible, second look procedures will certainly be necessary.[14] This will help to keep the cholesteatomatous sac in its entirety, and to perform a real "en bloc" resection. It seems therefore desirable to us that these distinct pathways and points of entrance should be taken into account in any classification concerning cholesteatomatous pathology.

Fig. 6. a. Image taken from a peroperative video recording, showing the cholesteatoma extending through anterior and posterior tympanic isthmus (arrows). b. The same view of the ossicles from superior: left ear.
1. Incus 2. Ext. ear canal 3. Cholesteatoma lateral from incus 4. Cholesteatoma in ATI 5. Cholesteatoma in PTI.

a

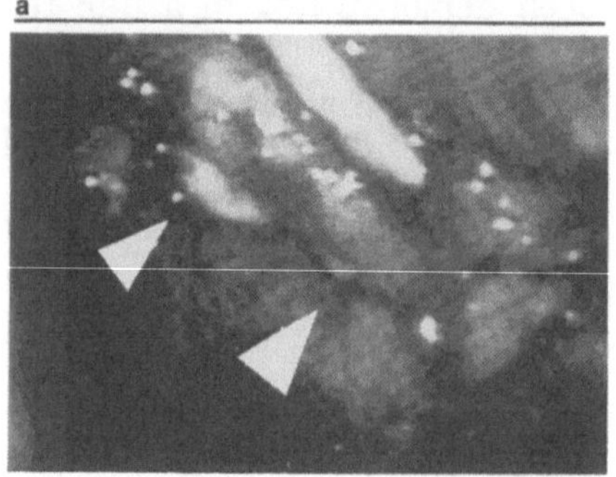

b

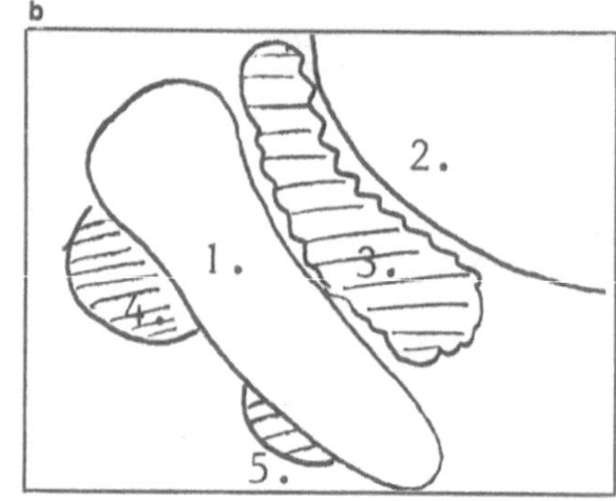

References:

1. PROCTOR B. The development of the middle ear spaces and their surgical significance. *J. Laryngol. Otol.* 78:631-47, 1964.
2. AIMI K. The clinical significance of epitympanic mucosal folds. *Arch. Otolaryng.* 94:499-508, 1971.
3. SMITH R. Tympanic membrane cholesteatoma (keratoma) in children with no prior otologic surgery. *Laryngoscope* 87 (2):237-44, 1977.
4. MARQUET J. Cholesteatoma or keratoma: Apathological approach. *Acta Otorhinolaryngol. Belg.* 34 (1):5-11, 1980.
5. RÜEDI L. Pathogenesis and surgical treatment of the middle ear cholesteatoma. *Acta Otolaryngol.* (Suppl.) 361:1-45, 1979.
6. MARQUET J. The incudo-malleal joint. *J. Laryngol. Otol.* 95:543-65, 1981.
7. SADÉ J. Retraction pockets and attic cholesteatomas. *Acta Otorhinolaryngol.* Belg. 34 (1):62-84, 1980.
8. SADÉ J. Atelectasis, retraction pockets and cholesteatoma. *Acta Otolaryngol.* 92 (5-6):501-12, 1981.
9. DAWES J.D. The postero-superior quadrant. *J. Laryngol. Otol.* 88 (10):955-67, 1974.
10. ZALIN H. The post-superior quadrant. *J. Laryngol. Otol.* 88 (10):969-74, 1974.
11. TOS M. Attic retractions following secretory otitis. *Acta Otolaryngol.* 89 (5-6):479-86, 1980.
12. IWANOGA M. Collagenase activity in cholesteatoma. *ORL J. Otolaryngol.* Relat. Spec. 45 (3):166-75, 1983.
13. BOEDTS D. Studie van het gedrag van het Trommelvliesepitheel in normale en pathologische toestanden. Aggregaatsthesis UIA, 1976.
14. MORGENSTEIN K.M. Cholesteatoma: pathological considerations in surgical planning. *Ann. Otol. Rhinol. Laryngol.* 83 (5):648-51, 1974.

Classification of allografts in middle ear surgery

D. Keusters, C. Van Laer, J.F.E. Marquet

Faced with numerous and various combinations in the surgical use of tympanic and ossicular allografts, a tympano-ossicular formula based on an ossicular code has been conceived. The use of such a formula makes any discussion on the subject easier and more comprehensive.

The five components making up the tympano-ossicular formula are written in capitals:
T: Tympanic membrane
M: Malleus
I: Incus
S: Stapes
W: Wall (posterior).

If one of these components is not used intact but is remodelled as a substitution prosthesis, or if only a part of it is used, it is indicated by small letters:
r: remodelled
p: partial

The origin of the material is also indicated by capital letters:
O: Original, i.e. ossicles or tympanic membrane that have not been separated either from their points of supply or from their natural points of attachment.
A: Autografts, i.e. material belonging to the patient but having been temporarily removed from the ear (i.e. for remodelling).
H: Allografts (Homografts), i.e. material obtained from a human donor, used after fixation in formaldehyde and preservation in Cialit.
P: Prosthesis.

During a second-stage operation, the formula between brackets and preceeded by the letter O, expresses the element left in situ during the second operation, but implanted in a first operation.

The plus sign indicates that arthroplasties have been carried out.

The joints have their own classification in numbers:
0: original
1: juxtaposition
2: mortesis
3: holes
4: juxtaposition + glue
5: mortesis + glue
6: holes + glue.

We translated the tympano-ossicular formula into numbers, so that it can be combined with the notation for joints. Each element of the tympano-ossicular chain has two number possibilities, because it is sometimes necessary to use two different materials to restore one element (figure 1).

Fig. 1

	O	O_p	A	A_p	A_r	H	H_p	H_r	P
T	1	2	3	4	5	6	7	8	9
M	1	2	3	4	5	6	7	8	9
I	1	2	3	4	5	6	7	8	9
S	1	2	3	4	5	6	7	8	9
W	1	2	3	4	5	6	7	8	9

Here we give an example of the most commonly used combinations:

— HT + OMIS (figure 2)
06 1 01 0 01 0 01
T + M + I + S

— HTMI + OS (figure 3)
06 0 06 0 06 1 01
T + M + I + S

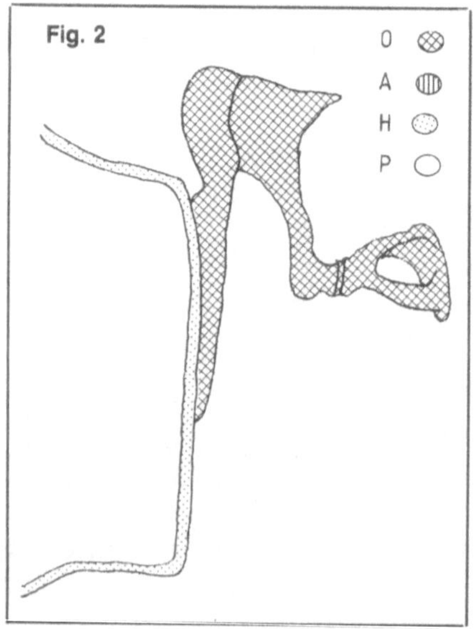

Fig. 2

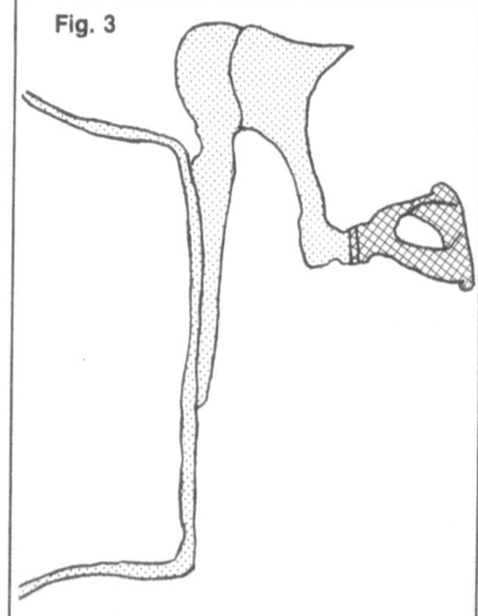
Fig. 3

— HTMIS$_p$ + OS$_p$ (figure 4)
06 0 06 0 06 1 72
T + M + I + S

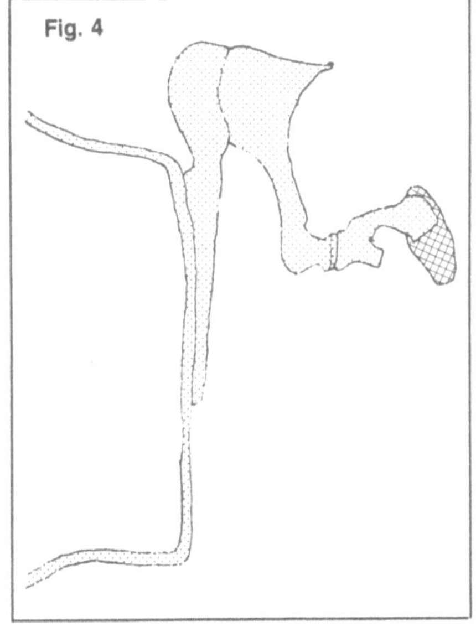
Fig. 4

— OTMI + PS +OS$_p$ (figure 6)
01 0 01 0 01 3 92
T + M + I + S

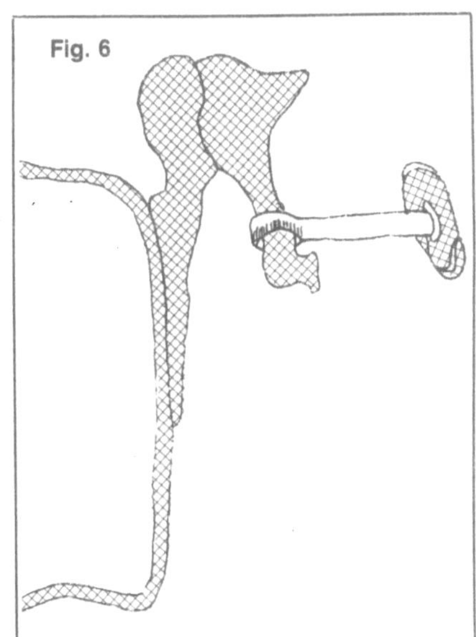
Fig. 6

— OTM + AI$_r$ +OS (figure 5)
01 0 01 3 05 3 01
T + M + I + S

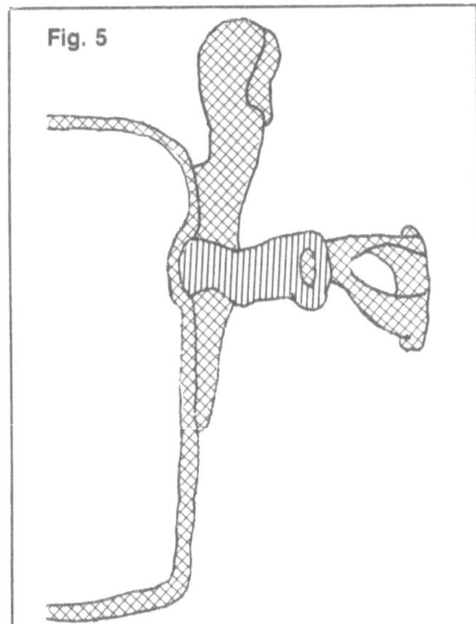
Fig. 5

Conclusion
The use of the tympano-ossicular formula in allograft middle ear surgery is indispensible for stating all the possible combinations succinctly and fully.

Literature:

MARQUET J. Twelve years' experience with homograft tympanoplasty. *Otolaryngol, clin. North Amer.* Vol. 10. Nr. 3, p. 581. Oct. 1977.
MARQUET J. Tympano-ossicular homografts in reconstructive middle ear surgery. Proceedings of the second Asia-Oceania congress of otorhinolaryngology p. 147, 1971.

Applying the language of "transplantese" to tympanoplasty

N.J. Frootko

Introduction

Otologists using tissue transplants to reconstruct the middle ear, have, like other transplant surgeons, needed to add a number of new words to their vocabulary in order to describe the types of grafts they use. This jargon has been called "transplantese" by Gorer[1] and there has been much debate and even more confusion over the terminology that will prove to be most appropriate, informative and etymologically accurate. Although no international nomenclature committee has been established, a new terminology has evolved and this can and should be applied to tympanoplasty.

Discussion

One of Peter Gorer's last works[1,2] was to overhaul the terminology used by those involved in transplantation research so that they could communicate to one another in a language that was etymologically correct and not in conflict with long established immunological terms. His sentiments were shared by Snell[3], and the proposed revisions of "transplantese" by these authors have subsequently been adopted internationally by the majority of transplant surgeons and researchers.

The genetic relationship between a donor and a recipient enables four types of graft to be defined:

Tissue transplanted from one part of the body to another in the same individual, e.g. a temporalis fascia or tragal perichondrial graft used to repair the tympanic membrane. Such grafts have been called "autografts" but there has been some debate about which adjective is most suitable. Gorer et al.[2] and Snell[3] favoured "autogenous" but "autologous" and "autogeneic" appear to have become the most popular adjectives used.

Tissue transplanted between genetically identical individuals, e.g. an incus graft between rats of the same inbred strain. Snell[3] originally suggested that these grafts should be called "isografts" and this is the term currently used. The adjectives related to this noun are "isologous" and "isogenic" and these were changed to "isogeneic" to cover all types of grafts between genetically uniform populations, i.e. inbred animal strains, monozygotic twins and the F_1 between inbred animal strains. Gorer et al.[2] suggested the term "syngeneic" and both "isogeneic" and "syngeneic" are the adjectives used today.

Tissue transplanted between genetically non-identical members of the same species, e.g. a preserved human cadaver acquired tympanomeatal graft used to repair the tympanic membrane, or a preserved human cadaver acquired incus used to repair an ossicular chain defect. The firmly established term "homograft", used to describe these grafts, was critisised by Gorer et al.[2] because "homos" (Greek = same) should always be used to denote some type of agreement or correspondence and there was no justification for using the word to mean "genetically different".

The term "allograft" (Greek allos = other or different) was therefore introduced and is the term currently used to describe these grafts. Although no objections were raised to the adjective "allogenic", the word sounded like "allergenic" and was changed to "allogeneic".

Tissue transplanted between members of different species, e.g. a preserved bovine pericardial graft used to repair a human tympanic membrane. The term "heterograft" previously used to describe these grafts, became inappropriate once the term "allograft" was adopted because "heteros and allos" have similar meaning. Gorer et al.[2] felt that the term "xenograft" was more explicit and this was introduced together with the adjective "xenogeneic".

The old and the new "transplantese" are shown in table 1.

Grafts of any genetic origin may be further defined according to

Table 1. Transplantese

Old terminology		**New terminology**		
Noun	**Adjective**	**Noun**	**Adjective**	**Definition**
Autograft	Autogenous	Autograft	Autologous or Autogeneic	Tissue transplanted from one part of the body to another in the same individual.
Isograft	Isologous or Isogenic	Isograft	Isogeneic or Syngeneic	Tissue transplanted between genetically identical individuals.
Homograft	Homologous	Allograft	Allogeneic	Tissue transplanted between genetically non-identical members of the same species.
Heterograft	Heterologous	Xenograft	Xenogeneic	Tissue transplanted between members of different species.

their new anatomical site, pattern of vascularisation and functional capacity. Grafts placed in an anatomical position normally occupied by such tissue are *"orthotopic grafts"* (Greek ortho = right or correct), e.g. a tympano-ossicular allograft used to reconstruct the tympanic membrane and ossicular chain. Sculptured ossicular bone grafts used to reconstruct the ossicular chain, placed in their normal anatomical site but not usually into their normal anatomical position should probably also be called "orthotopic" to avoid confusion. Those grafts placed in an unnatural recipient location are *"hetero-topic grafts"* (Greek heteros = other or different), e.g. a sculptured nasal septal cartilage graft to reconstruct the ossicular chain or outer attic wall.

A graft placed directly onto a vascular pedicle is a *"vascularised graft"*, e.g. a kidney transplant, whereas a *"free or non-vascularised graft"* vascularises indirectly from the recipient bed, e.g. a preserved dura mater graft used to repair the tympanic membrane.

Those grafts expected or intended to fulfil their normal physiological functional capacity are *"vital grafts"*, e.g. a kidney transplant, while *"static grafts"* serve a mechanical function that does not require "physiological viability". Such grafts act as a scaffolding or matrix onto and into which host tissues gradually extend. At present all tissue grafts used in tympanoplasty and tympanoplasty with mastoidectomy, are "free, non-vascularised grafts" and these latter distinctions therefore do not have to be made.

Conclusions

Because of the frequent use of tissue grafts in middle ear reconstructive surgery, otologists should aquaint themselves with the new terminology used to describe these grafts. In this short article the new "transplantese" has been outlined and it can quite easily be adapted to tympanoplasty.

References:

1. GORER P.A., *Ann. N.Y. Acad. Sci.* 87, 604, 1960.
2. GORER P.A., LOUTIT J.F., MICKLEM H.S. *Nature.* 189, 1024, 1961.
3. SNELL G.D., *Transplantation* 2, No 5, 655, 1964.

Ear surgery, CT in postoperative evaluation

B. Appel, J.F.E. Marquet

Introduction

Since there are a great number of otosurgical procedures, including the so-called "closed techniques", a postoperative control and follow-up by otoscopic examination only is insufficient. Radiology, polytomography, and the more recent highly performing computerized tomography with special bone review, are therefore very useful to control the postoperative status and to detect early or late complications.

Material and method

With a general electric CT/T 8.800 scanner with bone review program (pixel 0,25 mm/0.25 mm) we had the opportunity to examine many previously operated patients. The axial and coronal projections were used and contiguous slices of 1,5 mm thickness were chosen.

We classified the cases according to surgical techniques:

— translabyrinthine approach
— mastoidectomy
— posterior tympanotomy
— stapedectomy
— fenestration
— congenital middle ear surgery.

Translabyrinthine approach

This technique is used to remove acoustic neuromas, even very large ones, or even to practice neurectomies. After removal of the lesion, the original technique introduced by one of the authors consists in the closure of the translabyrinthine defect by a "cover", partially remodelled autogeneous cortical bone fitting perfectly in order to avoid cerebrospinal fluid leakage (figures 1, 2, 3).

Fig. 1. Man, 51 years old. Preoperative CT of a large left acoustic neuroma: axial view with bony filter for visualization of the enlarged left I.A.C. (*)

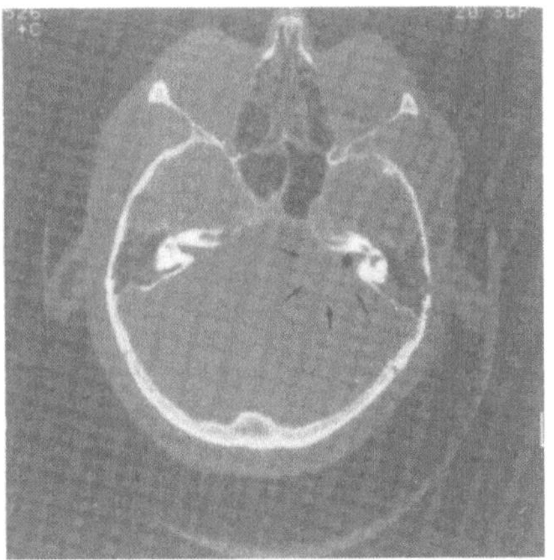

Fig. 2. Same patient. Postoperative axial view with normal reference. After removal of the tumor (ø = 2,2 cm) by translabyrinthine route a "cover" was used to close the bony defect in order to avoid C.S.F. leakage. ↗↗

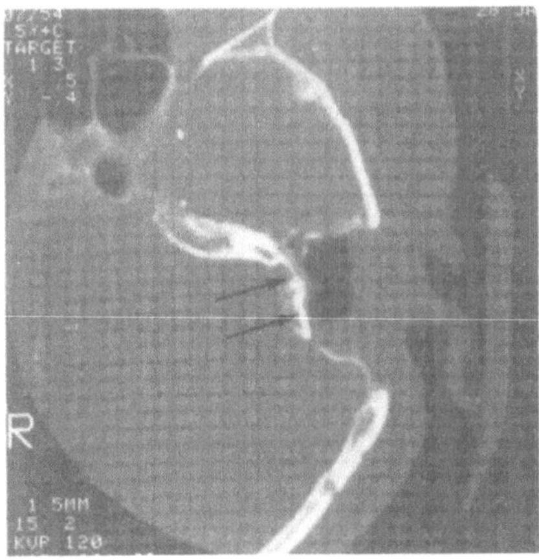

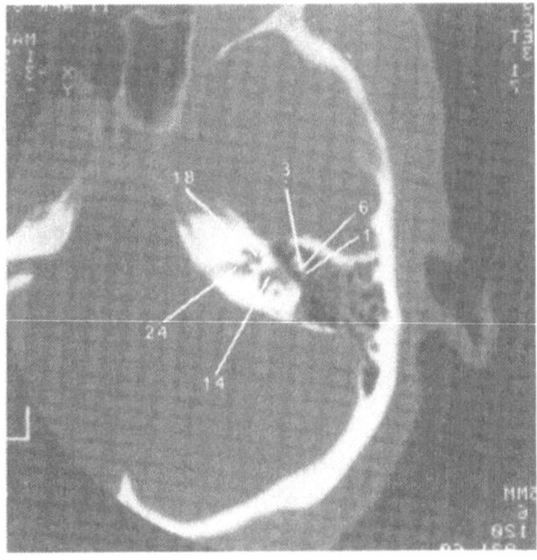

Fig. 3. Woman, 40 years old. Coronal slice of a "cover" (⇇) closing a translabyrinthine route after removal of an acoustic neuroma. And normal reference

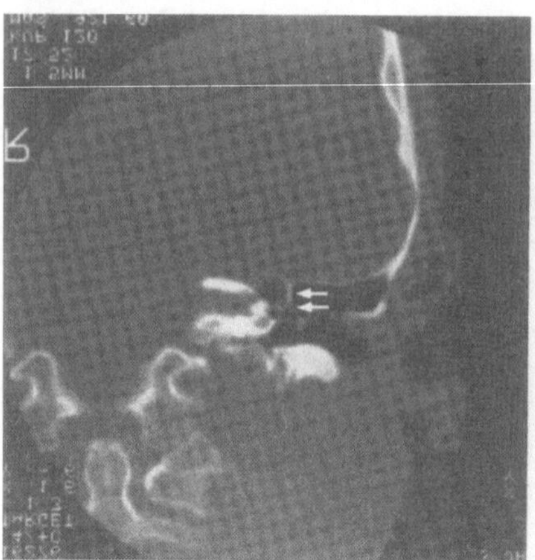

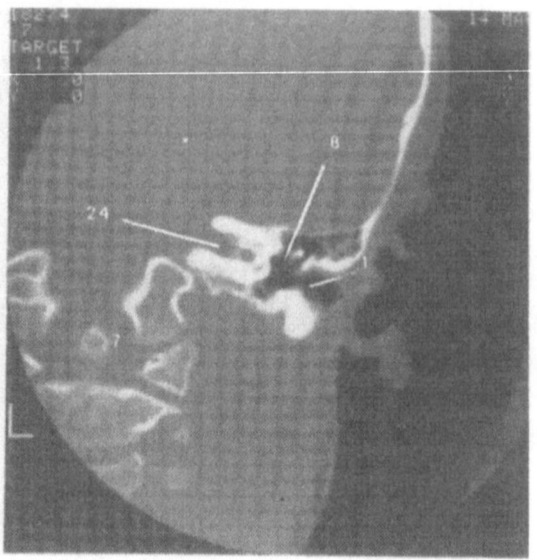

Postoperative CT is useful to control the position of the cover but also to detect residual as well as recurrent pathology (figure 4).

Fig. 4. Woman, 55 years old. Recurrence of a very large acoustic neuroma 5 years after primary surgery

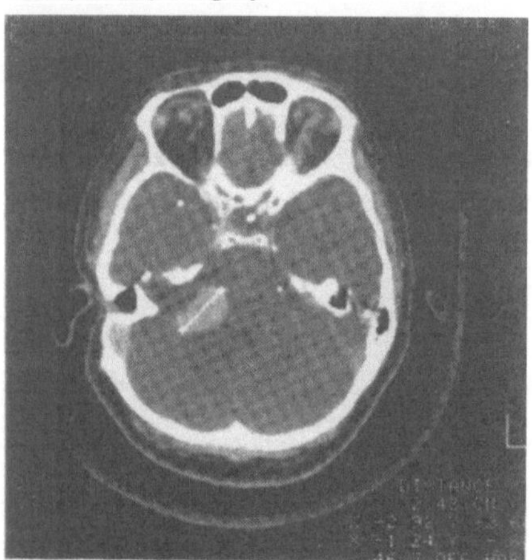

Mastoidectomy

This is performed for chronic middle ear otitis or cholesteatoma. Early postoperative CT is essential to establish the "status presens" to allow the evaluation of the follow-up including the complications (figure 5).

Posterior tympanotomy

This is the approach of choice for example to implant the monobloc tympano-ossicular allografts (HTMIS) and the variations of these allogeneous ossicular chains needed to reconstruct the columellar effect after eradication of the middle ear pathology (figure 6).

Stapedectomy

This is also illustrated on CT slices but shows only a nearly normal picture since the prosthesis cannot always be seen depending on the type of material used.

Fenestration

This was an old technique used for otosclerosis, and the case presented here has still a very good hearing 30 years after surgery (figure 7).

Congenital middle ear surgery

A preoperative CT is essential to discover the hypoplastic bone

Fig. 5. Man, 23 years old. Empty cavity 10 years after mastoidectomy for cholesteatoma. The inner ear (14,24) and the lateral semicircular canal (16) are intact. The postero-superior wall of the external auditory canal has been removed

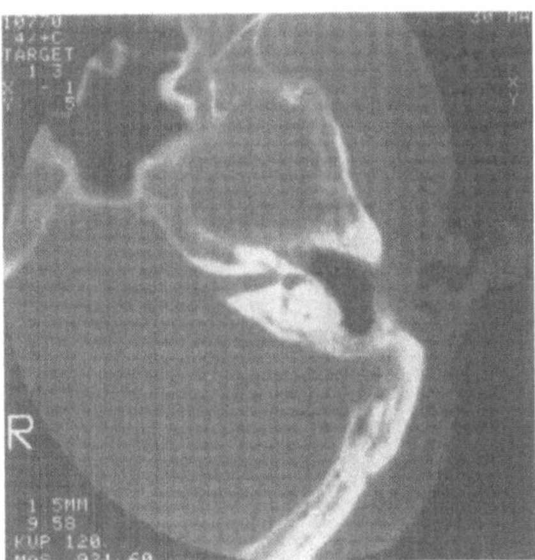

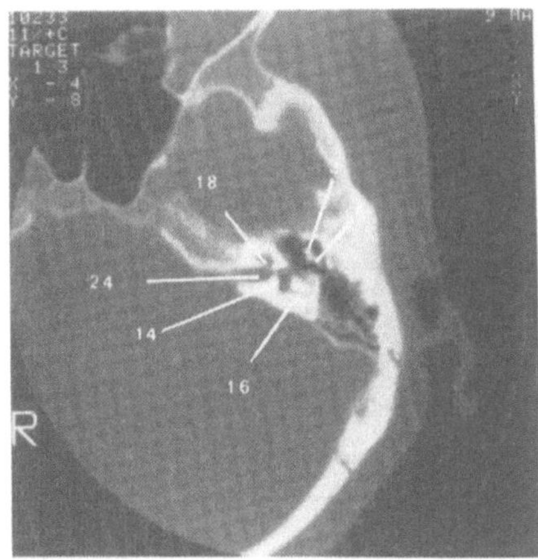

Fig. 6. Man, 40 years old. Posterior tympanotomy (★) and monobloc allogenous tympano-ossicular implant (HTMIS) with reconstruction of the posterior wall of the external auditory canal (AW).

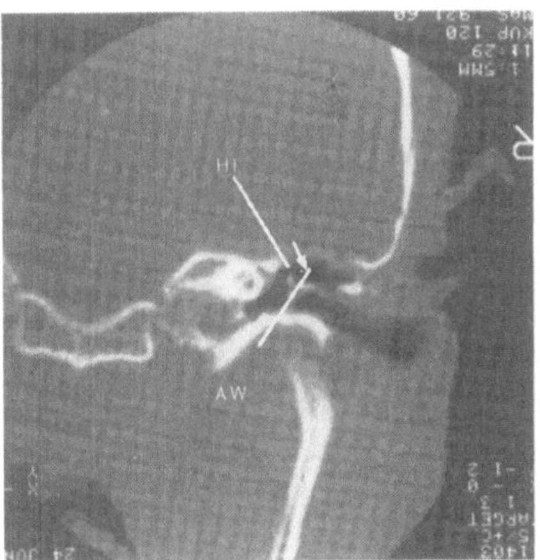

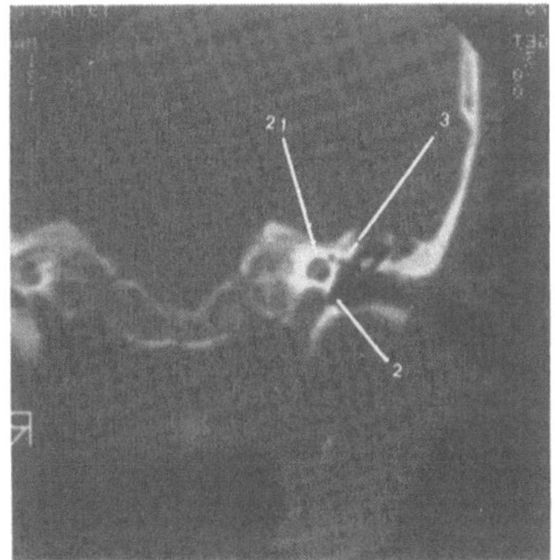

1. external auditory canal
2. tympanum
3. malleus
4. manubrium mallei
5. tendon of M. tensor tympani
6. incus
7. long process incudis
8. stapes
9. oval window
10. tegmen
11. antrum
12. atticum
13. Eustachian tube
14. vestibulum
15. aqueductus vestibuli
16. lateral semicircular canal
17. posterior semicircular canal
18. cochlea
19. basal turn cochleae
20. aqueductus cochleae
21. canalis facialis (first portion)
22. canalis facialis (second portion)
23. geniculate ganglion
24. internal auditory canal

Fig. 7. Woman, 55 years old. Fenestration surgery for otosclerosis still functional thirty years later. Open fenestra (←). Coronal view and normal reference

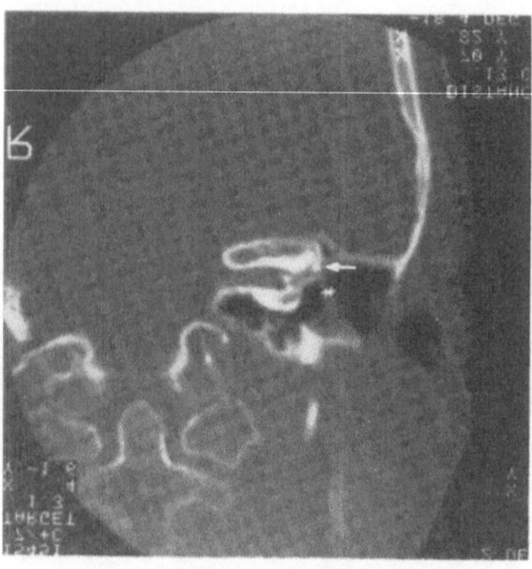

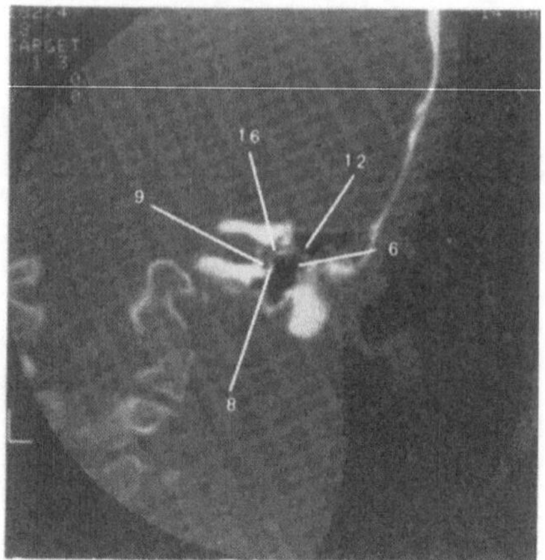

Fig. 8. Male, 6 years old. Congenital hypoplasia of the E.A.C. and the ossicular chain (↙). Preoperative axial view and same at immediate postoperative control. Implanting of an allogenous monobloc meato-tympano-ossicular graft (HWTMI) connected to the original stapes (OS) by a 4th ossicle, a remodelled cortical bony graft (AIr). Very good hearing, despite the fresh blood filling the middle ear.

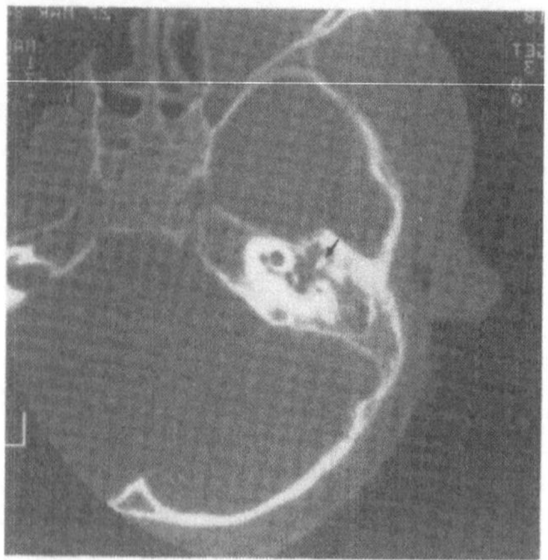

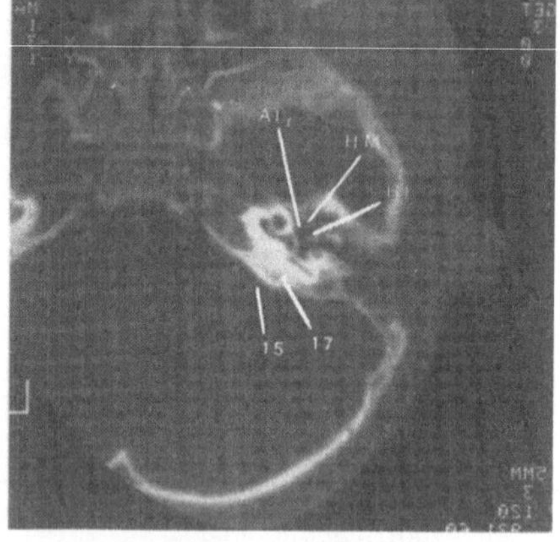

structures of the middle ear and any kind of malformation in order to determine if surgery is indicated or not (figure 8). In addition, the visualization of the facial nerve is indispensable because of its numerous anatomical abnormalities. Postoperative CT is useful for the so-called "status presens".

Conclusion

In our opinion, the preoperative CT is as absolutely necessary for diagnosis, as the postoperative CT is essential in order to have a reference for the follow-up. Therefore, we give the preference to the CT scan because of the better density discrimination compared with polytomography and because it gives the opportunity to discover possible petrous and intracranial complications.

Literature:

LLOYD G.A.S., DU BOULAY G.H., PHELPS P.D., PULLICINO P. The demonstration of the auditory ossicles by high resolution CT. *Neuroradiology* 18, 243-248, 1979.

MARQUET J., CLAUS E. Implants ossiculaires en oto-radiologie, V. Internationales Symposium für Radiologie in der Hals-Nasen-Ohrenheilkunde. Würzburg, 28-30 Sept. 1970.

MARQUET J., CLAUS E. Ossicular implants and radio-otology. Proceedings of the second Asia-Oceania Congress of Oto-rhinolaryngology, 358-365, 1971.

MARQUET J., VAN CAMP K.J., CRETEN W.L., DECRAEMER W.F., WOLFF H.B., SCHEPENS P. Topics in physics and middle ear surgery. *Acta Oto-rhino-laryngol. Belg.*, 27: 137-320, 1973.

MARQUET J., VAN CAMP K.J., DECRAEMER W., CRETEN W.L. Some physical considerations in the choice of techniques for ossiculoplasty. *Audiology*, 14: 82-92, 1975.

MARQUET J. Historical notes on homografts. *Otolaryngol, Clin. North Amer.* 10: 479-485, 1977.

MARQUET J. Homografts in tympanoplasty and other forms of middle ear surgery. Operative Surgery. Volume Ear, Nose and Throat. 2nd edition. Edit. J.C. Ballantyne. Butterworths London, 1976.

MARQUET J. Twelve years' experience with homograft tympanoplasty. *Otolaryngol, Clin. North Amer*, 10: 581-593, 1977.

MARQUET J. Congenital malformations and middle ear surgery. *J. Royal Soc. Med. Vol 74, Feb. 1981.*

PERKINS R. Human homograft otologic tissue transplantation: buffered formaldehyde preparation. *Trans. Amer. Acad. Ophtál. Otolaryng.*, 74: 278-282, 1970.

RUSSELL E.J. et al. Transverse axial plane anatomy of the temporal bone employing high spatial resolution computed tomography. *Neuroradiology*, 22: 185-191, 1982.

SOM P.M. et al. Computed tomography of glomus tympanicum tumors. *J. Computed Tomography*, 7(1): 14-17, Feb. 1983.

VALAVANIS A. et al. The current state of the radiological diagnosis of acoustic neuroma. *Neuroradiology*. 23: 7-13, 1982.

Complications in surgery for otospongiosis

Y. Schepens, Ph. Schepens, S. Vlaminck

After a post-mortem study on stapedectomies H.F. Schuknecht came to the conclusion that: "In at least half of the cases, the surgical techniques of stapedectomy were less than ideal. Surgeons who perform stapedectomies should be cognizant of the relevant surgical pathology, and adapt methods which will optimize functional results and minimize complications".

(Ann. ORL Vol. 88 part 2, 1979)

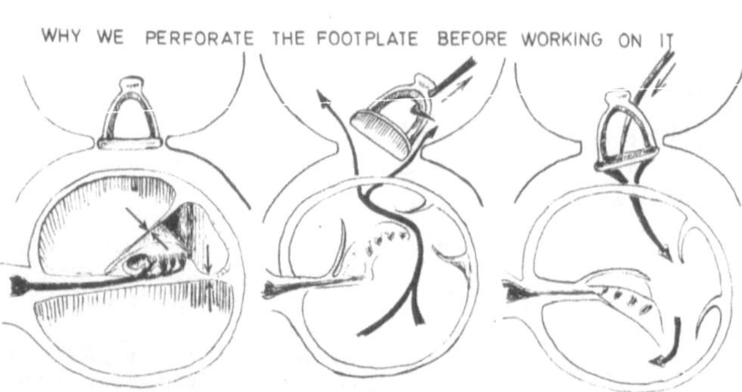

WHY WE PERFORATE THE FOOTPLATE BEFORE WORKING ON IT

Normal labyrinth before any work on the footplate. Membrana vestibuli and basilaris, between endolymph and perilymph are under equal pressure.

The stapes is extracted without previous perforation. It is removed like a cork from a bottle. Membrana vestibuli and basilaris burst. Result: a dead ear.

Before the decompression hole is made, hard pressure on the footplate may depress it into the labyrinth. Consequently, the membrana vestibularis is ruptured, and membrana basilaris is crushed.

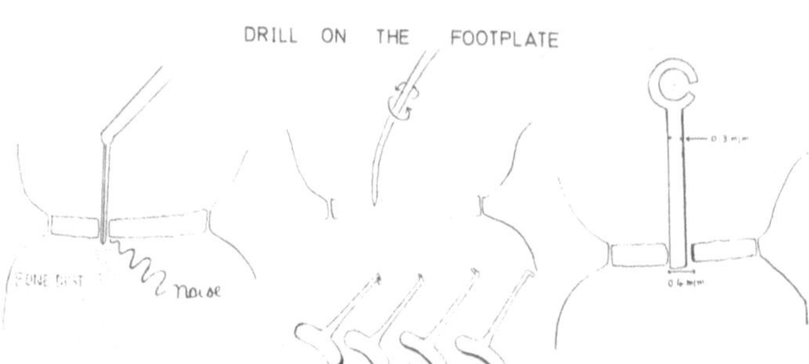

Using a drill on the footplate is another cause of labyrinth trauma. Noise, overheating and possibly bone dust in the labyrinth. To avoid this, the drill must turn slowly (150 R.P.M.), stopping every 10 seconds to clean with moist cotton and also for inspection.

If possible we make the first hole in the footplate by swivelling a needle without pressing. Then we introduce a very fine hook (0,1 mm) into the hole to enlarge it. DR. Marquet's hooks with different angles are very useful.

To avoid complications caused by total removal of the stapes, we prefer to make a well calibrated 0,4 mm hole in the footplate, allowing the introduction of a 0,3 mm teflon piston.

(The annals of O.R.L. p. 47 suppl. 29 vol. 85. July/Aug. 1976)

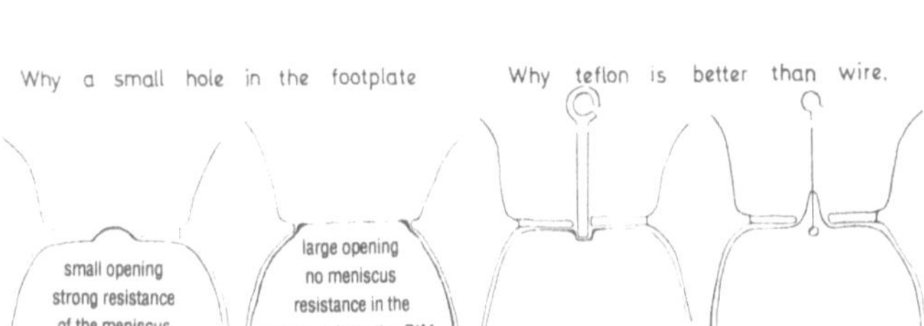

The surface tension of the perilymph is an obstacle to the penetration into the labyrinth of foreign particles.
This resistance only exists in a small opening of the footplate, so that the smaller the opening, the greater the resistance of the perilymph meniscus to accidental penetration of foreign particles (blood, bone chips, etc).

Van Camp, Greten and Marquet
(ACTA OTOLARYNGOL. 75: 61-63, 1973)

These authors have also demonstrated that the perilymphatic meniscus reacts differently towards Teflon or Wire.
Teflon is not wettable, so that the meniscus remains below the prosthesis.
Metal adheres to, and attracts the meniscus outwards.
Consequently, the endothelium from the vestibular side which attempts to close the opening in the footplate follows the perilymph meniscus under the teflon piston.
Whereas with the metal prosthesis, it goes along the metal where it is joined by the fossula ovalis tissue, and can thus create adhesions, fixing the metal prosthesis in the middle ear.

GELFOAM-WIRE PROSTHESIS CAN CAUSE 3 KINDS OF COMPLICATIONS
(J.L.Sheehy 1976)
(J.H. Perkins The Laryngosc number 3)

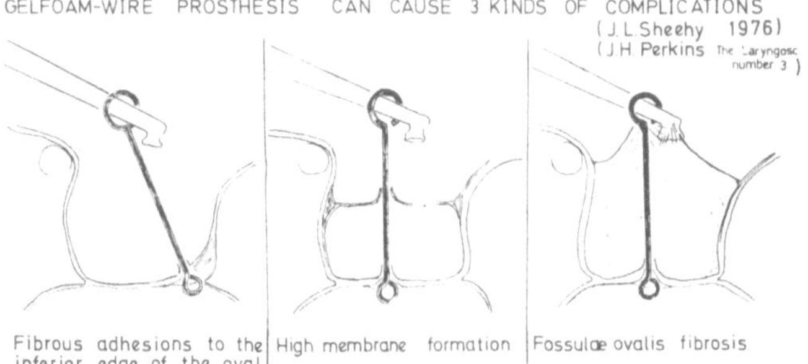

Fibrous adhesions to the inferior edge of the oval window.	High membrane formation	Fossulae ovalis fibrosis

One can imagine that gelfoam hydrated above by blood, and underneath by perilymph, disintegrates rapidly.
The blood fibrin which hydrates the gelfoam can become organised and fix the prosthesis with fibrosis.
If the perilymphatic pressure is strong enough, the liquid comes up through a cuff along the metal, causing a fistula.

WHICH FOOTPLATES ARE APT TO FLOAT

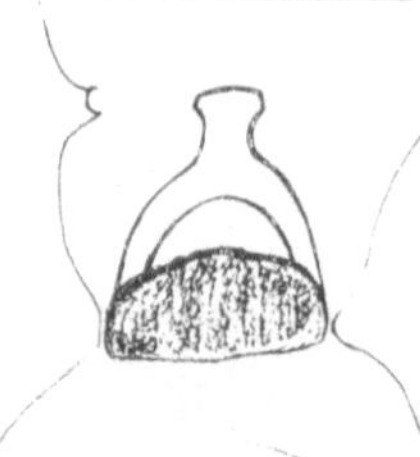

Footplates thick in the center but only slightly fixed at the edges.

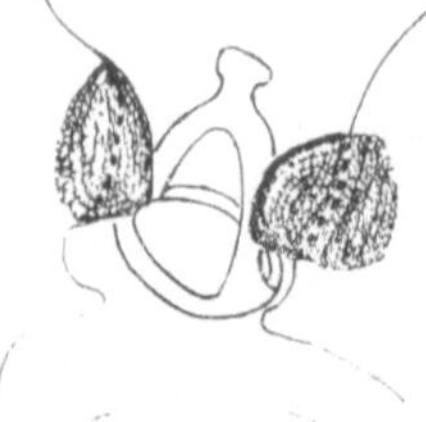

Footplates which could be normal, but are fixed by an otospongiotic mass overhanging the window.

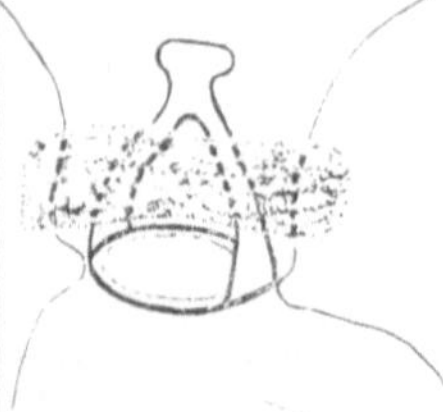

Footplates which could be normal, hidden under an otospongiotic mass invading the fossula ovalis (oval niche)

AFTER UNFORTUNATE / MANOEUVRES:
THERE ARE TWO KINDS OF FLOATING FOOTPLATE

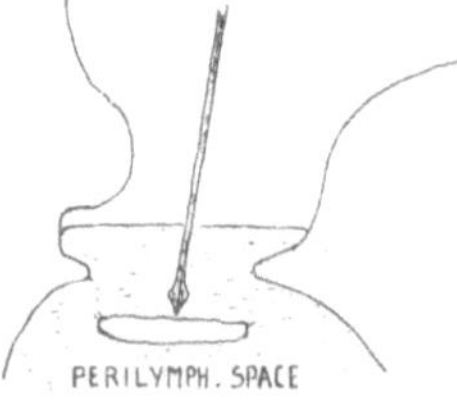

Those of which the annular ligament has been ruptured entirely, and which can float adrift.

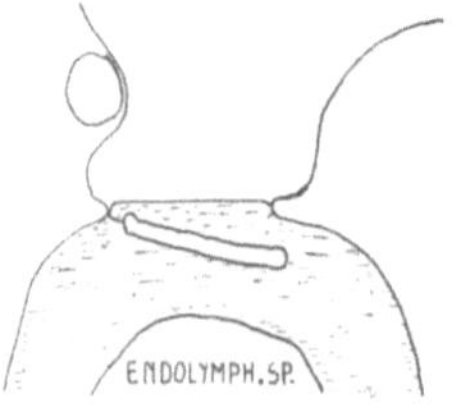

Those of which the annular ligament has not been entirely ruptured, and which remain moored.

Thick footplate, very frail crura - danger of floating footplate.

When separating the incudo-stapedial joint, the crura can break and become detached from the footplate

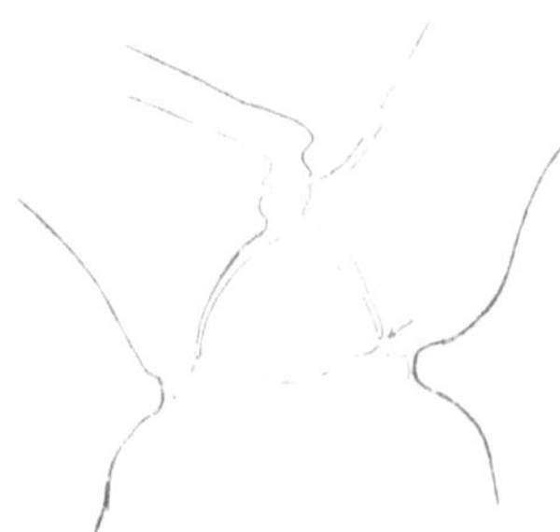

If the edges of the footplate are not well fixed, when attempting to perforate it, the footplate can sink into the vestibule.

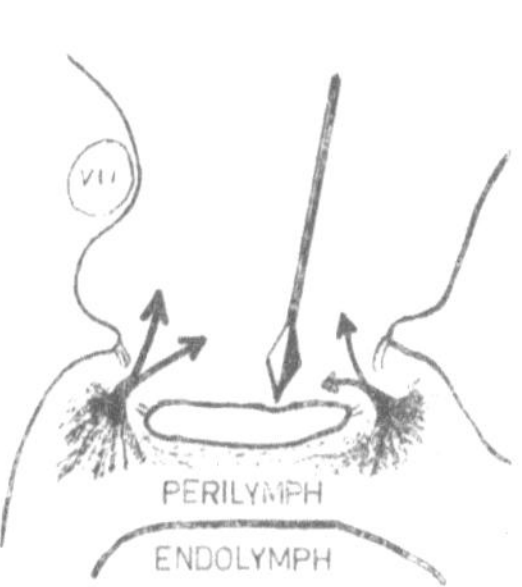

Possible consequence, rupture of the annular ligament, perilymph overflows.

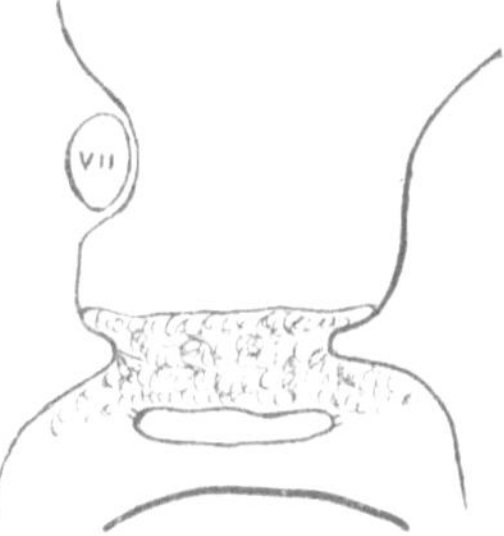

The footplate is depressed.
Blood clouds the perilymph, the footplate is invisible.

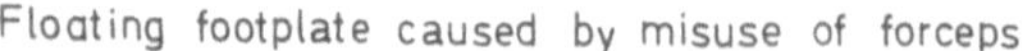

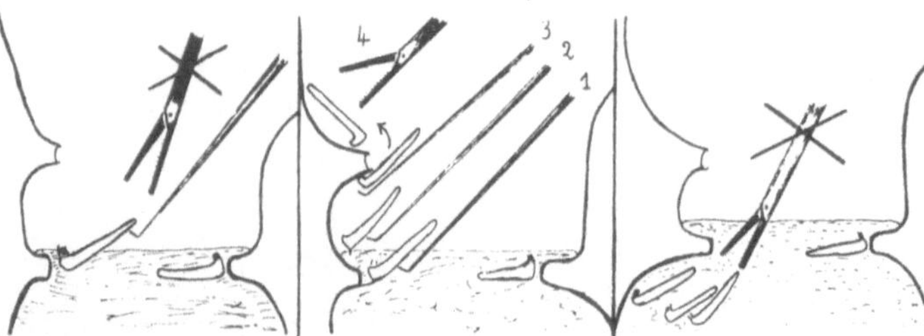

The hook must extract the footplate fragments and pull them away from the limits of the oval window.
Forceps must always be used away from the window.

We never use forceps in the window.

Used in the oval window, they will not be able to remove anything, but can push floating footplate fragments deeper and deeper.

POSSIBLE COMPLICATIONS DUE TO SUCTION OF PERILYMPH

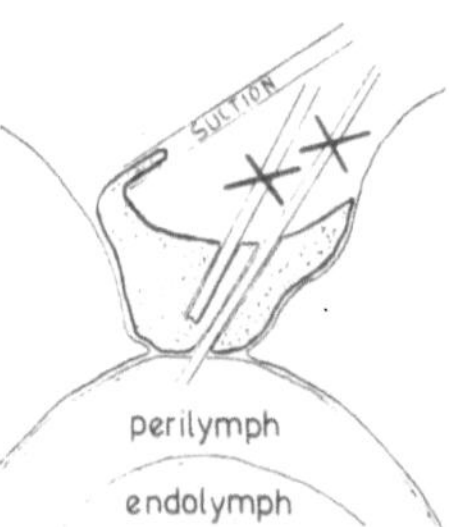

To avoid this, we never place the suction tube above or in the open labyrinth; we give the clot time to organise itself.

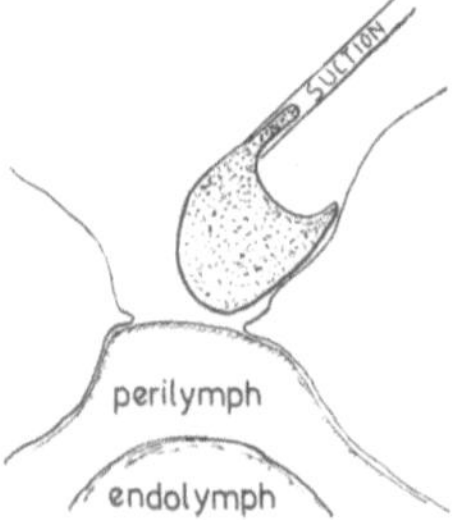

Suck it out by its edges, pull it out gently.
The perilymph remains and prevents the fibrinous organisation of the labyrinth.

FOOTPLATE SINKS INTO THE LABYRINTH BY MISUSE OF THE SUCKER.

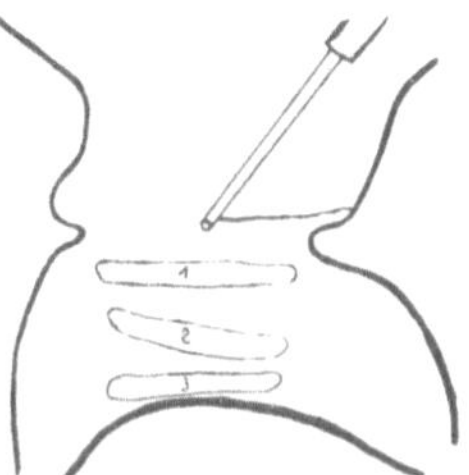

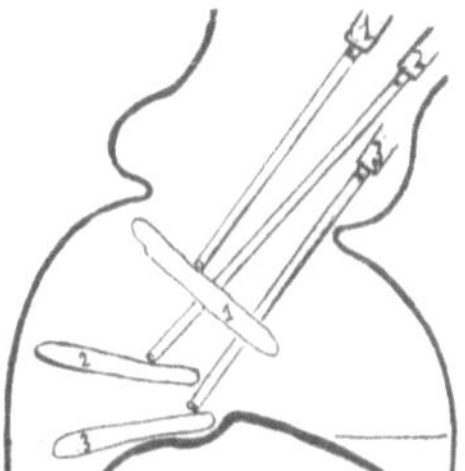

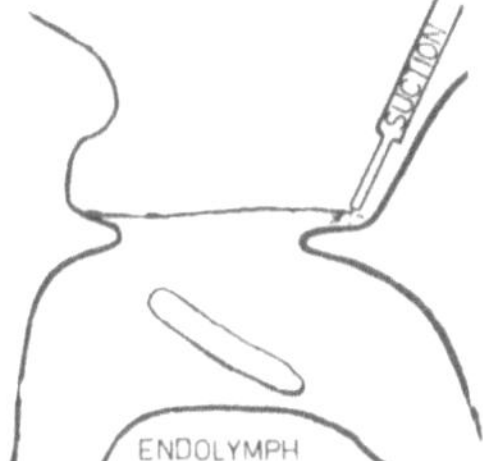

We do not suck the perilymph in the labyrinth, because the footplate sinks in, and can disappear.

Consequently we do not try to remove the footplate by suction. It is impossible

Excess perilymph must always be sucked out, beyond the labyrinth.

Footplate pushed into the labyrinth, by misuse of the hook.

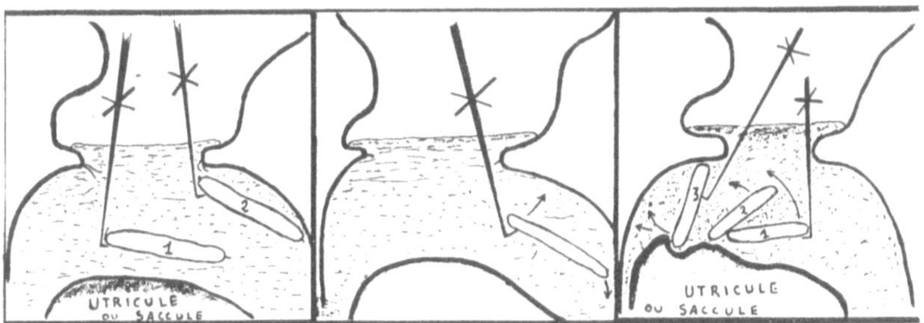

We do not work on the footplate in the labyrinth with hooks. We risk rupturing the moorings, push the footplate too far, loose it, and unnecessarily irritate the labyrinth.

CRURA REMOVED, FOOTPLATE SUNK IN: WHAT TO DO ?

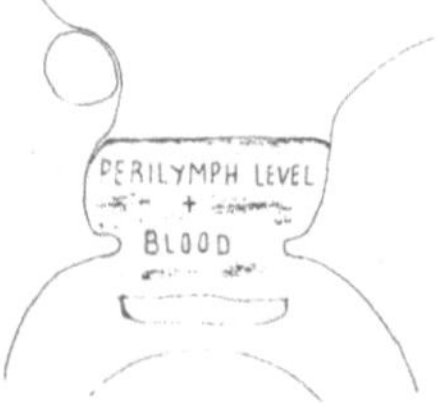

Blood clouds the perilymph.
Footplate invisible.
No manoeuvres. We wait for bleeding.

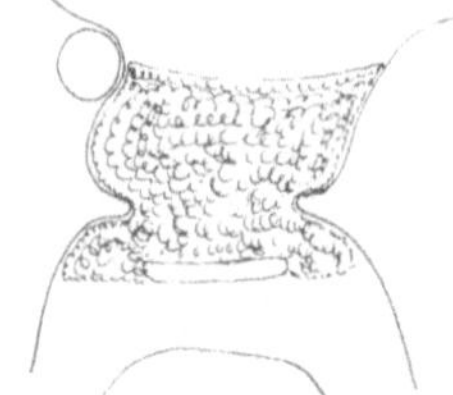

Blood invades the perilymphatic space and overflows into the fossula.

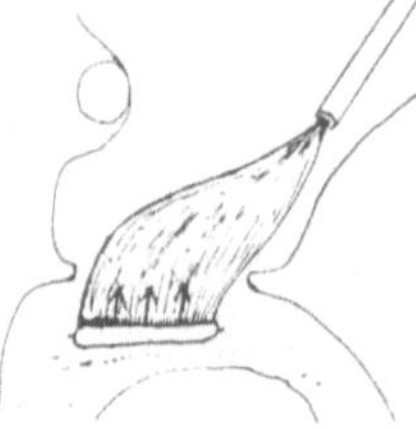

We wait until the blood is well clotted. Then we suck out the clot by one of its extremities, far from the window.

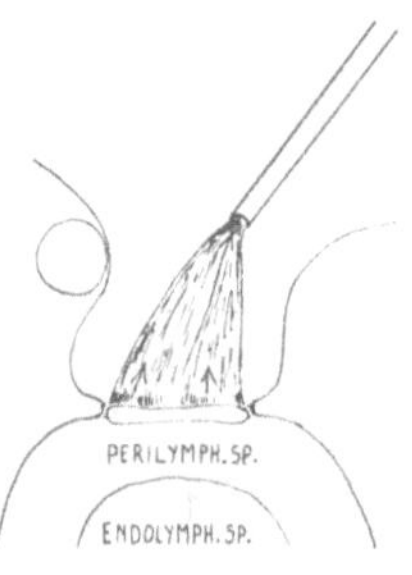

We do it carefully and sometimes the footplate comes away with the clot.

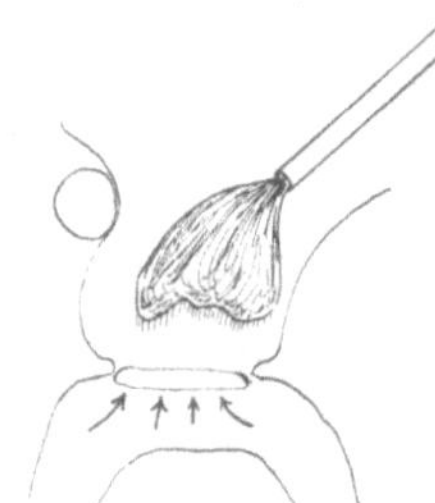

If the perilymph rises it supports the footplate which has a chance of remaining in place and is also mobile.

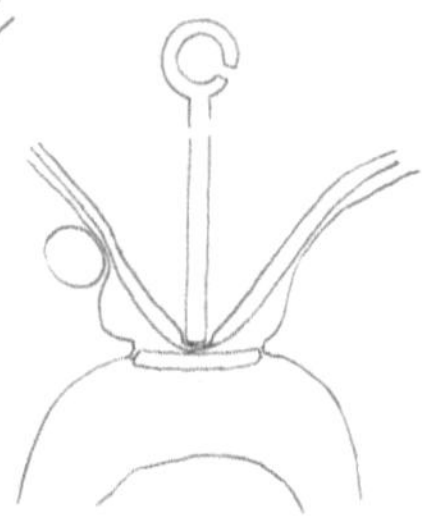

Then we apply a vein or a fascia graft, not too deeply into the oval window. For that reason we place a shorter piston (4 mm).

SLIPPED OFF PISTON

Through graft retraction the piston is pushed off the incus.	Partial necrosis of the incus by constant rubbing of the prosthesis.	The piston slips off.

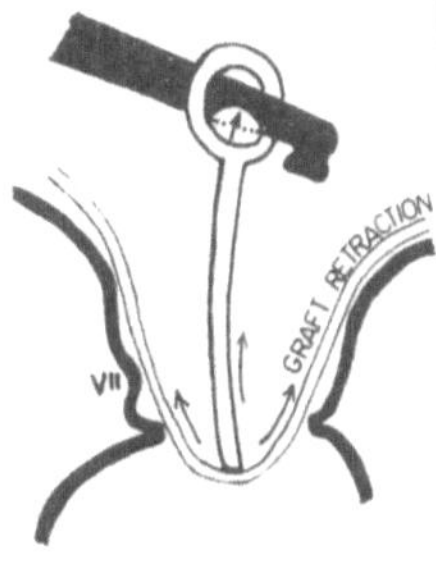

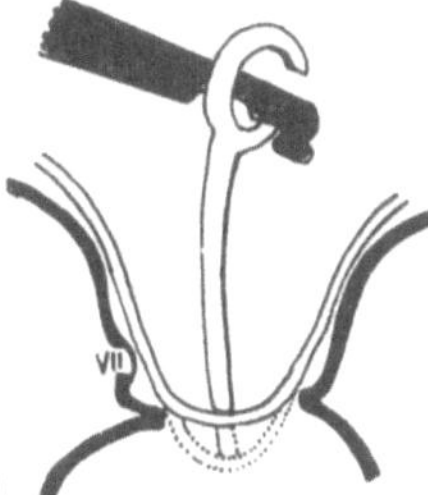

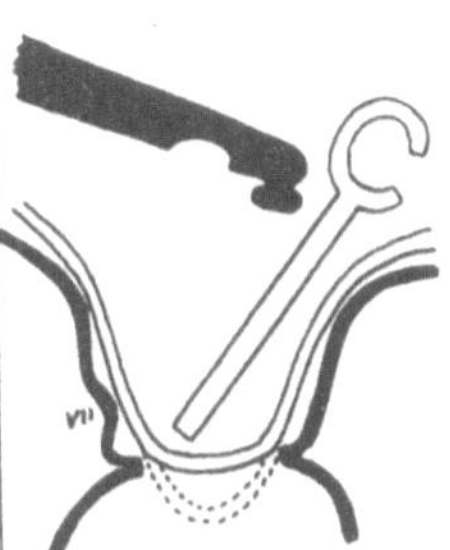

VERY THICK FOOTPLATES : 3 KINDS

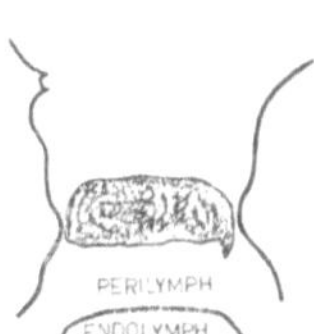

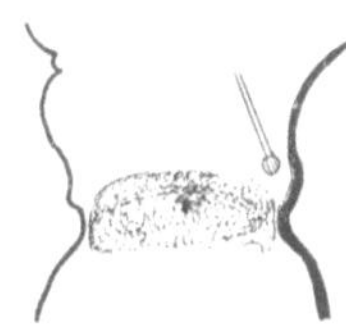

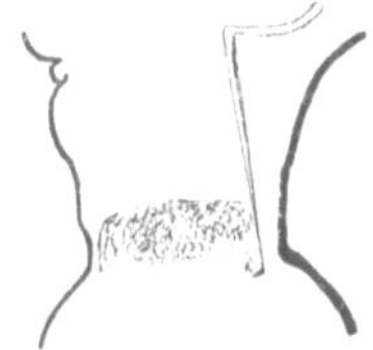

First kind.

What to do ?

Footplate very thick in its center with only slight peripheral fixation. In this case the crura are free. Danger of floating footplate.

We enlarge the fossula on the side of the promontory by drilling a hole beyond the annular ligament.

We introduce a hook into the drilled hole, lift up the footplate and pull it out.

Footplate not incorporated under an otospongiotic mass

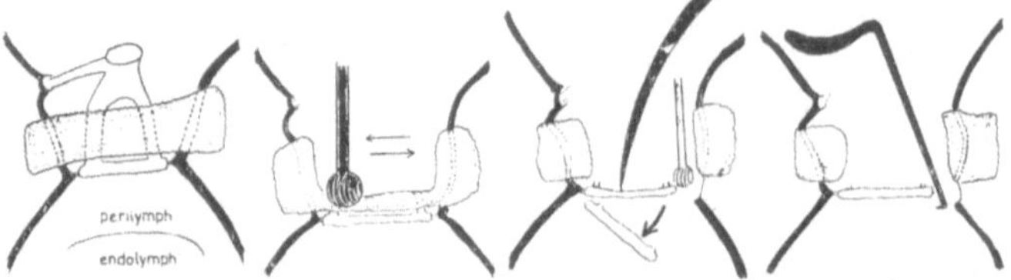

If the footplate is under an otospongiotic mass, but not incorporated in it,

We drill a large area so as to see the former limits of the annular ligament, we watch carefully for perilymph to appear.

Side of the

We do not try to perforate such a footplate with a needle because we risk pushing it into the labyrinth. Instead, we drill a hole near the annular ligament on the promontory.

We introduce a hook into the hole, lift up the footplate and pull it out. There may be an overhang on the side of the facial. Be careful, the footplate does not get caught on to it.

Footplate incorporated in an otospongiotic mass

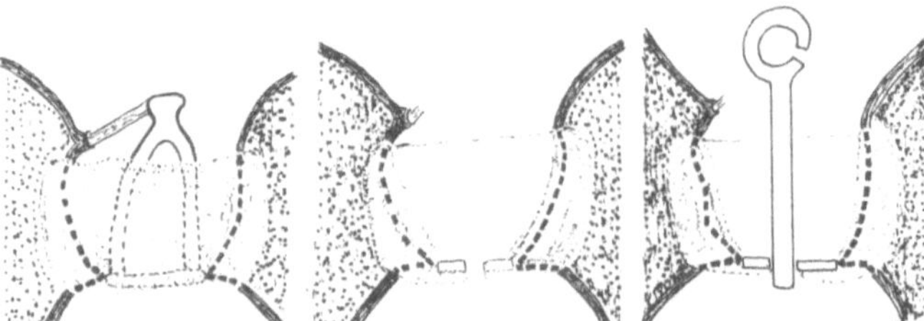

Otospongiotic mass invades almost the entire fossula ovalis.

We drill a large funnel shaped area and make a hole on the thinnest part at the bottom.

Then a piston is slipped into the hole. To prevent perilymph from leaking, the hole must be well judged.

Constant rubbing of the piston on the incus can cause total necrosis of the long process

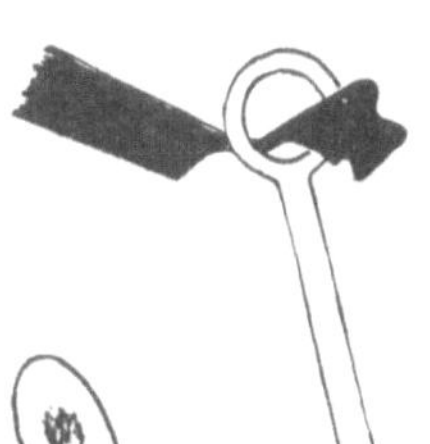

The piston slips off with the processus lenticularis in its ring.

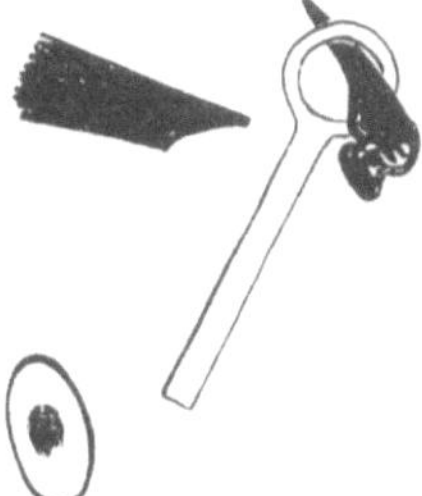

A piston between the oval window and the manubrium mallei is a simple method to restore conduction.

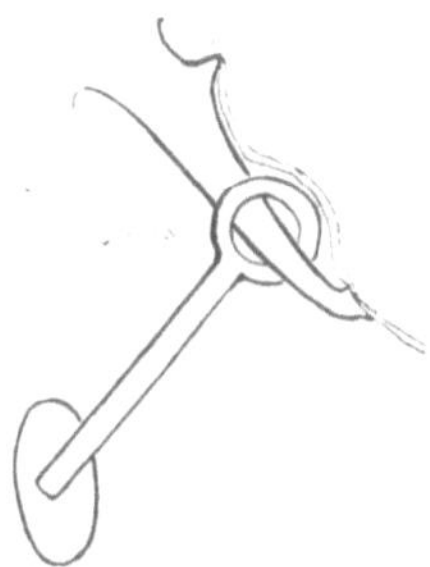

ACCIDENT BY CERTAIN BADLY FINISHED PROSTHESIS

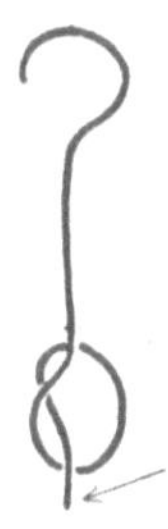

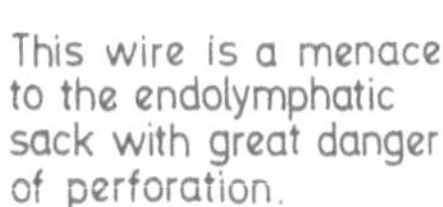

This wire is a menace to the endolymphatic sack with great danger of perforation.

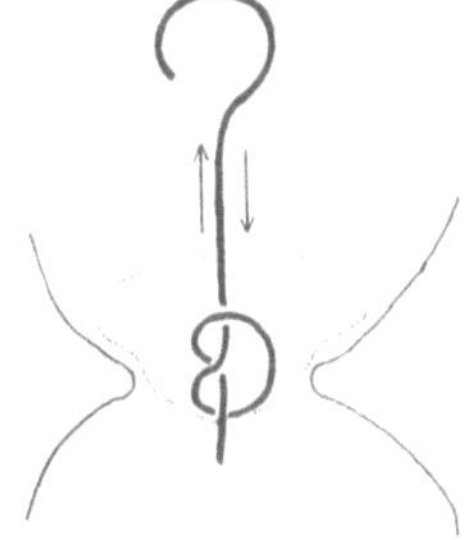

The sack is perforated, resulting in a dead ear.

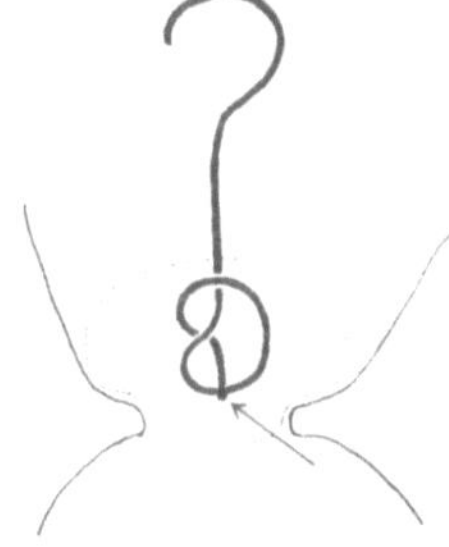

Examine carefully such a prosthesis. Do not place it too deeply in the oval window.

(Laryngoscope vol LXXXVI Sept 1976 p 1328)

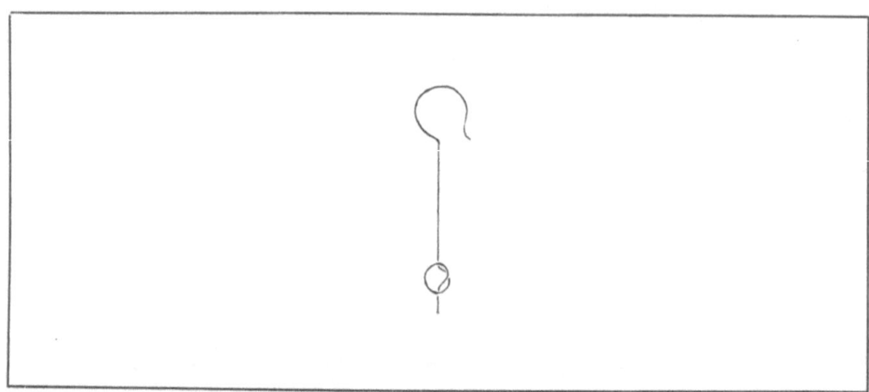

This was originally a gelfoam/wire prosthesis.

The prosthesis having been placed too deeply in the oval window, its terrible point caused damage to the inner ear. We did an exploration of this ear as the patient complained of vertigo.

The perilymph gusher

The perilymph gusher is a complication due to a too large communication between the cerebrospinal and the perilymphatic liquid, so that the pressure against the footplate is increased from 1 to 10 mmHg.

— There are 3 possible routes:
— the ductus vestibularis along the endolymphatic canal,
— the lamina cribrosa, through the porus acusticus internus - perineural route,
— the ductus cochlearis.

When the footplate is too widely open, a flow of perilymph floods the middle and external ear and can overflow to the outside. If a small safety hole has been made in the footplate, the flooding is less important and easier to control.

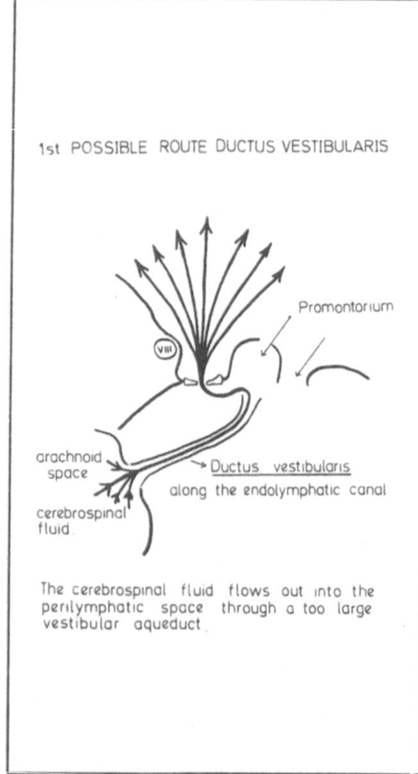

The cerebrospinal fluid flows out into the perilymphatic space through a too large vestibular aqueduct.

HERE IS THE DESCRIPTION OF THE FIRST CASE I SAW IN 1958.

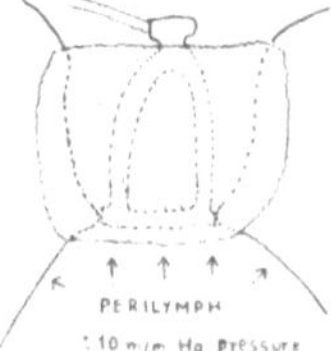

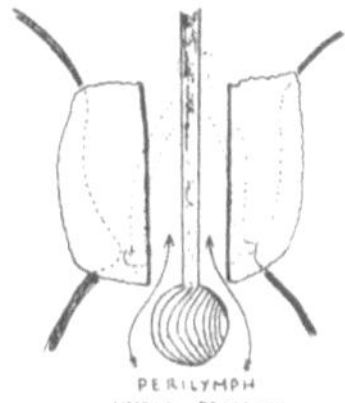

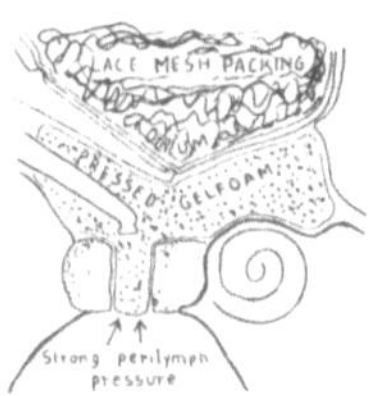

The stapes structures had disappeared in an otospongiotic mass. Only the capitulum stapedis was visible; the facial nerve was invisible.

In this case the mistake was to drill a 2 mm. hole in the shape of a long, narrow funnel.
The observation of such a hole was impossible whilst drilling.
The perilymphatic liquid escaped by a very wide funnel.
The decompression of the labyrinth was brutal, result: a dead ear.

The rate at which the cerebro-spinal liquid was escaping could cause vital problems.
A sucker was applied so as to see the hole. Gelfoam was then applied loco dolenti, so as to fill the middle ear. The flow was stopped, the drum replaced and compressed with packing. The patient recovered after 2 weeks vertigo but his hearing was lost.

HOW TO AVOID A PERILYMPH GUSHER? By making a safety hole with a fine needle, we avoid hyperpressure complications. The smaller the hole, the less complications.

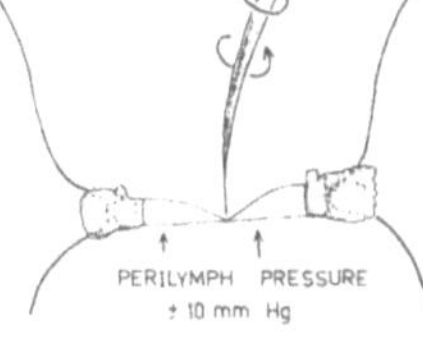

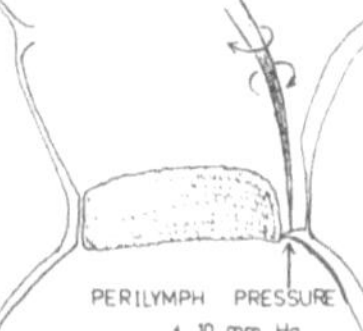

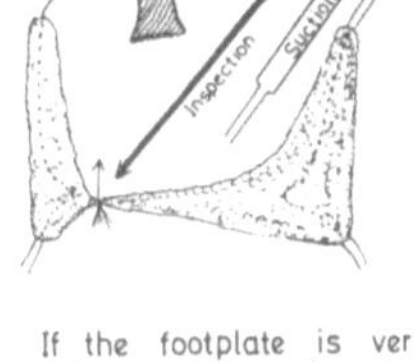

If the footplate is thin in the center but very fixed at the edges, we place a fine needle on the thinnest side. We swivel the needle very gently between the fingers without pushing, and make a safety hole. We look carefully for perilymph to appear.

If the footplate is thick in the center and only slightly fixed at the edges, we drill very carefully on the promontory on the side of the footplate. We try to preserve a thin layer of bone above the perilymph, make a safety hole and look out for perilymph.

If the footplate is very thick, includes the stapes and fills the fossula ovalis, we always use the same technique, drilling on the entire surface of the footplate sub-inferiorly at 150 R.PM. Minimum noise and heating.
We do not press hard, and stop every five seconds to inspect the footplate and look out for escaping perilymph.

IN CASE OF ACCIDENTAL PERILYMPH GUSHER: WHAT TO DO ?

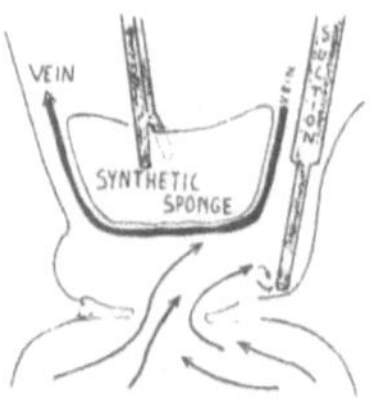

In one hand the sucker, far from the hole. In the other hand introduction of a plug consisting in synthetic sponge, wrapped in a piece of vein.

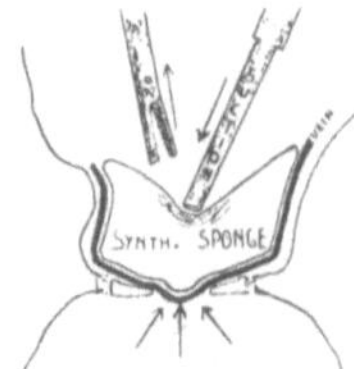

The plug is applied on the hole by means of a forceps. The forceps is replaced by the sucker and then removed.
The sucker maintains the vein, pressed into the hole.

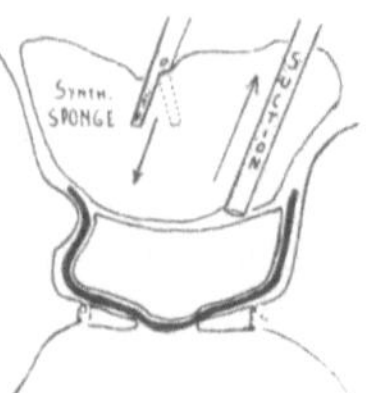

Then, a larger piece of sponge is placed by the forceps on top of the first, and compresses it.
The sucker replaces the forceps to compress the new packing.

Carcinoid of the middle ear

J.J. Manni, U.J.G.M. Van Haelst, K. Kubat, E.H.M.A. Marres

Introduction

Carcinoid tumour is a very unusual primary tumour of the middle ear. A tumour is called an apudoma when it originates from the APUD cell system (figure 1). APUD is the abbreviation for Amine Precursor Uptake and Decarboxyation, characteristic of these cells. The APUD cell has a high intracellular concentration of amines and the capacity for endocrine activity as well as the

Fig. 1. Proposed embryologic derivation of the cells of the APUD cell system (Pearce, 1974).

- Neural crest derivated cells (C-cells, adrenal medullary and paraganglionic cells, melanoblasts)
- Neural tube and ridge derivated cells (pineal, adenohypophysis, hypothalamic neurosecretory cells)
- Neuro-endocrine programmed ectoblast (gastro-entero-pancreatic axis, parathyroid, placental endocrine cells)

production of a variety of polypeptide hormones. At the present time, 40 types of APUD cells have been recognized, responsible for the production of 35 more or less biologically active polypeptide hormones and a number of amines.[1] The embryogenesis of the APUD cell is still controversial.

The middle ear carcinoid was first reported in 1980[2] and a review of the literature revealed two other cases.[3,4] The purpose of this paper is to present another case of carcinoid of the middle ear, with the longest reported follow-up to date.

Case report

In 1975, a 51-year old female patient presented with a persistent hearing loss of the left ear after an upper respiratory tract infection. Otitis media with effusion was diagnosed and the treatment consisted of myringotomy. One year later she returned with the same complaints. Otoscopy revealed hyperaemia and bulging of the posterior part of the left eardrum (figure 2). Radiography demonstrated decreased aeration of the left mastoid. Audiometry revealed a conductive hearing loss of 20 dB. On exploration, a tumour was found, which completely encased the ossicular chain without evident destruc-

Fig. 2. Bulging of the posterior part of the left tympanic membrane

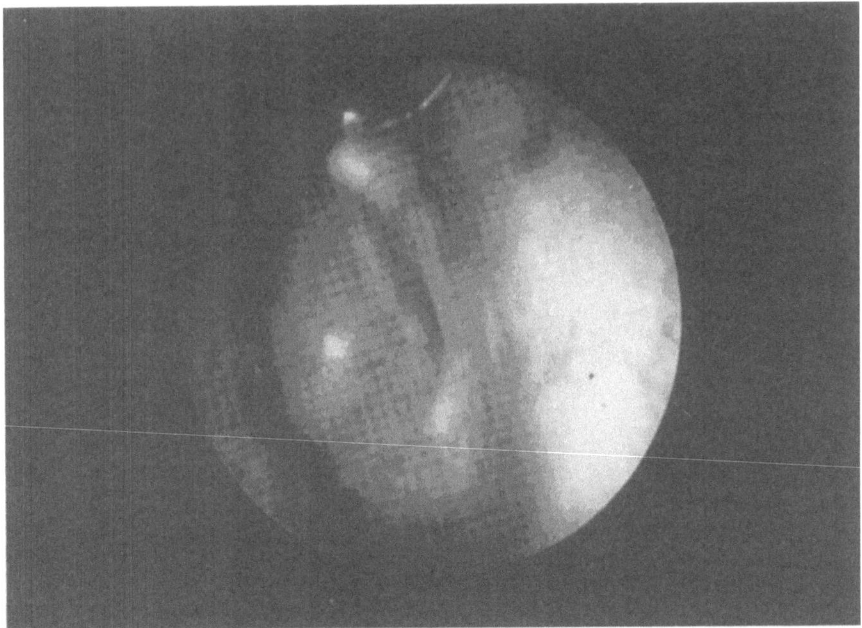

tion. Radical mastoidectomy was performed with complete removal of the tumour.

Histopathological findings

Light microscopy. The tumour consisted of large columnar or cuboidal cells arranged in solid sheets or in other areas in a more trabecular-acinar pattern. The nuclei were usually oval with small nucleoli. Mitotic figures were seldom seen. The cytoplasms showed fine eosinophilic granules with negative reaction for PAS and Alcian Blue staining. However, the granules were strongly positive with Grimelius staining for argyrophilia (figure 3). Within the lumina of the tubules PAS and Alcian Blue staining revealed positive reaction indicating the presence of glycoproteins.

Electron microscopy revealed large numbers of small, round or oval neurosecretory granules with a diameter of 120-300 nm with an electron-dense core and a distinctive limiting membrane (figure 4). In seven years follow-up the patient remained free of

Fig. 3. Black argyrophitic granules in many tumour cells. Silver impregnation after Grimelius (1340x)

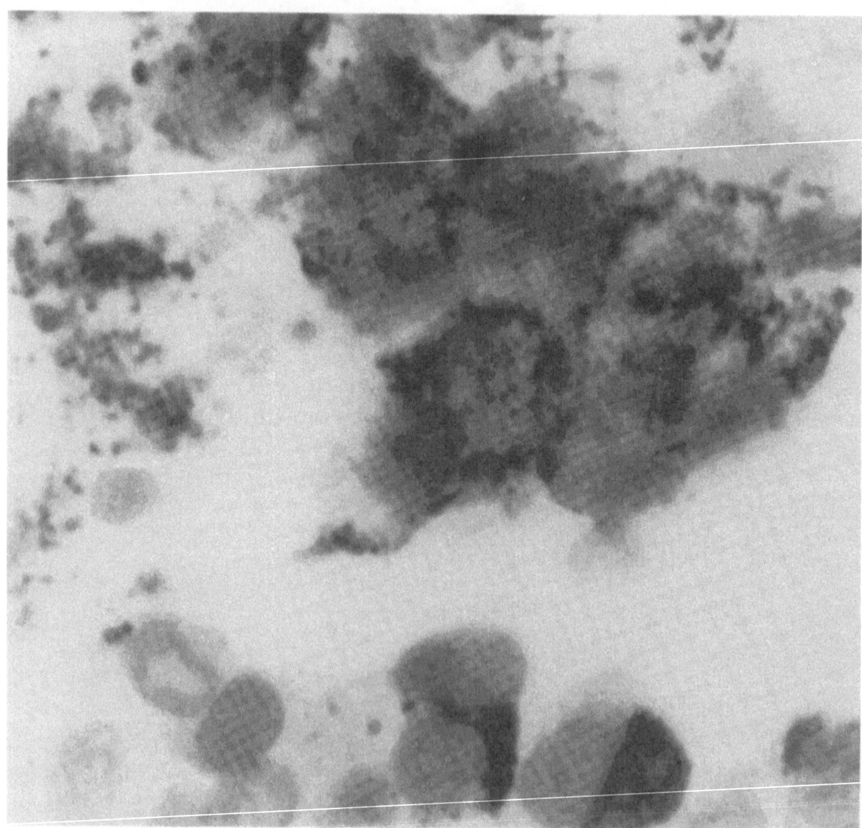

Fig. 4. Electron micrograph. (12.500x). Large numbers of neurosecretory granules with a diameter of 120-300 nm. Lumen and microvilli projections characteristic for the subclassification "composite carcinoid tumour"

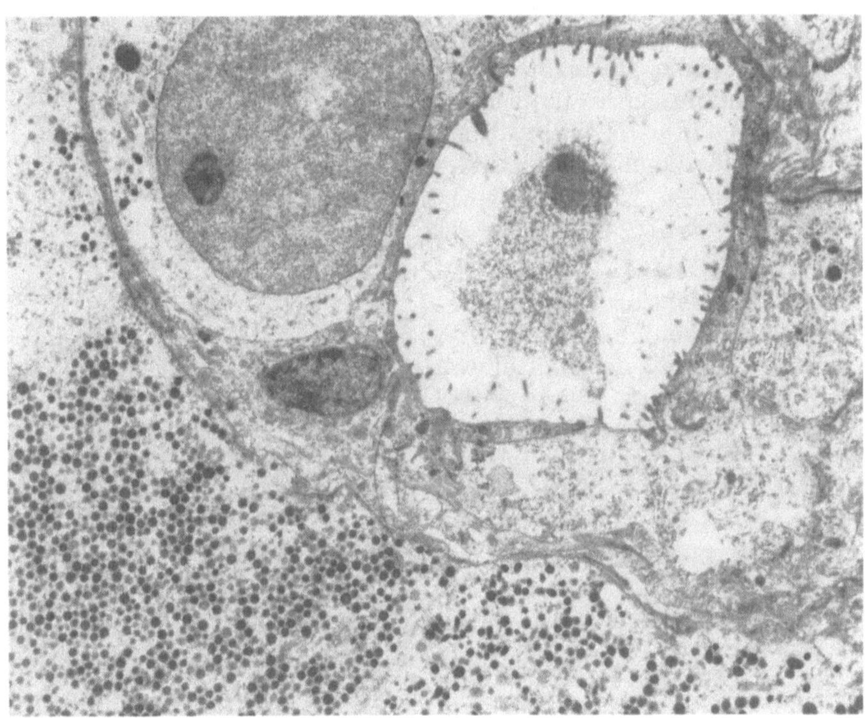

recurrent disease. She never manifested symptoms consistent with carcinoid syndrome or elevated levels of urinary 5-Hydroxy-indolacetic acid.

Discussion

Carcinoids are thought to arise from the entero-chromaffin (Kulchitsky) cells.[5] This member of the APUD cell system is distributed throughout the primitive fore-, mid- and hindgut.[6] The middle ear is a foregut derivate. The most distinctive property of the foregut apudoma is uptake and decarboxylation of 5-Hydroxy tryptophan (5-HT), the immediate precursor of serotonine. This property allows the cells to be identified histochemically, since the decarboxylated amines form highly fluorescent derivates with gaseous formaldehyde.[7]

The cells may also be identified by their characteristic argyrophilia and/or argents affinity. The foregut derived tumours, which include the middle ear, are usually argyrophilic with Grimelius stain.[6]

The differential diagnosis of middle ear apudomas includes: adenomatous tumour,[8,9] jugulo-tympanic paraganglioma and low grade adenocystic carcinoma. The Grimelius stain for argyrophilic granules is essential. Electron microscopy will reveal characteristic intra-cytoplasmic membrane-bound neurosecretory granules, while formaldehyde-induced fluorescence indicating the presence of 5-HT will further confirm the diagnosis of carcinoid.

The clinical course of the reported cases of carcinoid of the middle ear is benign, but the rarity of the disorder does not allow accurate assessment. The recently described carcinoids of the larynx appear to be clinically malignant and not sensitive to irradiation.[10] The treatment of choice for carcinoid of the middle ear appears to be radical surgery.

A new case will be reported in the Journal of Laryngology and Otology,[11] bringing the number of reported cases up to five.

References:

1. PEARCE A.G.E. The APUD cell concept and its implications in pathology. *Pathol. Ann.* 9, 27-41, 1974.
2. MURPHY G.F., PILCH B.Z., DICKERSON G.R. et al. Carcinoid tumor of the middle ear. *Am. J. Clin. Path.* 73, 816-823, 1980.
3. JNOUE S., TANAKA K., KAMAL S. Primary carcinoid tumor of the ear. *Virchows Arch.* 396, 357-363, 1982.
4. FRIEDMANN J., GALEY F.R., HOUSE W.F. et al. A mixed carcinoid tumour of the middle ear. *J. Laryngol. Otol.* 97, 465-470, 1983.
5. MENGEL Ch.E. The carcinoid syndrome. *Holland's cancer medicine,* ed. Lea Fabiger, Philadelphia, 1982.
6. WILLIAMS E.D., SANDLER M. The classification of carcinoid tumors. *Lancet* 1, 238-239, 1963.
7. ENERBÄCK L. Specific methods for detection of 5-hydroxytruptamine in carcinoid tumors. *Virchows Arch.* 385, 35-43, 1973.
8. DERLACKI E.L., BARNEY Ph.L. Adenomatous tumours of the middle ear and mastoid. *Laryngoscope* 86, 1123-1135, 1976.
9. HYAMS V.J., MICHAELS L. Benign adenomatous neoplasm of the middle ear. *Clin. Otol.* 1, 17-26, 1976.
10. BLOK Ph. H.H.M., MANNI J.J., VAN DEN BROEK P. et al. Carcinoid Apudoma of the larynx. *Laryngoscope,* to be published.
11. TANGE R.A., VAN DER BORDEN J., SCHIPPER M.E.J. A case of carcinoid tumour in the middle ear. *J. Laryng. Otol.*, 98, 1021-1027, 1984.

Formaldehyde-formed fascia graft in tympanoplasty

A. Robier, D. Goga, Y. Capelier, B. Arbeille-Brassart

Repair of tympanic membrane defects by autologous tissue grafts has become an established otologic practice. The main difficulty with total perforations is their relatively high incidence in the postoperative period of graft perforation, graft lateralization and anterior canal sulcus blunting (W. Hicks et al. 1979). Frequently, the fascia is dehydrated, prior to sealing the defect of the tympanic membrane.

In 1975, R. Perkins drew our attention to the presence of denaturation in protein moiety of the dehydrated temporalis fascia with supra physiological heat.

P.M. Shenoi (1982) shows with scanning electron microscopy that physiological heat on the collagen matrix seems, at first, to produce generalized swelling of the fibres, the denatured protein is drawn into "dome"-shaped structures with circular defects like "craters". To present the complications, R. Perkins proposed the formaldehyde-formed fascia graft. The fascia is pulled onto a mould shaped like the medial external auditory canal and the tympanic membrane. The fascia is dried, using a small electric dryer. The dried fascia and mould are placed in a solution bath of buffered formaldehyde 4 % pH 5,6 for about six minutes, then placed in three successive rinsing baths. The dried, shaped graft is now ready for implantation. We have realized electron microscopic observations of the preparation and the study of 65 perforations treated with formaldehyde-formed fascia grafts.

Materials and methods

Autogenous temporalis fascia from five patients undergoing tympanoplasty was obtained through a postauricular incision. Each time, three specimens were studied under scanning electron microscope: a fresh fascia, a dried fascia and a formaldehyde-formed fascia (FFF). Sixty-five chronic otitis were treated with FFF.

In 57 cases the tympanic membrane presented a total or a subtotal perforation, in 8 cases the perforation was associated with an extensive immigration of squamous epithelium over the perforation edge. In each case the remanent tympanic membrane and annulus were removed. Ten ears were draining one week before surgery and inflammatory phenomena were seen in the middle ear cleft in 40 cases. In 21 cases the surgery found no ossicular defect, 44 cases had ossicular defects involving either the absence of the long process of the incus or absence of both the long process of the incus and stapes crura, in each case there was a functional malleus. Closed technique tympanoplasty and, if necessary, ossicular reconstruction with homograft were performed.

Results

The scanning electron microscopy confirms "the unit stability" of the formaldehyde-formed fascia as described by Perkins in 1975 (figures 1, 2, 3).

Our anatomical results are as follows:

— postoperative perforation: 0 % (0),

— lateral displacement: 3 % (2),

Fig. 1. Fresh fascia: healthy collagen fibres are seen

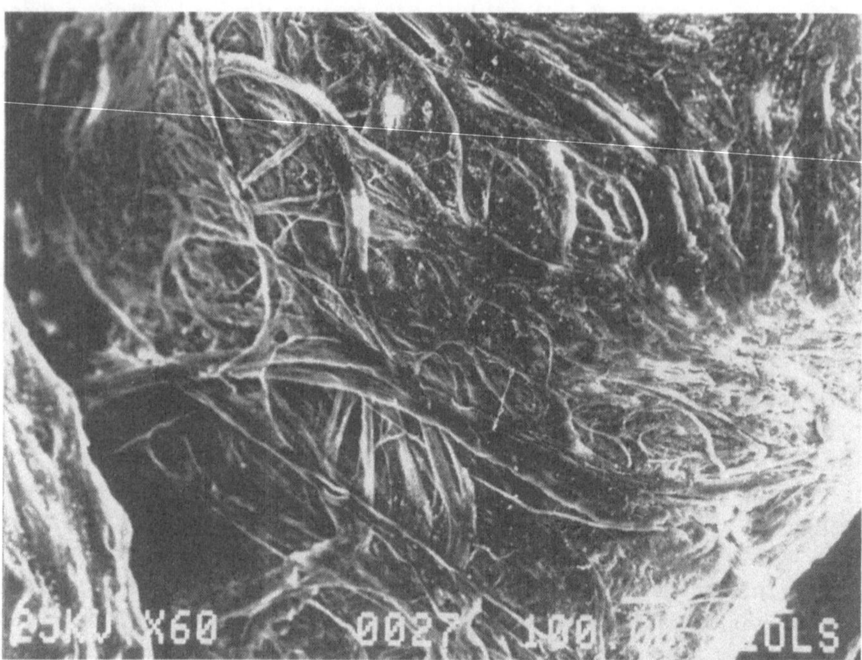

Fig. 2. Dried fascia: considerable swelling of collagen fibres is clearly visible

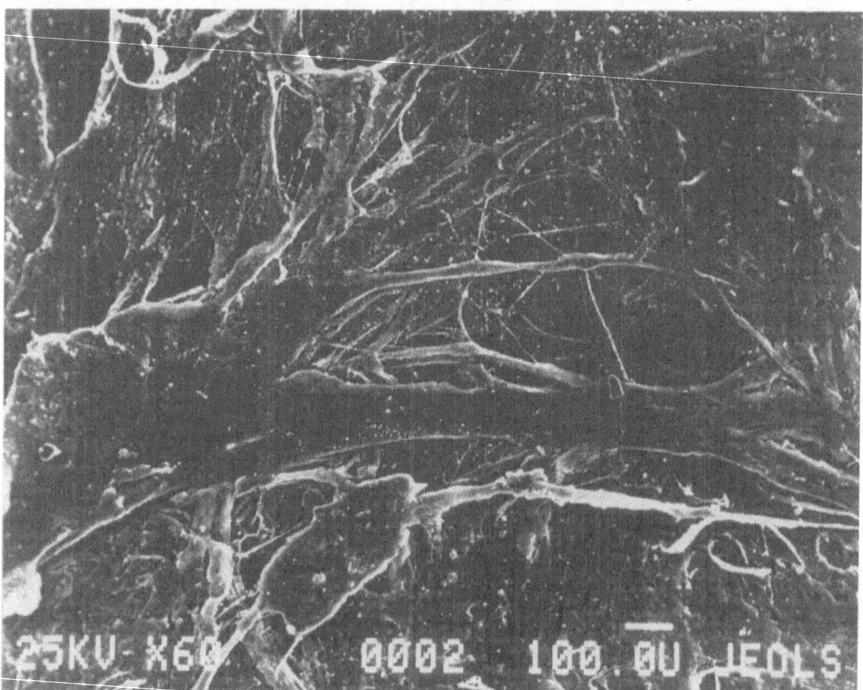

Fig. 3. Formaldehyde-formed fascia: amorphous material is the outstanding feature, normal collagen fibres are no longer visible, there are no defects

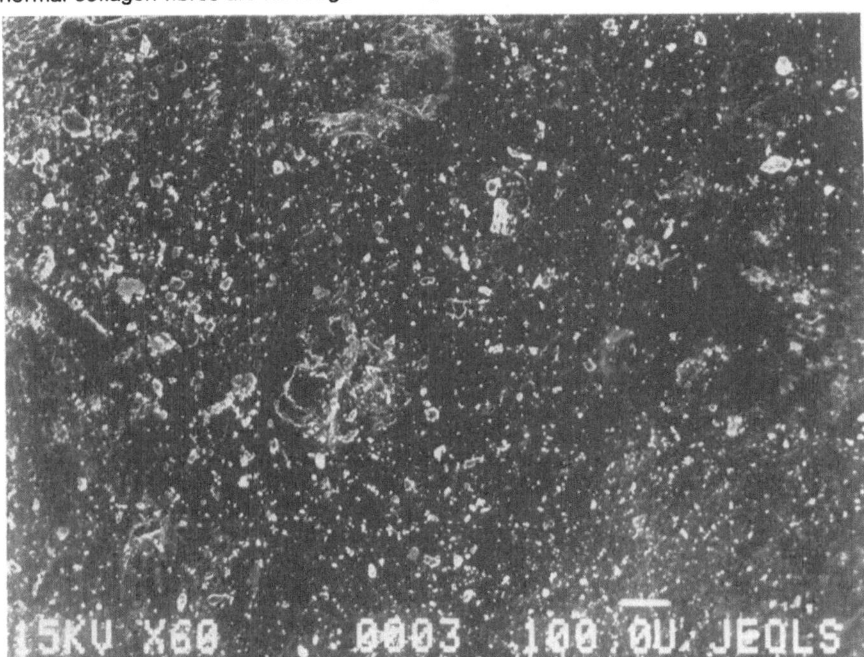

— anterior blunting: 1,5 % (1), (follow-up range: 2 - 1 year).

There were 21 cases of total perforations of the tympanic membrane with no associated ossicular defects. In these cases the postoperative air-bone gap was ⩽ 15 dB in 76 % (mean gain 10 dB).

Discussion

These results can be compared with others in the literature.

F.F.F.	N° Perforation	N° Displacement
PERKINS	(41) 98 %	
HICKS	(130) 96,4 %	94,2 %
FOMBEUR	(80) 92 %	
TOURS	(65) 100 %	95,5 %

ANATOMICAL RESULTS

F.F.F.	Post op A - B gap ⩽ 10 dB	⩽ 15 dB	⩽ 20 dB
PERKINS		71 %	
HICKS			78 %
FOMBEUR	97 %		
TOURS		76 %	

FUNCTIONAL RESULTS

Conductive hearing loss and autosomal dominant proximal symphalangism

ABSTRACT
C.W.R.J. Cremers, E.J.J.M. Theunissen, W. Kuypers

A father and his 13- and 10-year old sons were referred for an otological examination. A conductive hearing loss, suspected to have a congenital origin, had been diagnosed. Deafness was noted in the older son at school age. Proximal symphalangism was present in the hands and feet of the father and also his sons. Otoscopy was normal. Conductive hearing loss, ranging from 15 to 40 dB, was found. Stapedial reflexes could not be elicited. Exploratory tympanotomy in the older son with a 40 dB bilateral loss revealed a congenitally fixed stapes and an incus fixed in the fossa incudis. Surgical intervention in the right ear resulted in normal hearing. The first histological report of a stapes in this syndrome revealed a normal suprastructure and a rather normal footplate, except for the posterior part, which was largely thickened. In this area the annular ligament fracture resulted from bony fixation in the oval window niche. Incudal fixation had not been described earlier for this syndrome. Stapes surgery for all cases with this syndrome reported in the literature has been successful.

Computer processing of data in middle ear surgery

N. Gómez Estancona, I. de la Torre, U. Ruiz, L. Muñiz, J.R. Urruticoechea, A. Urruticoechea, N. Arenaza

A protocol for computer processing of data in exploratory tympanotomy, myringoplasty, tympanoplasty, simple mastoidectomy, radical mastoidectomy, reconstruction of an open cavity, muscle flaps and tympanoossicular graft is presented here.

We have developed an informatic solution based on RDBMS in

which each protocol is a data base.

The data included in the RDBMS can be consulted and compared in any way we like; this means that we can get hundreds of details of information, classified by any concept, in one single process of data, always with the possibility of consulting anything we like. Anyone can benefit from data processing technology, even if one is not a programmer.

OPERATION
Exploratory tympanotomy (1)
Myringoplasty (2)
Tympanoplasty (3)
Simple mastoidectomy (4)
Radical modified (5)
Radical mastoidectomy (6)
Revision tympanoplasty (7)
Revision radical mastoidectomy (8)
Antrostomy (9)
Tympano-ossicular graft (10)
Muscle flaps (11)
Another (12)
FINDINGS
External auditory canal
Normal (1)
Narrow (2)
Wide (3)
Dry (4)
Wet (5)
Polypus in external auditory canal (6)
Granulations (7)
Tympanic membrane
Normal (1)
Thick (2)
Wide (3)
Promontory (4)
Adhered to ossicles (5)
Tympanosclerosis (6)
Perforation small (7)
Perforation kidney shaped (8)
Perforation wide (9)
Perforation attic (10)
Perforation marginal (11)
Attical depression (12)
Another (13)
Tympanic cavity
Dry (1)
With mucous (2)
With pus (3)
Cholesteatoma cavity (4)
Cholesteatoma sinus tympani (5)
Cholesteatoma ossicles (5)
Cholesteatoma malleus handle (6)
Cholesteatoma oval window (7)
Cholesteatoma congenital (8)
Normal mucosa (9)
Mucosa inflammatory (10)
Mucosa metaplasia (11)
Mucosa granulations (12)
Eustachian tube normal (13)
Eustachian tube closed (14)
Tympanosclerosis ossicular chain free (15)
Tympanosclerosis malleus or incus fixation (16)
Tympanosclerosis stapes fixation (17)
Round window normal (18)
Round window inflammatory (19)
Round window with tympanosclerosis (20)
Fibrous tissue with partial mobilization of the ossicular chain (21)
Malleus normal (22)
Malleus absent (23)
Malleus necrosis of the handle (24)
Malleus necrosis of the head (25)
Incus normal (26)
Incus necrosis of the long handle (27)
Incus absent (28)
Stapes normal (29)
Stapes head necrosis (30)
Stapes crural necrosis (31)
Stapes footplate only present (32)
Footplate with otosclerotic focus (33)
Facial nerve normal (34)
Facial nerve dehiscence of the 2nd portion (35)
Facial nerve with granulation tissue (36)
Facial nerve dehiscence of the 3rd portion (37)
Facial nerve swelling (38)
Another finding (39)
Attic normal (40)
Attic mucosa inflammatory (41)
Attic mucosa with granulations (42)
Cholesteatoma medial (43)
Cholesteatoma anterior (44)
Tympanosclerosis (45)
Another finding (46)
Antrum normal (47)
Antrum big (48)
Antrum small (49)
Antrum mucosa inflammatory (50)
Antrum mucosa with granulations (51)
Antrum cholesteatoma (52)

Antrum fistula lateral semicircular canal (53)
Antrum fistual lateral semicircular canal
Antrum cover by cholesteatoma (54)
Antrum another finding (55)
Mastoid normal ebony (56)
Mastoid sclerosed (57)
Mastoid pneumatized few (58)
Mastoid pneumatized many (59)
Mastoid cells retrofacial (60)
Mastoid cells perilabyrinthine (61)
Mastoid mucosa inflammatory (oedematous) (62)
Mastoid mucosa with granulations (63)
Mastoid cholesteatoma (64)
Mastoid osteitis (65)
Mastoid another finding (66)
Lateral sinus normal (67)
Lateral sinus dehiscent (68)
Lateral sinus protruded (69)
Lateral sinus with granulations (70)
Lateral sinus thrombosed (71)
Lateral sinus another finding (72)
Dura not exposed (73)
Dura low (74)
Dura very low (75)
Dura dehiscent (76)
Dura with granulations (77)
Dura another finding (78)
Revision surgery
Tympanic membrane displaced (1)
Epithelial cyst (2)
Cholesteatoma (3)
Strands of tissue (4)
Inadequate ventilation (5)
Failure of sound transmission (6)
Another finding (7)
Another finding (8)
Surgical approach
Permeatal (1)
Endaural approach (2)
Postaural (3)
Combined (4)
Another (5)
Bone dissection
Antrostomy (1)
Antro-atticotomy (2)
Mastoidectomy (3)
Posterior tympanotomy (4)
Atticotomy by endaural approach (5)
Partial removal of canal wall (6)
Total removal of canal wall (7)
Another (8)

LESIONS REMOVAL
Tympanic membrane
Removal of the margin of the tympanic perforation (1)
Removal of the epithelial layer (2)
Superior tympanomeatal flap (3)
Complete removal tympanic membrane (4)
Removal tympanosclerosis plates (5)
Removal the inferior part of the tympanic membrane (6)
Removal of the meatal and tympanic skin (7)
Attic and tympanic cavity
Removal of mucosa (1)
Removal of the stapes footplate (2)
Removal of the stapes arch (3)
Removal of the malleus (4)
Removal of the head of the malleus (5)
Removal of the incus (6)
Removal of a piece of incus (7)
Cholesteatoma removal (8)
Osteitis removal (9)
Granulations removal (10)
Removal of the bone covering the oval window niche (11)
Mastoid cavity
Mucosa removal (1)
Cholesteatoma removal (2)
Osteitis (3)
Mastoid cell drilling (4)
Problems
Footplate mobilization (1)
Perilymph leak (2)
Lateral sinus exposition (3)
Middle fossa dura plate exposition (4)
Opening through the posterior canal wall (5)
Retrofacial cells present (6)
Perilabyrinthine cells present (7)
Horizontal semicircular canal injured (8)
Lateral sinus injured (9)
Dura injured (10)
Facial nerve exposed (11)
Facial nerve injured (12)
Tympanic membrane perforation (13)
Ossicular chain luxated (14)
Another (15)
RECONSTRUCTION
Tympanic membrane
Without (1)
Underlay (2)
Overlay (3)
Skin graft meatal (4)
Skin graft retroauricular (5)
Graft
Autograft fascia (6)
Autograft perichondrium (7)
Autograft periostal (8)
Autograft fat (9)
Autograft vein (10)
Heterograft tympanic membrane with skin (11)
Heterograft tympanic membrane with skin (12)
Posterior canal wall
Without (1)
Replaced the same posterior canal wall (2)
With cartilage (3)
With bone (4)

With muscle flap and meatal skin (5)
With bone paste (6)
Another (7)
Ossicular chain
Without (1)
Tympani stapes (2)
Malleus stapes (3)
Malleus footplate (4)
Malleus vestibule (5)
Incus footplate (6)
Incus vestibule (7)
Tympanic membrane and ossicular chain (8)
Graft
Bone
Autograft (1)
Heterograft (2)
Cartilage
Autograft (3)
Heterograft (4)
Polyethylene and perichondrium (5)
Fat (6)
Polyethylene (7)
Teflon (8)
Wire and:
Teflon (9)
Fat Gelfoam (10)
Homograft
Tympanic membrane and ossicular chain (1)
Tympanic membrane and malleus (2)
Tympanic membrane, malleus and incus (3)
Another (4)
Interesting things
Gelfoam in middle ear (1)
Middle ear Teflon sheet (2)
Middle ear Sylastic sheet (3)
Stapes fixed (4)
Stapes mobile (5)
Stapes partially mobile (6)
Bleeding (7)
Eustachian tube obstructed (8)
Eustachian tube non-obstructed (9)
Another (10)
Packing
With Gelfoam (1)
With spongostan (2)
With gauze (3)
With rayon (4)
With fat (5)
Another (6)
Drain grummet (7)
Drain retroauricular (8)
Mastoid drain (9)
Suture silk (10)
Suture intradermic (11)
Suture another (12)

EVOLUTION
Secretion
Earache (1)
None (2)
Sporadic (3)
Steady (4)
Hearing
Same (5)
Better (6)
Worse (7)
Tinnitus
Same (8)
None (9)
Increased (10)
Decreased (11)
Dizziness
None (12)
Same (13)
Worse (14)
Headache
None (15)
Same (16)
Worse (17)
External auditory canal
Dry (18)
Wet (19)
Middle ear
Dry (20)
Wet (21)
Cholesteatoma (22)
Tympanic membrane
Intact (23)
Perforation (24)
Neotympany
Normal (25)
Thickness (26)
Perforated (27)
Blunting (28)
Lateral displacement (29)
Inclusion cholesteatoma (30)

Facial nerve function							
Facial nerve							
Frontalis %	0 50	10 60		20 70	30 80	40 80	
Orbicularis oculi %	0 60	10 70		20 80	30 90	40 100	50
Orbicularis oris %	0 60	10 70		20 80	30 90	40 100	50
Rest	0 60	10 70		20 80	30 90	40 100	50
Synkinesia			0^{+}				0^{++}
Hemispasm			0^{+}				0^{++}

Postoperative hearing

Pure tone audiometry

	Bone curve right ear							**Bone curve left ear**						
	125	250	500	1000	2000	4000	8000	125	250	500	1000	2000	4000	8000
0	0	0	0	0	0	0	0	0	0	0	0	0	0	0
10	0	0	0	0	0	0	0	0	0	0	0	0	0	0
20	0	0	0	0	0	0	0	0	0	0	0	0	0	0
30	0	0	0	0	0	0	0	0	0	0	0	0	0	0
40	0	0	0	0	0	0	0	0	0	0	0	0	0	0
50	0	0	0	0	0	0	0	0	0	0	0	0	0	0
60	0	0	0	0	0	0	0	0	0	0	0	0	0	0

	Aircurve right ear							**Aircurve left ear**						
	125	250	500	1000	2000	4000	8000	125	250	500	1000	2000	4000	8000
0	0	0	0	0	0	0	0	0	0	0	0	0	0	0
10	0	0	0	0	0	0	0	0	0	0	0	0	0	0
20	0	0	0	0	0	0	0	0	0	0	0	0	0	0
30	0	0	0	0	0	0	0	0	0	0	0	0	0	0
40	0	0	0	0	0	0	0	0	0	0	0	0	0	0
50	0	0	0	0	0	0	0	0	0	0	0	0	0	0
60	0	0	0	0	0	0	0	0	0	0	0	0	0	0
70	0	0	0	0	0	0	0	0	0	0	0	0	0	0
80	0	0	0	0	0	0	0	0	0	0	0	0	0	0
90	0	0	0	0	0	0	0	0	0	0	0	0	0	0
100	0	0	0	0	0	0	0	0	0	0	0	0	0	0
110	0	0	0	0	0	0	0	0	0	0	0	0	0	0
120	0	0	0	0	0	0	0	0	0	0	0	0	0	0

Air-Bone Gap — Superimposed 0 — Decreased 0 — Increased 0

Hearing — Same — Low frequencies increased — Low frequencies decreased — High frequencies increased — High frequencies decreased

Postoperative hearing 3 months 6 months 1 year 2 years 3 years

Computer processing of data in stapedectomy

N. Gómez Estancona, I. de la Torre, U. Ruiz, L. Muñiz,
J.R. Urruticoechea, A. Urruticoechea, N. Arenaza

A protocol of data processing is presented here for the surgical operations of stapedectomy.

We have developed an informatic solution based on RDBMS in which each protocol is a data base.

The data included in the RDBMS can be consulted and compared in any way we like; this means that we can get hundreds of details of information, classified by any concept, in one single process of data, always with the possibility of consulting anything we like.

Anyone can benefit from data processing technology, even if one is not a programmer.

OPERATION
Exploration of the middle ear (a)
Stapedius mobilization (b)
Stapedectomy (c)
Total removal of footplate (1)
Partial removal of footplate (2)
Another (3)
Revision (4)
Another operation (d)
FINDINGS
Malleus
Normal (1)
Fixed (2)
Fixed partially (3)
Congenital malformation (4)
Another feature (5)
Incus
Normal (1)
Ankylosis (2)
Handle small (3)
Handle long (4)
Necrosis of the long handle (5)
Dislocated (6)
Missing (7)
Congenital malformation (8)
Another feature (9)
Stapes
Fixed (1)
Partially fixed (2)
Another feature (3)
Oval window
Normal (1)
Wide (2)
Narrow (3)
Otosclerotic focus
Anterior (1)
Posterior (2)
Ringshaped (3)
Vestibular (4)
Footplate itself (5)
Obliterating partially (6)
Obliterating (7)
Length Incus-footplate (mm): 4, 4,5, 5, 5,5.
Round window
Normal (1)
Obliterated (2)
Obliterated partially (3)
Strands in middle ear
Mucous membrane thick
Mucous membrane normal
TECHNIQUE
Chorda tympani nerve
Injured (1)
Cut (2)
Bony annulus
Removed (1)
Untouched (2)
Removal of footplate
Shafted pick fracture (1)
Hook removal (2)
Drilling footplate (3)
Drilling facial nerve (4)
Drilling promontory (5)
Promontory footplate (6)
PROSTHESIS
Piston
Wire (1)
Wire-teflon (2)
Polyethylene tube
Vein (3)
Perichondrium (4)
Wire
Fat (5)
Gelfoam (6)
Length of prosthesis: 3,5, 4, 4,5, 5, 5,5, 6, 6,5, 7

Window sealing
Gelfoam (1)
Fat (2)
Perichondrium (3)
Any (4)
ACCIDENTS
Piece of footplate into the vestibule (1)
Bleeding into the vestibule (2)
Vertigo (3)
Floating footplate (4)
Dry vestibule (5)
Perilymph fistula (6)
Perforation of the tympanic membrane (7)
Another (8)
DATE OF SURGICAL OPERATION
Day
Month
Year
COMPLICATIONS FOLLOWING SURGERY
Vertigo (1)
Chorda symptoms (2)
Acute otitis media (3)
Acute external otitis (4)
Tinnitus (5)
Perforation of tympani membrane (6)
Oval window fistula (7)
POSTOPERATIVE HEARING
Pure Tone audiometry
Yes
No
REVISION FINDINGS
Prosthetic malfunctions (1)
Prosthesis on the border of footplate (2)
Prosthesis small (3)
Prosthesis long (4)
Anatomical obstacles (5)
Fistula (6)
Granuloma (7)
Depressed footplate (8)
Another (9)

Digital subtraction angiography in the diagnosis of carotid body tumors

ABSTRACT

P. Parizel, H. Vereycken, T. Stadnik, J. Van Nueten,
J. de Moor, A. De Schepper

In the neck region, the use of intravenous digital subtraction angiography is limited by several factors, which are specific to the technique and the region of interest, such as poor spatial resolution, motion artifacts, vascular superpositions and the large amount of contrast medium needed. Nevertheless, intravenous digital subtraction angiography provides a good alternative as a screening method in high-risk patients and in the preoperative evaluation of the major extracerebral vessels.

In the evaluation of vascular and space occupying pathology intra-arterial angiography remains necessary but digital registration allows the use of smaller catheters, less selective injections, reduced amount, concentration and injection of contrast medium and should thus replace the conventional film-screen combination in nearly all circumstances.

The advantages and disadvantages of conventional and digital subtraction angiography in the diagnosis of carotid body tumors are discussed and illustrated in four patients.

Data processing in otosclerosis at the Jean Causse Otology Clinic

J.R Causse, J.B. Causse

The application of data processing techniques to patients' files is particularly recommended in otospongiotic otosclerotic disease, since the parameters defining history, symptoms, operation and follow-up to surgery are relatively simple, easily identifiable, accurate and limited in number.

— **Data processing** involves three basic aspects:

— *Computer:* our first computer, purchased in 1972, was an IBM 3/6, rapidly replaced by an IBM 32. Our future computer will be an IBM 36.

— *Data collected:* in fact, data was collected from 1959 to January 1984 from:

o 27 700 stapedectomies
o 180 000 otology out-patients.

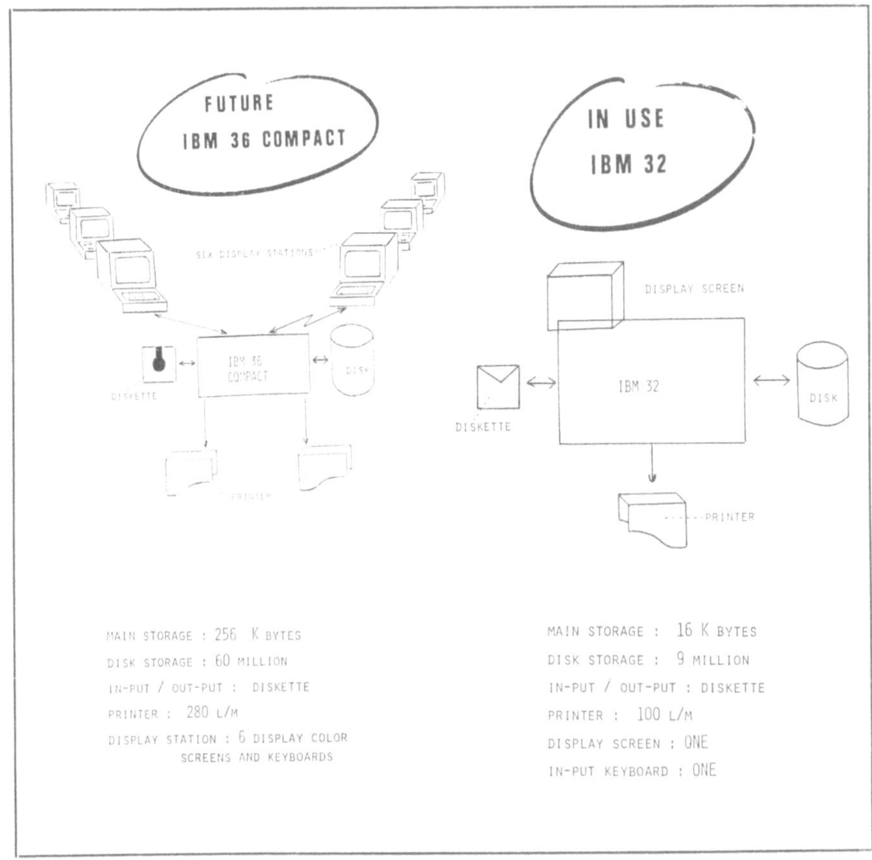

— *Parameter processing system:* we started in 1970 on two bases:

○ first, only a significantly wide range of parameters allows accuracy, sharpness, variety and reliability in the information given;

○ second, data processing in stapes surgery must be based not only on the intra-operative data, but also on the extensive study of collected data showing various aspects of the patients' status.

Only a wide range of parameters can provide accuracy, sharpness, variety and reliability. Checking-off selected items never requires much time: just 15' for the first consultation; 8' for subsequent consultations; 3' for the operation; 4' for postoperative check-ups.

Methodical processing provides a correct frame of each case (example: 1).

— **Resulting information:** computerized data provide immediate and precise information in each case.

— *Files for in-patients and out-patients.* For instance, a flash of stapedectomy: (example 2)

— *Statistical data concerning medical and surgical problems:* data processing allows objectivity, rapidity and validity

○ *in the evalution of functional results* in stapedectomy and medical therapy. Example:

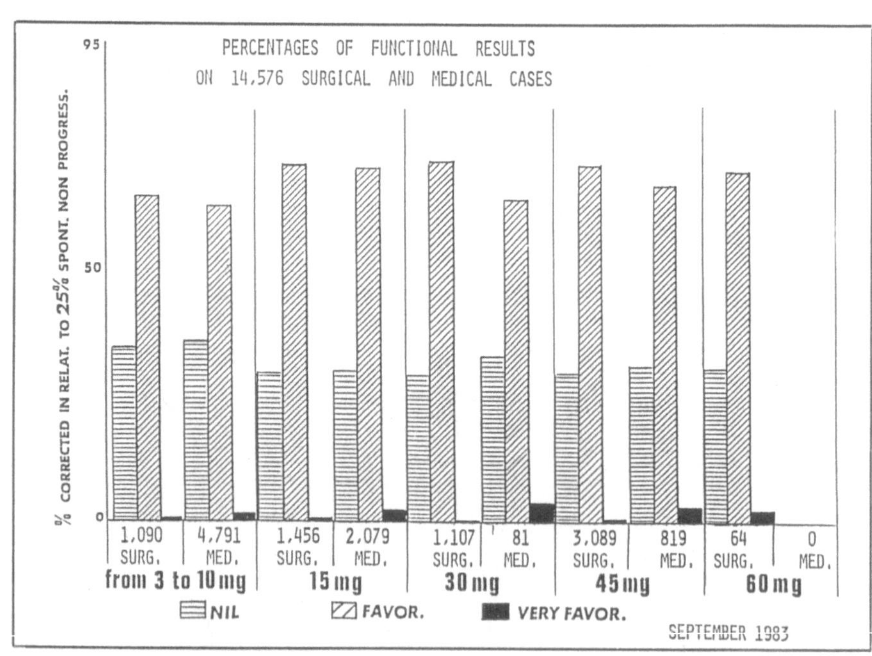

Example 1

J. CAUSSE ET COLLABORATEURS

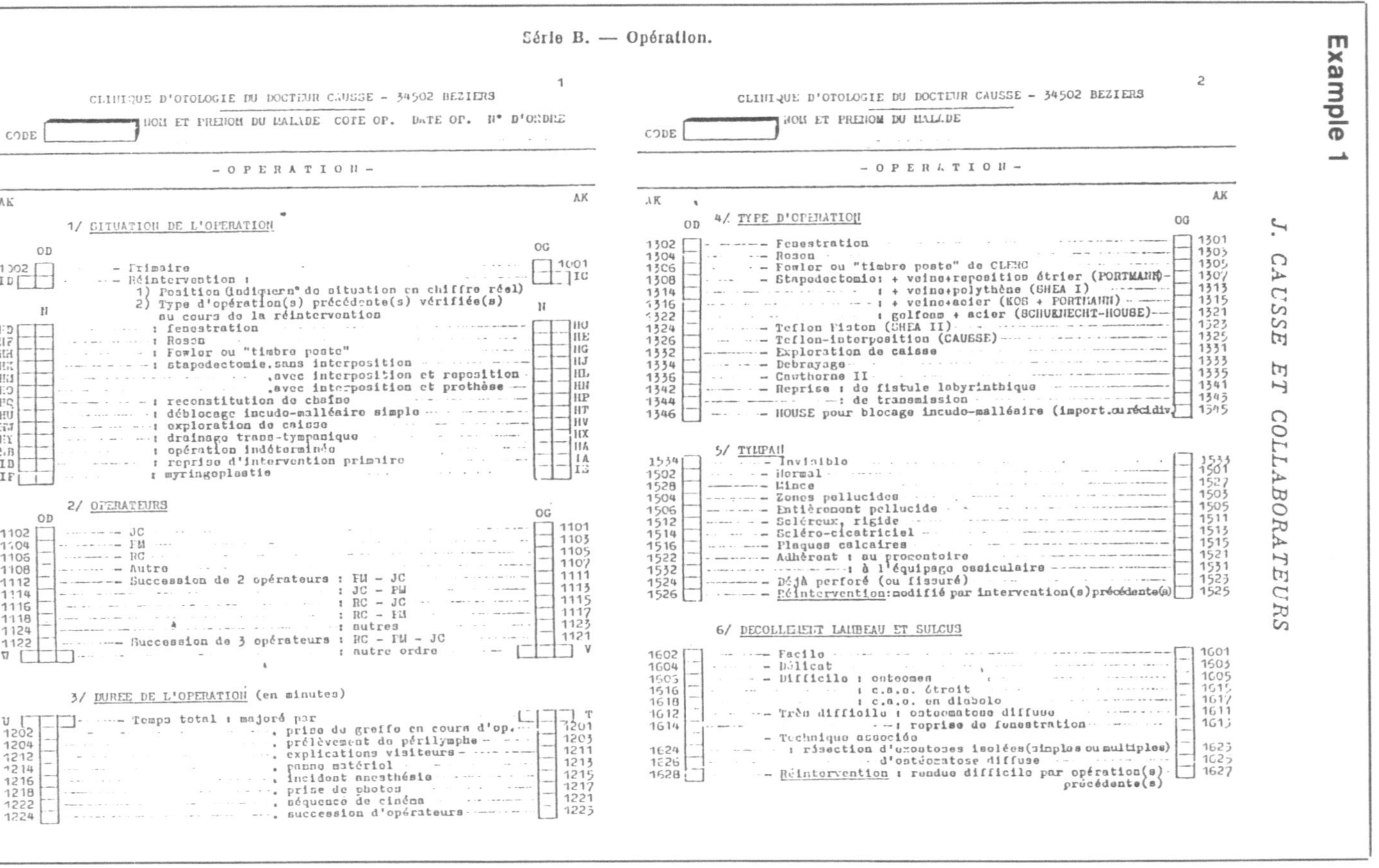

Série B. — Opération.

1

CLINIQUE D'OTOLOGIE DU DOCTEUR CAUSSE - 34502 BEZIERS

CODE [ ] NOM ET PRENOM DU MALADE COTE OP. DATE OP. N° D'ORDRE

- O P E R A T I O N -

AK — AK

1/ SITUATION DE L'OPERATION

OD		OG	
1302	- Primaire		1001
ID	- Réintervention :		IC
	1) Position (indiquer* de situation en chiffre réel)		
	2) Type d'opération(s) précédente(s) vérifiée(s) au cours de la réintervention		
N		N	
HD	: fenestration		HO
HF	: Roson		HE
HH	: Fowler ou "timbre poste"		HG
HK	: stapedectomie,sans interposition		HJ
HM	,avec interposition et reposition		HL
HO	,avec interposition et prothèse		HN
HQ	: reconstitution de chaîne		HP
HU	: déblocage incudo-malléaire simple		HT
HW	: exploration de caisse		HV
HY	: drainage trans-tympanique		HX
IB	: opération indéterminée		IIA
ID	: reprise d'intervention primaire		IA
IF	: myringoplastie		IE

2/ OPERATEURS

OD		OG
1102	- JC	1101
1104	- FM	1103
1106	- RC	1105
1108	- Autre	1107
1112	- Succession de 2 opérateurs : FM - JC	1111
1114	: JC - FM	1113
1116	: RC - JC	1115
1118	: RC - FM	1117
1124	: autres	1123
1122	- Succession de 3 opérateurs : RC - FM - JC	1121
W	: autre ordre	V

3/ DUREE DE L'OPERATION (en minutes)

U	- Temps total : majoré par	T
1202	. prise du greffe en cours d'op.	1201
1204	. prélèvement de périlymphe	1203
1212	. explications visiteurs	1211
1214	. panne matériel	1213
1216	. incident anesthésie	1215
1218	. prise de photos	1217
1222	. séquence de cinéma	1221
1224	. succession d'opérateurs	1223

2

CLINIQUE D'OTOLOGIE DU DOCTEUR CAUSSE - 34502 BEZIERS

CODE [ ] NOM ET PRENOM DU MALADE

- O P E R A T I O N -

AK — AK

4/ TYPE D'OPERATION

OD		OG
1302	- Fenestration	1301
1304	- Roson	1303
1306	- Fowler ou "timbre poste" de CLERC	1305
1308	- Stapedectomie: + veine+reposition étrier (PORTMANN)	1307
1314	: + veine+polythène (SHEA I)	1313
1316	: + veine+acier (KOS + PORTMANN)	1315
1322	: golfoam + acier (SCHUKNECHT-HOUSE)	1321
1324	- Teflon Piston (SHEA II)	1323
1326	- Teflon-interposition (CAUSSE)	1325
1332	- Exploration de caisse	1331
1334	- Debrayage	1333
1336	- Cawthorne II	1335
1342	- Reprise : de fistule labyrinthique	1341
1344	: de transmission	1343
1346	- HOUSE pour blocage incudo-malléaire (import.ou récidiv.)	1345

5/ TYMPAN

1534	- Invisible	1533
1502	- Normal	1501
1528	- Mince	1527
1504	- Zones pellucides	1503
1506	- Entièrement pellucide	1505
1512	- Scléreux, rigide	1511
1514	- Scléro-cicatriciel	1513
1516	- Plaques calcaires	1515
1522	- Adhérent : au promontoire	1521
1532	: à l'équipage ossiculaire	1531
1524	- Déjà perforé (ou fissuré)	1523
1526	- Réintervention:modifié par intervention(s)précédente(s)	1525

6/ DECOLLEMENT LAMBEAU ET SULCUS

1602	- Facile	1601
1604	- Délicat	1603
1606	- Difficile : ostoomes	1605
1616	: c.a.e. étroit	1615
1618	: c.a.e. en diabolo	1617
1612	- Très difficile : ostoomatose diffuse	1611
1614	: reprise de fenestration	1613
	- Technique associée	
1624	: résection d'exostoses isolées(simples ou multiples)	1623
1626	d'ostéomatose diffuse	1625
1628	- Réintervention : rendue difficile par opération(s) précédente(s)	1627

Example 2

```
760755              DEP▬▬▬ PIERRETTE              CPTE RENDU OP.              15.05.76

SITUATION DE L OP.
        OR. GAUCHE -PRIMAIRE -OPERATEUR : JC -TPS TOT 50MN -ANESTHESIE : GENERALE -PREMEDICATION -
            TYPE D OP. : TI -
C.A.E.  :
      TYMPAN: NORMAL -
      DECOL. LAMBEAU & SULCUS : FACILE -
      RESEC. POSTERO-SUP. C A E : GOUGE -CURETTE -DIMENSION RESECT: MODEREE  -
      CORDE OU TYMPAN : NORM. SOUPLE, MINCE -
CAISSE :
        ABORD : DIRECT -ETROIT -
        ETAT LIBRE -
        FACIAL :. PROCI. -MASQ PRESQ TOT. F.O. NIV. 2EME PORTION -RAP. FACIAL AVEC : LONG ENCL. COURT -PROMONT. COURT -
            BR: COURT -
      FOSSE OVALE ET PROMONTOIRE : FOSSE OVALE ETROITE -PROFONDE -REMANIEE TOTAL -VIRTUELLE -
        PROMONTOIRE SURELEVE EN DOME -
      MUCOPERIOSTE : TRES EPAIS ET EXTREM. VASCULAR. -
      CHAINE OSSICUL. : MARTEAU : NORMAL, MOBILE -
        ENCLUME NORMALE -MOBILE -GRELE -PLONGEANTE -AVASCULAIRE ET SECHE -
        BRANCHES ETRIER : TRES SOLIDES -
        TENDON MUSCLE ETR. NORMAL -
      TYPE LESIONS STAPEDOVEST. : IX B -
ES. STAPEDOVESTIB. ASSOC.
        AUCUNE -
      TEMPS STAPEDO-VESTIBULAIRE :
      TYPE DE FEN. RONDE INVISIBLE -
      ABORD LESIONS STAPED. VESTIB. ABOMINABLE -
      HEMOST. AU DEMUCOP. : DIFF. AV. ADRENAL. + ATTENTE MS BONNE -
      DESARTICUL. INCUDO-STAP. : FACILE
      SECT. BRANCHES : SECT. PREMIERE DES 2 BRANCHES -
      ATTAQUE LES. PLATIN. : MICROFRAISAGE : AU MICROF. DE 2/10MM -SECTEUR -BIEN AIR -
      TACTIQUE PLATIN. RECALIB.   5/9B AU MICROFORET -
      DIFFIC. EXECUT. TPS PLATIN. : ABOMINABLE -
      RESULT. PLATIN. : PLATINECTOMIE IMPOSSIBLE -
PERILYMPHE : EN DEBUT D OP PRESSION HABITUELLE -EN FIN D OPERATION CONSERVEE -PURE -
TRANSMISSION :
      FERMET. DE LA F/O : VEINE MINCE DE LARG. SUFF. -
      INVAGINATION : MODEREE -
TRANSMISSION : -SUR ENCLUME : PISTON DE TEFLON 6/10E LONG : 425 -XOMED MODELE JC
      COULISSEMENT : TB, EXCEL. -
INC. OU ACCID. PER-OP: PLATINE FLOT. -
      TECHN. COMPLEMENTAIRE PAS -
LAMBEAU : NORMAL -MECHAGE C A E : POPE EAR WICK -ANTIBIOTIC. LOCAL. : PAS -
RESERVES :
        EXTREMES -
            POUR CONDIT. ANATOMIQUES IMPORTANCE -ACTIVITE -INCIC. OP. -MANOEUV. PLATIN. -
            CONDITIONS AUDIOMETRIQUES RESERVE COCHLEAIRE MAUVAISE -ETAT GENERAL -VASCULAIRE -
DIAGN. DEFINITIF RETENU :
        OTOSPONGIOSE -
```

o *in comparison of operative techniques.* For instance: Long-term success of various techniques

15 YEAR STAPEDECTOMY STATISTICAL DATA
EVALUATION OF LONG-TERM SUCCESS OF 16,822 STAPEDECTOMIES PERFORMED
BETWEEN JANUARY 1ST 1960 AND JANUARY 1ST 1975
ACCORDING TO THE TECHNIQUE USED

TYPE OF OPERATION	NUMBER	LONG-TERM SUCCESS (5 TO 15 YEARS)	
		NUMBER	PERCENT.
- STAPEDECTOMIES			
+ VEIN + STAPES REPOSITION (PORTMANN)	859	791	92,08
+ VEIN + POLYTHENE STRUT (SHEA I)	1 050	963	91,71
+ VEIN + STEEL WIRE (KOS + PORTMANN)	13 *	12	92,30
+ GELFOAM + STEEL WIRE (SCHUKNECHT-HOUSE)	10 *	7	70,00
- TEFLON PISTON (SHEA II)	174	162	93,10
- TEFLON INTERPOSITION (CAUSSE)	14 716	14 444	98,15
TOTAL :	16 822	16 379	97,36
- REVISION-OPERATIONS			
CONDUCTION	173	96	55,50
PERILYMPH FISTULA	7 *	6	85,72

* NOT SIGNIFICANT (TOO FEW CASES)

Bone conduction improvement with regard to frequency and to the type of operation performed.

AVERAGE DECIBEL IMPROVEMENT IN BONE CONDUCTION
ONE YEAR AFTER THE OPERATION
ACCORDING TO THE FREQUENCY AND TO THE TYPE OF OPERATION PERFORMED
STATISTICAL DATA FROM 1977 THROUGH 1983
IN 6,724 STAPEDECTOMIES/STAPEDOTOMIES

	200 Hz	500 Hz	1000 Hz	2000 Hz	4000 Hz
0,8MM SMALL FENESTRA LOCATED AT THE POST. 1/3 OF THE FOOTPLATE	8,487	10,641	12,948	16,350	9,102
ABLATION OF COMPLETE POSTERIOR 1/3 OF THE FOOTPLATE	9,633	11,166	13,166	14,166	2,833

o *Research:* The flexibility of the computer and the reliability of its memory make computed data remarkably helpful for research, provided that data processing is correctly programmed. Two examples:

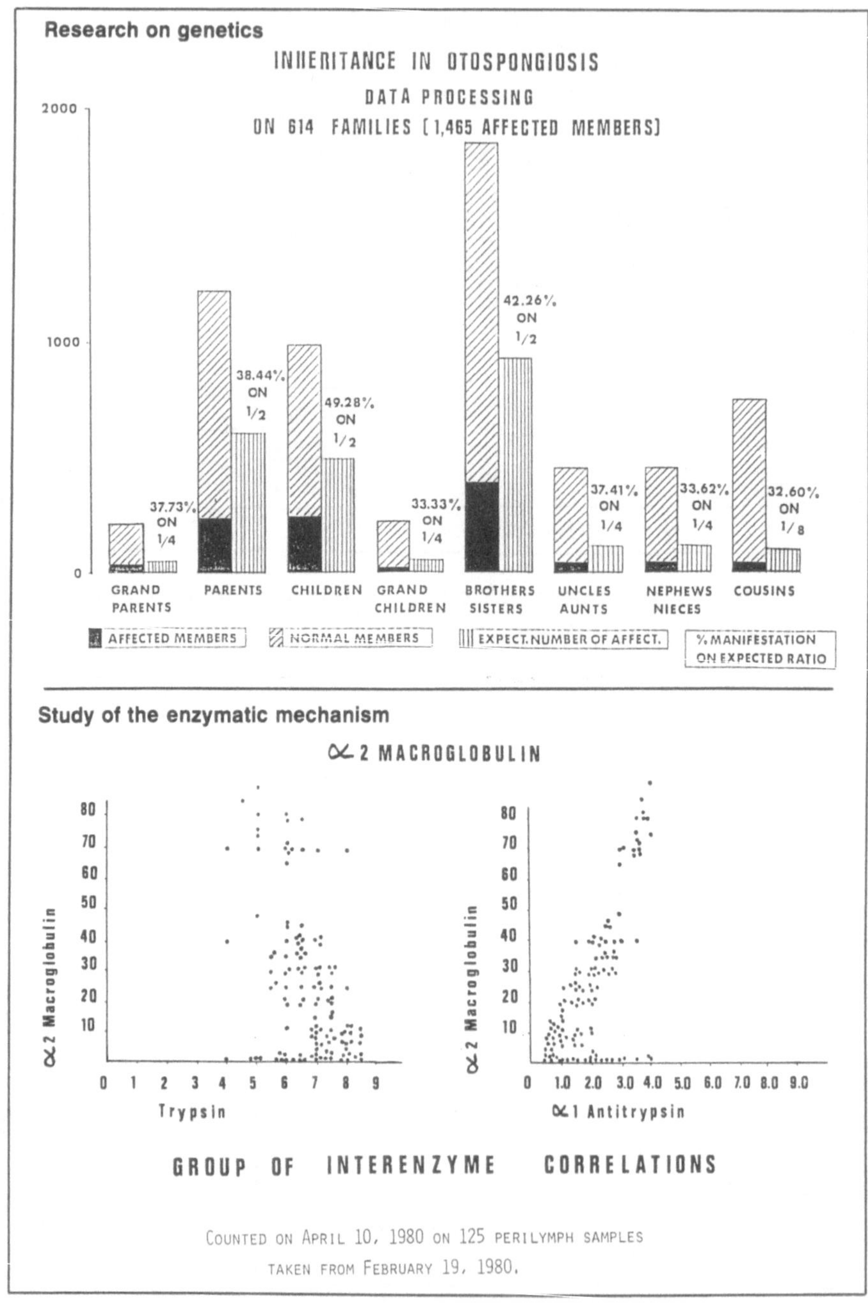

The International Medical Classification Code of Diseases (ICD) in audiological practice

ABSTRACT

T. Spillmann, N. Dillier

We have developed a system of classification using a relatively short list of code numbers derived from the international code. This enables us to determine the frequency with which any one audiological or otological diagnosis is made, as well as the frequency of combinations of these diagnoses. It is hoped that this system will help the user to determine the relationship between disease entities in an audiological caseload. Furthermore, it may render possible a comparison of diagnoses and therapeutic results between different centers.

Liste of authors

Dr. F. Abes 317
AZA, Dept. of ENT
Wilrijkstraat 10
B-2520 Edegem

Dr. M. Andrea
Faculdada de Medicina
Servicio ORL
Lisboa, Portugal

Dr. K. Aoki 344,363
Dept. of ENT
The Jikei Univ. School of Medicine
3-25-8 Nishishinbashi, Minato-ku
Tokyo 105, Japan

Dr. B. Appel 376
Dept. of Radiology
Middelheim Ziekenhuis
Lindendreef 1
B-2020 Antwerpen

Dr. B. Arbeille-Brassart 398
Electron Microscopy Department
CHU Bretonneau
F-Tours

Dr. N. Arenaza 402,407
Dept. of ORL
Hospital of Galdácano
Bilbao
Spain

Dr. B. Ars 233,316
Avenue du Polo 68, Bte 02
B-1150 Bruxelles

Dr. D. Austin 57
Austin Otologic Center
55 East Washington
Chicago 60602 (U.S.A.)

Dr. M. Bagot D'Arc 261
Clinique Universitaire XX Tripode
Service ORL
Place Amolie Raba Léon
F-33076 Bordeaux

Dr. B. Bael 338
MISA - Dept. of ENT
Oosterveldlaan 24
B-2610 Wilrijk

Dr. Z. Bankowski 15
Executive Secretary C.I.O.M.S.
Avenue Apia
CH-1211 Genève

Prof. J.P. Bebear 261
Clinique Universitaire XX Tripode
Service ORL
Place Amélie Raba Léon
F-33076 Bordeaux

Dr. J. Bel 290
Otology Clinic
F-34325 Béziers Cedex

Dr. R. Bertrand 298
4915 De Salaberry
Suite 105
C DN - Montréal H4J 1H8

Dr. A. Bismuth 273
Centre Hospitalier Emile-Roux
F-95600 Eaubonne

Dr. C. Bismuth 273
Centre Hospitalier Emile-Roux
F-95600 Eaubonne

Prof. C.D. Bluestone 163
Dept. of ENT, Children's Hospital
125 de Soto Street
Pittsburgh, Pennsylvania 15213 (U.S.A.)

Dr. D. Boedts 245
Rode Beukendreef 13
B-9831 Deurle

Dr. R. Boniver 261
Rue de Bruxelles 21
B-4800 Verviers

Dr. Y. Capelier 398
ENT Department
CHU Bretonneau
F-Tours

Dr. J. B. Causse 290,409
2, Avenue Alphonse Mas,
BP. 4225
F-34325 Béziers Cedex

Dr. J.R. Causse 290,409
2, Avenue Alphonse Mas
BP. 4225
F-34325 Béziers Cedex

Dr. R. Cezard 290
Otology Clinic
F-34325 Béziers Cedex

Prof. R. Charachon 68
Centre Hospitalier Régional
Université de Grenoble,
BP. 217 X
F-38043 Grenoble Cedex

Dr. E. Chiossone 120
Fundacion Venezolana de Otologica
Apartado 62.277
Caracas 106 (Venezuela)

Dr. J. Claes 328,365
AZA, Dept. of ENT
Wilrijkstraat 10
B-2520 Edegem

Dr. E.V. Claus 328
Dept. of Radiology
Medisch Centrum
St.-Jacobsmarkt 49
B-2000 Antwerpen

Dr. C.W.R.J. Cremers 402
St.-Radboudziekenhuis
Ph. van Leydenlaan 15
P.O. Box 9101
NL-6500 HB Nijmegen

Dr. M.N. Daouk 310
King Faisal Specialist Hospital
P.O. Box 3354
Riyadh 11211
Saudi Arabia

Dr. J.D.K. Dawes 201
The Royal Victoria Infirmary
Queen Victoria Road
GB-Newcastle upon Tyne NE1 4LP

Dr. F. Debruyne 308
Kapucijnenvoer 7
B-3000 Leuven

Dr. G. Declercq 333
University Hospital
B-9000 Gent

Dr. M. De Cock 301
AZA, dept. of ENT
Wilrijkstraat 10
B-2520 Edegem

Dr. C. Deguine 284
134 Bd. de la Liberté
F-59000 Lille (Nord)

Dr. M. De Haen 338
MISA
Oosterveldlaan 24
B-2610 Wilrijk

Dr. J. Delaruelle 338
Medical Institute St.-Augustinus
Oosterveldlaan 24
B-2610 Wilrijk

Dr. I. de la Torre 402,407
Dept. of ORL
Hospital of Galdácano
Bilbao
Spain

Dr. J. de Moor 408
Department of Radiology
Oosterveldlaan 24
B-2610 Wilrijk

Dr. A. De Schepper 408
Department of Radiology
Oosterveldlaan 24
B-2610 Wilrijk

Prof. H. Diamant 155
University of Umeå
Dept. of ORL
S-90187 Umeå

Dr. N. Dillier 415
Audiology Division
ENT Department, University Hospital
CH-8091 Zürich

Prof. I. Eliachar 250,257
ENT Department,
Rambam Medical Center
Haifa, Bat-Galim
Israel

Dr. K. Enatsu 52
Dept. of ORL
Miyazaki Medical College
5200 Kihary, Kiyotaka-Cho
Miyazaki-Gun, Miyazaki Prefecture
Japan

Dr. S. Esaki 363
Dept. of ORL
The Jikei Univ. School of Medecine
3-25-8 Nishishinbashi, Minato-ku
Tokyo 105
Japan

Dr. L. Feenstra 300
Academisch Ziekenhuis
Vrije Universiteit
De Boelelaan 1117
NL-Amsterdam

Prof. U. Fisch 183
University of Zürich
Dept. of ENT
Rämistrasse 100
CH-8091 Zürich

Dr. G. Flottorp 270
Dept. of ENT
University of Oslo
Rikshospitaal
N-Oslo 1 (Norway)

Dr. W. Frank 215
Dept. of ENT
Allgemeines Krankenhaus
D-Hamburg

Dr. N.J. Frootko 215,374
8 Worminghall Road
GB-Ickford, Bucks

Dr. N.B. Gagnon 261
Université de Montréal
Dept. of ENT
Hôpital Notre Dame
1851 Est Sherbrooke
CAN-Montréal Que H2L 4K8

Dr. R. Gamoletti 108
Second ENT Clinic
University of Parma
Via Rondani 8
I-Parma

Dr. G. Gates 273
University of Texas
Health Service San Antonio
Curl drive
San Antonio, Texas 78284, USA

Dr. M.C.H. Gersdorff 72,310
U.C.L.
Avenue Hippocrate 10
B-1200 Bruxelles

Dr. A.G. Gibb 177
Dept. of ENT, Ninewells Hospital
11 Dudhope Terrace
GB-Dundee DD3 6HG

Dr. W. Kuypers 402
Dept. of ORL
University of Nijmegen
NL-Nijmegen

Dr. P. Kylén 269
Karolinska Institutet
Sodersjukhuset
S-10067 Stockholm 38

Dr. G. Lacher 133
25 rue Detroits
F-33200 Bordeaux Caudéran

Dr. M. Lachman 266
30 Bd. Maxime Gorki,
Stains
F-93240 St.-Denis

Dr. S.G. Lesinski 129
Otology and Neuro-Otology
629 Oak Street, Suite 201
Cincinnati Ohio 45206 (U.S.A.)

Dr. M. Lorré 328
Edelinckstraat 9
B-2000 Antwerpen

Dr. J.-P. Maisin 72,310
U.C.L.
Avenue Hippocrate 10
B-1200 Bruxelles

Dr. A.J. Maniglia 186
Miami Beach Florida
P.O. Box 016960 (D 48A)
Miami, Florida 33101 (U.S.A.)

Dr. J.J. Manni 238,394
Sint Radboudziekenhuis
Ph. van Leydenlaan 15
NL-6500 HB Nijmegen

Dr. L. Manolidis 209,213
Ahepa Hospital
Aristotelian University Dept. of ENT
Dimitriou Gounari Street 1
Thessaloniki (Greece)

Dr. J.F.E. Marquet 20,139,150
Fruithoflaan 91/12 233,301,317,328
B-2600 Berchem 335,365,371,376

Prof. E.H.M.A. Marres 58,394
Rijksuniversiteit Limburg
Dept. of Otolaryngology
St.-Annadal Hospital
NL-Maastricht

Dr. A. Mazzoni 126
Ospedali Riuniti
Division ORL
I-24100 Bergamo

Prof. U. Mercke 230
University Hospital of Lund
Dept. of ENT
S-221 85 Lund

Dr. P. Michaux 290
Otology Clinic
F-34325 Béziers Cedex

Dr. T. Minatògawa 134
Dept. of ENT
Hyogo Medical College
1-1 Mukogawa-cho
Nishinomiya, Hyogo, 663 (Japan)

Dr. I. Miyajima 347
Dept. of ORL
The Jikey Univ. School of Medecine
3-25-8 Nishishinbashi, Minato-ku
Tokyo 105 (Japan)

Dr. H. Miyake 117
Tokai University School of Medecine
Tokyo Hospital
1-2-5 Yoyogi Shibuya-Ku
Tokyo 151 (Japan)

Dr. N. Mizorogi 359
Dept. of ORL
The Jikey Univ., School of Medicine
3-25-8 Nishishinbashi, Minato-ku
Tokyo 105 (Japan)

Dr. J. Moeneclaey 233,317
ENT Laboratory
University of Antwerp
B- 2000 Antwerpen

Dr. T. Morimitsu 52
Dept. of ENT
Miyazaki Medical College
5200 Kihary, Kiyotake-ChO
Miyazaki-Gun, Miyazaki Prefecture

Dr. H. Moriyama 344
Dept. of ORL
The Jikey Univ., School of Medicine
3-25-8 Nishishinbashi, Minato-ku
Tokyo 105 (Japan)

Dr. U. Muñiz 402,407
Dept. of ORL
Hospital of Galdácano
Bilbao
Spain

Dr. M. Münzel 215
Allgemeines Krankenhaus Hamburg
Eissendorfer Pferdeweg 52
D-2100 Hamburg 90

Dr. K. Murata 145
Kinki University, 380 Nishiyama,
Sayama-Cho Minami-Kawachi
Osaka 589 (Japan)

Dr. M. Nagai 52
Dept. of ORL
Miyazaki Medical College
5200 Kihary, Kiyotaka-Cho
Miyazaki-Gun, Miyazaki Prefecture
Japan

Dr. P. Savary 65
ENT
Côte du Palais 44
Quebec, Que Gir 4H8 (Canada)

Dr. Ph. Schepens 381
St.-Jozef Kliniek
B-8700 Bruges

Dr. Y. Schepens 381
Spinolarei 19
B-8000 Bruges

Dr. J.J. Shea 37,299
Shea Clinic
1080 Madison Avenue,
P.O. Box 40 049
Memphis, Tennessee 38104 (U.S.A.)P

Dr. A. Shinkawa 117
Tokai University School of Medecine
Tokyo Hospital
1-2-5 Yoyogi Shibuya-Ku
Tokyo 151
Japan

Dr. G.D.L. Smyth 161
Royal Victoria Hospital
ENT Department
Grosvenor Road
Belfast BT1 26 BA (Ireland)

Dr. T. Spillmann 415
Audiology Division
ENT Department, University Hospital
CH-8091 Zürich

Dr. P. Spiritus 338
MISA
Oosterveldlaan 24
B-2610 Wilrijk

Dr. T. Stadnik 408
Dept. of Radiology
University Hospital
B-2000 Antwerpen

Dr. H. Steinbach 228
University of Tübingen
D-4700 Tübingen

Prof. J.M. Sterckers 205
Head of ORL, CHU-Cochin
27, rue de Faubourg St. Jacques
F-75014 Paris (France)

Prof. J.-I. Suzuki 193
Dept. of ORL
Teikyo University School of Medecine
2-11-1 Kaga
Itabashi-ku, Tokyo 173, (Japan)

Dr. I. Sziklai 222
Szeged University of Medical Science, Dept. of ENT
Lenin krt 111
H-6701 Szeged Pg 422

Dr. E.J.J.M. Theunissen 402
St. Radboudziekenhuis
Ph. van Leydenlaan 15
NL-6500 HB Nijmegen

Prof. M. Tos 170
Kobenhavns Amts Sygehus I Gentofte
ENT Departement
Niels Andersens vej 65,
DK-2900 Hellerup

Dr. Y. Umetani 134
Dept. of ENT
Hyogo Medical College
1-1 Mukogawa-cho
Nishinomiya, Hyogo, 663
Japan

Dr. A. Urruticoechea 402,407
Dept. of ORL
Hospital of Galdácano
Bilbao
Spain

Dr. J.R. Urruticoechea 402,407
Dept. of ORL
Hospital of Galdácano
Bilbao
Spain

Dr. K.J. Van Camp 271
RUCA
Groenenborgerlaan 171
B-2020 Antwerpen

Dr. P. Van Cauwenberge 333
Eeuwfeestlaan 56
B-9720 De Pinte

Dr. P. Van de Heyning 139,328
AZA, Dept. of ENT
Wilrijkstraat 10
B-2520 Edegem

Prof. P. van den Broek 31
Sint Radboudziekenhuis
Ph. van Leydenlaan 15
NL-6500 HB Nijmegen

Dr. J.G.M. Van Haelst 394
Sint Radboudziekenhuis
Ph. van Leydenlaan 15
NL-6500 HB Nijmegen

Dr. C. Van Laer 371
AZA, Dept. of ENT
Wilrijkstraat 10
B-2520 Edegem

Dr. J. Van Nueten 408
Dept. of Radiology
University Hospital
B-2000 Antwerpen

Dr. H. Vereyken 408
Dept. of Radiology
University Hospital
B-2000 Antwerpen

Dr. L. Vergnon 273
Centre Hospitalier Emile-Roux
F-95600 Eaubonne

Dr. S. Vlaminck 381
St.-Jozefkliniek
B-8000 Bruges

Dr. A.R. Welch 201
Dept. of ORL
University
GB-Newcastle upon Tyne

Prof. M. Wigand 81
Klinik und Poliklinik für HNO
Waldstrasse 1
D-8520 Erlangen

Dr. S.R. Wullstein 61
Praxisklinik
Oberer Neubergweg, 10a
D-8700 Wütrzburg

Prof. K. Yamashita 329,332
Kanazawa Medical University
Uchinada Ishikawa 920-02 (Japan)

Dr. C. Zini 108
Second ENT Clinic
University of Parma
Via Rondani 8
I-Parma

Dr. B. Zoller 290
Otology Clinic
F-34325 Béziers Cedex